Contents

Section III: Endocrinology & Infertility

a LANGE medical book

Handbook of Gynecology & Obstetrics

First Edition

Edited by

JEANETTE S. BROWN, MD
Assistant Clinical Professor
Department of Obstetrics, Gynecology,
and Reproductive Sciences
University of California School of Medicine
San Francisco, California

WILLIAM R. CROMBLEHOLME, MD
Professor and Vice-Chairman
Department of Obstetrics, Gynecology,
and Reproductive Sciences
Magee-Womens Hospital
University of Pittsburgh
Pittsburgh, Pennsylvania

APPLETON & LANGE
Stamford, Connecticut

0-8385-3608-5

97 98 99 / 9 8 7 6 5 4 3

Prentice Hall International (UK) Limited, *London*
Prentice Hall of Australia of Pty. Limited, *Sydney*
Prentice Hall Canada, Inc., *Toronto*
Prentice Hall Hispanoamericana, S.A., *Mexico*
Prentice Hall of India Private Limited, *New Delhi*
Prentice Hall of Japan, Inc., *Tokyo*
Simon & Schuster Asia Pte. Ld., *Singapore*
Editora Prentice Hall do Brasil Ltda., *Rio de Janeiro*
Prentice Hall, *Upper Saddle River, New Jersey*

ISBN: 0-8385-3608-5
ISSN: 1062-5704

Acquisitions Editor: Martin J. Wonsiewicz
Production Editor: Charles F. Evans

 printed on recycled paper

PRINTED IN THE UNITED STATES OF AMERICA

/ *Contents*

Section VII: Fetal Assessment

Section VIII: Labor, Delivery, & Postpartum Care

The Authors

Janice L. Andreyko, MD
Assistant Clinical Professor, Department of Obstetrics, Gynecology, and Reproductive Sciences, University of California School of Medicine, San Francisco.

Joseph A. Bachicha, MD
Assistant Professor, Department of Obstetrics and Gynecology, Northwestern University School of Medicine, Chicago.

Valerie L. Baker, MD
Fellow, Reproductive Endocrinology and Infertility, Department of Obstetrics, Gynecology, and Reproductive Sciences, University of California School of Medicine, San Francisco.

Jeanette S. Brown, MD
Assistant Clinical Professor, Department of Obstetrics, Gynecology, and Reproductive Sciences, University of California School of Medicine, San Francisco.

David Chelmow, MD
Assistant Professor, Department of Obstetrics and Gynecology, Tufts University Medical School, New England Medical Center, Boston.

Patricia L. Collins, MD, PhD
Assistant Professor, Department of Reproductive Biology, Case Western Reserve University School of Medicine, and Department of Obstetrics and Gynecology, MetroHealth Medical Center, Cleveland.

C. Andrew Combs, MD, PhD
Assistant Professor, Division of Maternal-Fetal Medicine, Department of Obstetrics and Gynecology, University of Cincinnati, Cincinnati.

Bonnie A. Coyne, MD
Staff Perinatologist, Department of Obstetrics and Gynecology, Mercy Hospital, Pittsburgh.

Mitchell D. Creinin, MD
Fellow in Family Planning, Department of Obstetrics, Gynecology and Reproductive Sciences, University of California School of Medicine, San Francisco.

William R. Crombleholme, MD
Professor and Vice-Chairman, Department of Obstetrics, Gynecology, and Reproductive Sciences, Magee-Womens Hospital, University of Pittsburgh, Pittsburgh.

Bonnie J. Dattel, MD
Associate Professor, Director of Perinatal Research, Department of Obstetrics and Gynecology, Eastern Virginia Medical School, Norfolk.

Rosemary Delgado, MD
Staff Physician, Department of Obstetrics and Gynecology, Kaiser Permanente Medical Center, Santa Clara, California.

Jonathan S. Friedes, MD
Staff Physician, Harvard Community Health Plan, Boston.

Steven A. Friedman, MD
Assistant Professor, Department of Obstetrics and Gynecology, University of Tennessee, Memphis.

Elena A. Gates, MD
Assistant Clinical Professor and Associate Director of Residency Program, Department of Obstetrics, Gynecology, and Reproductive Sciences, University of California School of Medicine, San Francisco.

Ruth B. Goldstein, MD
Associate Professor, Department of Radiology and Department of Obstetrics, Gynecology, and Reproductive Sciences, University of California School of Medicine, San Francisco.

Deborah G. Grady, MD, MPH
Assistant Professor, Departments of Medicine and Epidemiology, University of California School of Medicine, San Francisco.

Susan Jan Hornstein
Consultant for centers on violence against women, San Francisco.

Sarah J. Kilpatrik, MD, PhD
Assistant Professor, Department of Obstetrics, Gynecology, and Reproductive Sciences, University of California School of Medicine, San Francisco.

Audrey S. Koh, MD
Clinical Instructor, Department of Obstetrics, Gynecology, and Reproductive Sciences, University of California School of Medicine, San Francisco.

Abner P. Korn, MD
Assistant Professor, Department of Obstetrics, Gynecology, and Reproductive Sciences, University of California School of Medicine, San Francisco.

David K. Levin, MD
Assistant Chief of Service, Department of Obstetrics and Gynecology, Kaiser Permanente Medical Center, Santa Clara; Clinical Assistant Professor, Department of Gynecology and Obstetrics, Stanford University School of Medicine, Palo Alto.

Lesley R. Levine, MD
Director of Residency Program, Department of Obstetrics and Gynecology, Kaiser Permanente Hospital, Oakland; Clinical Instructor, Department of Obstetrics, Gynecology, and Reproductive Sciences, University of California School of Medicine, San Francisco.

Elizabeth G. Livingston, MD
Assistant Professor, Department of Obstetrics and Gynecology, Duke University Medical Center, Durham.

Carol A. Major, MD
Assistant Professor, Department of Obstetrics and Gynecology, University of California Irvine Medical Center, Irvine.

Maureen P. Malee, MD, PhD
Assistant Professor, Obstetrics and Gynecology, Division of Maternal-Fetal Medicine, University of Iowa School of Medicine, Iowa City.

David N. Marinoff, MD
Perinatologist, Alta Bates Medical Center, Berkeley; East Bay Perinatal Medical Associates, Oakland.

Karen K. Smith McCune, MD, PhD
Assistant Professor, Department of Obstetrics, Gynecology, and
Reproductive Sciences, and Fellow, Department of Microbiology
and Immunology, University of California School of Medicine,
San Francisco.

Nancy Milliken, MD
Assistant Professor, Department of Obstetrics, Gynecology, and
Reproductive Sciences, University of California School of Medi-
cine, San Francisco.

Thomas J. Musci, MD
Assistant Professor, Department of Obstetrics, Gynecology, and
Reproductive Sciences, University of California School of Medi-
cine, San Francisco.

Michael L. Pearl, MD
Fellow, Division of Gynecologic Oncology, Department of Ob-
stetrics and Gynecology, University of Michigan Medical Center,
Ann Arbor.

Thomas L. Pinckert, MD
Assistant Professor, Director of Clinical Genetics, Department of
Obstetrics and Gynecology, Georgetown University Hospital,
Washington, D.C.

Anne C. Regenstein, MD
Assistant Clinical Professor, Department of Obstetrics, Gynecology, and Reproductive Sciences, University of California School
of Medicine, San Francisco.

Patricia A. Robertson, MD
Assistant Clinical Professor, Department of Obstetrics, Gynecology, and Reproductive Sciences, University of California School
of Medicine, San Francisco.

Lisa G. Sandles, MD
Gynecologic Oncologist, Department of Obstetrics and Gynecology, Division of Gynecologic Oncology, Kaiser Permanente Medical Center, San Francisco.

Elizabeth C. Saviano, RNC, MSN
Nurse Practitioner II, Faculty Obstetrics and Gynecology Group,
University of California School of Medicine, San Francisco.

Kris Strohbehn, MD
Assistant Professor, Department of Obstetrics and Gynecology, Tufts University Medical School, New England Medical Center, Boston.

Shari Thomas, MD
Director of Urogynecology and Assistant Professor, Department of Obstetrics and Gynecology, King Drew University Medical Center, and Assistant Professor, Department of Obstetrics and Gynecology, University of California School of Medicine, Los Angeles.

Victoria L. Tishman, MD
Assistant Professor, Department of Obstetrics and Gynecology, Duke University School of Medicine, Durham.

Cheryl K. Walker, MD
Assistant Clinical Professor, Department of Obstetrics, Gynecology, and Reproductive Sciences, University of California School of Medicine, San Francisco.

Dilys M. Walker, MD
Assistant Professor, Department of Obstetrics, Gynecology, and Reproductive Sciences, University of California School of Medicine, San Francisco.

Preface

The *Handbook of Gynecology & Obstetrics* is a completely new handbook. It is current, concise, and clinically relevant. Expert faculty, clinicians, and residents have collaborated to provide pertinent and practical information for the reader. Each chapter includes a list of suggested readings for further in-depth study.

The *Handbook* has been written in a unique format with greater emphasis on gynecology. This break from tradition reflects the importance of gynecology in virtually all aspects of medical training and practice. The majority of students, residents, and practitioners care for female patients, and therefore a broad understanding of gynecology is essential. The *Handbook* is a superb resource covering subjects in general gynecology, endocrinology, infertility, and gynecologic oncology. Specifically, evaluation and management of common clinical problems such as the abnormal Pap smear, ectopic pregnancy, pelvic mass, and sexually transmitted diseases are reviewed. Issues pertaining to the mature woman are contained in chapters on menopause, urinary incontinence, and pelvic relaxation. Also included are current topics on women and AIDS and ethical issues in women's health care.

The *Handbook* is also an ideal quick reference for major topics and problems in obstetrics. It was written with the reader in mind, whether that user is a medical student, nurse practitioner or midwife, resident or family physician. The unique maternal demands of pregnancy and the dynamics of the evolving fetal compartment are reviewed in the chapters on physiology and fetoplacental development. The focus of the clinician's early assessment of the pregnant patient is addressed in the chapters on prenatal care and genetic screening. While the vast majority of pregnancies proceed to term without difficulty, the clinician can also be challenged to manage the wide range of complications that may attend pregnancy. The Handbook provides a current resource for the major obstetric, surgical, and medical complications of pregnancy including multiple gestation, placenta previa and abruption, hypertensive disorders, and infectious diseases. The application of new technologies to the estimation of fetal well-being is considered in the chapters on antepartum and intrapartum fetal assessment. Finally, the culmination of pregnancy, the emergence of the newborn infant through the process of labor and delivery, is presented with an overview of the physiologic return to the non-pregnant state in the post-partum period.

The *Handbook of Gynecology & Obstetrics* was envisioned, in theory, to be a rapid and informative reference for the novice clinician in the area of women's health care. It is hoped that, in practice, it will complement and foster the clinical development of a provider of health care to women.

San Francisco, California   Jeanette S. Brown, MD
June, 1992   William R. Crombleholme, MD

Section I:
Anatomy & Physiology of the Female Reproductive System

Embryology & Anatomy of the Female Urogenital Tract | 1

William R. Crombleholme, MD

Understanding the physiology and pathophysiology of the female reproductive system requires knowledge of embryonic development and normal anatomy. This chapter reviews early developmental changes to provide such an anatomic foundation.

EMBRYOLOGY

Urinary System

The permanent kidneys develop in 3 stages. In the first stage, the pronephros develops at the end of the pronephric duct, which runs caudally to open into the cloaca. The pronephros is nonfunctional and degenerates, but most of its duct remains as part of the second stage of kidney development, the mesonephros (Figure 1–1). The mesonephros develops from cells located medially to the pronephric duct in the nephrogenic cords. The cells develop into mesonephric tubules that grow laterally to connect with the pronephric duct, which now becomes the mesonephric (wolffian) duct. The medial end of each mesonephric tubule forms a mesonephric corpuscle as a result of invaginated blood capillaries. However, like the pronephros, the mesonephros degenerates except for the mesonephric duct, which persists. In the third and final stage of kidney development, the **metanephros** develops from the metanephric diverticulum or ureteric bud and the adjacent mesoderm, which is called the metanephrogenic mass. The ureteric bud grows

1

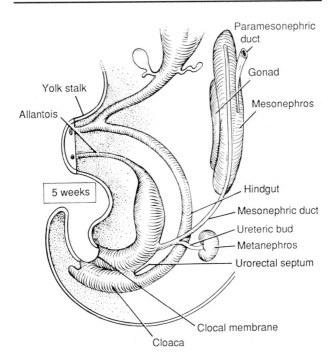

Figure 1-1. Left lateral view of urogenital system in relation to the hindgut at about 5 weeks. The paramesonephric duct does not appear until the sixth week but is shown here to indicate its position and downgrowth. *(Reproduced, with permission, from Pernoll ML [editor]: Current Obstetric & Gynecologic Diagnosis & Treatment, 7th ed. Appleton & Lange, 1991.)*

dorsally from the mesonephric duct near its entry into the cloaca. It continues to grow during development, eventually forming the ureter, renal pelvis, renal calices, and collecting tubules of the permanent kidney. The metanephrogenic mass, which caps the ureteric bud, gives rise to the nephrons of the permanent kidney.

Genital System

The cloaca becomes divided by a sheet of mesenchyme called the urorectal septum (Figure 1-1). This septum arises in the angle between the allantois and the hindgut. The urorectal septum eventually fuses with the cloacal membrane to form the perineal body. This fusion also divides the cloaca into 2 parts, the rectum dorsally and the urogenital sinus ventrally.

The urogenital sinus has 3 parts: a vesicourethral canal, a pelvic portion, and a phallic portion (Figure 1–2). The vesicourethral canal, which is continuous with the allantois, develops into the urinary bladder. The caudal portions of the mesonephric ducts become incorporated into the dorsal wall of the bladder so that the ureters come to eventually open into the bladder lumen. The pelvic portion of the urogenital sinus is incorporated into the development of the vagina, and the phallic portion into the development of the external genitalia.

Gonadal development at the indifferent stage begins with a proliferation of cells medial to the mesonephros called the gonadal ridge. Further growth leads to the development of an outer cortex and an inner medulla. In females (XX chromosomes), the cortex differentiates into the ovary and the medulla regresses. As the mesonephros regresses, the medially developing ovary becomes suspended by its own mesentery, the mesovarium.

Lateral to the mesonephros and parallel to it, longitudinal invagination of coelomic epithelium forms the paramesonephric (müllerian) ducts. The cranial ends remain open to the peritoneal cavity to form the fimbriated ends of the uterine (fallopian) tubes. The caudal ends of the paramesonephric ducts fuse in the midline ventral to the mesonephric ducts to form the uterovaginal primordium (Figure 1–2). The uterovaginal primordium develops into the epithelium and glands of the uterus, with adjacent mesenchyme forming stroma and myometrium. From the pelvic portion of the urogenital sinus, paired sinovaginal bulbs grow into the caudal end of the uterovaginal primordium to form the **vagina.**

Vestigial remnants of the mesonephric duct and mesonephric tubules may persist into adult life. A few tubules and a portion of the mesonephric duct may persist in the broad ligament between the ovary and tube and is called the **epoöphoron.** Similar vestiges in the broad ligament closer to the uterus are called the **paroöphoron.** Portions of the mesonephric duct may persist in the broad ligament, along the lateral margin of the uterus and the lateral wall of the upper vagina. This remnant is called Gartner's duct and may result in Gartner's duct cysts. Additionally, remnants of the cranial end of the paramesonephric duct that are not incorporated into the fimbria of the uterine tube may persist as hydatids of Morgagni.

Ventral to the phallic portion of the urogenital sinus, the geni-

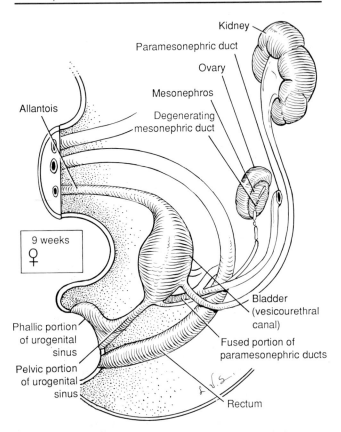

Figure 1–2. Female reproductive tract at an early stage of sexual differentiation (about 9 weeks). *(Reproduced, with permission, from Pernoll ML [editor]:* Current Obstetric & Gynecologic Diagnosis & Treatment, *7th ed. Appleton & Lange, 1991.)*

tal tubercle develops. Lateral to the cloacal membrane, the labio-scrotal swellings and urogenital folds develop. After the perineal body forms, the urogenital membrane develops ventrally then ruptures to create the urogenital opening. As the genital tubercle elongates to form a phallus, a urethral groove forms on its ventral surface that communicates with the urogenital opening. The phallus becomes the clitoris, and the unfused urogenital folds become the labia minora. The labioscrotal folds form the labia majora but fuse anteriorly to form the mons pubis. The phallic portion of the urogenital sinus ultimately forms the vestibule into which the urethra and vagina open.

ANATOMY

External Genitalia

The female reproductive system has both external and internal components. As shown in Figure 1–3, the external genitalia are readily visible on inspection of the vulva: mons pubis (veneris), labia majora, labia minora, clitoris, vestibule, external urethral meatus, Skene's glands (paraurethral glands), Bartholin's glands (vulvovaginal glands), hymen, fourchette, perineal body, and fossa navicularis.

The mons pubis is an elevation of fatty tissue over the area of the symphysis pubis that develops from the genital tubercle. It is the region immediately above the labia and is usually covered with coarse pubic hair. It is innervated by the ilioinguinal and genito-femoral nerves with its blood supply coming from the external pudendal artery.

The labia majora are the raised longitudinal folds of skin just lateral to the labia minora, which merge with the mons pubis superiorly. They consist of connective and areolar tissue and are homologous to the scrotum. The round ligaments of the uterus end in a fibrous insertion in the superior portion of the labia majora. The labia majora are innervated by the ilioinguinal and pudendal nerves superiorly and by the femoral cutaneous nerve posteriorly. Their blood supply is derived from the internal and external pudendal arteries.

The labia minora are narrow elongated folds of skin medial to the labia majora that surround the vaginal orifice laterally. Superior to the clitoris, the labia minora fuse to form the clitoral hood or prepuce and to form the frenulum of the clitoris inferiorly.

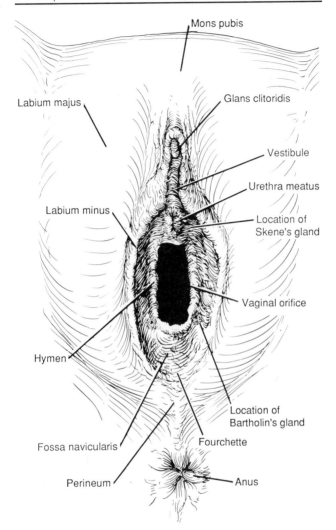

Figure 1-3. External female genitalia. *(Reproduced, with permission, from Benson RC:* Handbook of Obstetrics & Gynecology, *8th ed. Lange, 1983.)*

Posteriorly the labia merge at the fourchette. Innervation is provided by the ilioinguinal, pudendal, and hemorrhoidal nerves. The external and internal pudendal arteries provide their blood supply.

The clitoris is the homologue of the penis in the male. It is usually about 2–3 cm long and is located superior to the urethral meatus beneath the fused portions of the labia minora, which form its prepuce. The clitoris is composed of erectile tissue that is attached to the periosteum of the symphysis, and its terminal portion, the glans clitoridis, is richly innervated with sensory endings. This innervation is derived from the hypogastric and pudendal nerves as well as pelvic sympathetics. Its vascular supply is from the internal pudendal artery.

The roughly triangular area superior to the vaginal orifice and medial to the superior portions of the labia minora is the vestibule. The urethral meatus opens onto this area. Also in the vestibule, just inferior and lateral to the urethral meatus, are the orifices of the paraurethral ducts or Skene's ducts. All 3 of these structures are supplied by the internal pudendal artery and innervated by the pudendal nerve. The vestibule represents the mature structure in the adult female of the urogenital sinus of the embryo and also extends posteriorly. It remains medial to the labia minora but is bounded inferiorly by the fourchette, a low ridge of tissue where the labia majora and labia minora converge. The narrow portion of the vestibule between the fourchette and the vaginal orifice is the fossa navicularis. These posterior structures are supplied by the pudendal and inferior hemorrhoidal arteries and innervated by the corresponding nerves.

The vaginal orifice is demarcated from the vestibule by the hymen. The hymen is a membrane composed of connective tissue that is moderately elastic and partially (and rarely completely) occludes the vaginal canal. In newborns and infants the central aperture may range from only a pinpoint to a few millimeters in diameter. With childhood physical activity or the onset of puberty and menstruation, this aperture can enlarge so that first coitus is not necessarily accompanied by "tearing." As with the other structures in the posterior vestibule, innervation and vascular supply are from the pudendal and inferior hemorrhoidal arteries and nerves.

Just inside the vagina are two small openings, one on each side. A narrow duct, about 1–2 cm long, connects the opening to a small mucous-producing gland, the vulvovaginal or Bartholin's gland. These glands provide lubrication during coitus and are supplied by the internal pudendal artery and corresponding nerve.

Internal Genitalia

The internal genitalia, shown in Figures 1–4 and 1–5, consist of the vagina, cervix, uterus, fallopian tubes, and ovaries.

The vagina is a thin muscular canal that lies between the bladder arteriorly and the rectum posteriorly. It averages 8–10 cm in length and 4 cm in diameter. The cervix protrudes into the upper vagina such that recesses form between the cervix and the vault of the vagina called fornices. Innervation of the vagina is derived from the pudendal and hemorrhoidal nerves and the pelvic sympathetic chain. Its blood supply is from the vaginal artery, a branch of the descending uterine artery, and the middle hemorrhoidal and internal pudendal arteries.

The cervix is the lower portion of the uterus that extends into the upper vagina. Overall, the cervix is about 2–4 cm long with

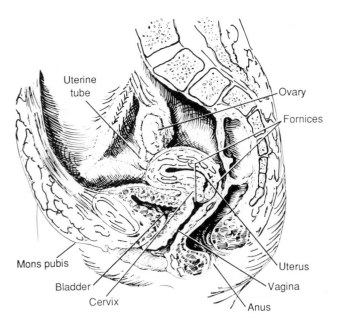

Figure 1–4. Midsagittal view of the female pelvic organs. *(Reproduced, with permission, from Benson RC:* Handbook of Obstetrics & Gynecology, *8th ed. Lange, 1983.)*

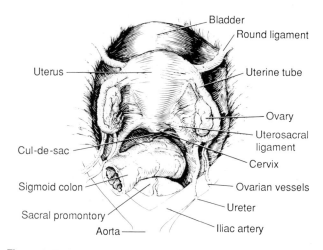

Figure 1–5. Superior view of the female pelvic organs. *(Reproduced, with permission, from Benson RC:* Handbook of Obstetrics & Gynecology, *8th ed. Lange, 1983.)*

half of its length above the level of the vaginal vault. The vaginal portion is about 2.5 cm in outside diameter with a central canal that connects the vagina with the uterine cavity. The external cervical os is the vaginal opening of the endocervical canal, and the internal os is at the junction between the cervix and the corpus of the uterus. Innervation of the cervix is derived from the second, third, and fourth sacral nerves and the pelvic sympathetic plexus. Its vascular supply is provided by the cervical artery, which is a branch of the descending uterine artery.

The uterus is a muscular pear-shaped organ that lies between the bladder and the rectum (Figure 1–5). In the nonpregnant state, the uterus is 6–8 cm long. From the upper or fundal portion of the uterus 4 tubular structures arise, 2 on each side. Anteriorly, the round ligaments arise and extend to the sidewall of the pelvis to end in the labia majora. Posteriorly, the uterine tubes arise to extend posterolaterally to end with their fimbria on the medial side of the broad ligament. Inferiorly, from the posterior aspect of the uterus at the junction of the uterus and cervix, fibrous supports originate to insert into the periosteum of the sacrum called the uterosacral ligaments. Innervation of the uterus is provided by the lower thoracic as well as lumbar and sacral roots. The blood supply is principally from the uterine artery, a terminal branch of the hypogastric artery, with branches to the upper cervical region, the uterine corpus and fundus, and some terminal branches anastomose with branches of the ovarian arteries.

The uterine tubes extend about 10–12 cm posterolaterally from the cornu of the uterus. The fimbriated end is open to the peritoneal cavity but is near the ovary to capture the released ovum at the time of ovulation. The tubes are enclosed in a peritoneal fold called the mesosalpinx, which is part of the broad ligament. Each tube is divided into segments of varying diameters. As mentioned above, the terminal portion is open and fimbriated. The distal 2–3 cm of the tube, just before the fimbriated end, is the infundibulum. The middle 6–8 cm of the tube is called the ampulla and is connected to the uterus by the isthmic portion, which is usually 1–2 cm long. The part of the tube passing through the uterine wall and connecting the tube with the uterine cavity (about 1 cm long) is the interstitial portion. Innervation is similar to that of the uterus. The vascular supply of the proximal portions of the tube is through the terminal branches of the uterine artery, whereas the distal portions are supplied by branches of both the uterine and ovarian arteries.

The ovaries are whitish, ovoid, firm structures suspended from the medial aspect of the broad ligament by the mesovarium and from the posterolateral aspect of the uterus by the suspensary ligament of the ovary. In women of reproductive age, each ovary is approximately $1.5 \times 3 \times 3.5$ cm and hangs freely in the peritoneal cavity. Innervation is from the dorsal roots of T10 and L1 as well as fibers from the pelvic and lumbar sympathetic plexuses. The ovarian arteries arise from the aorta and reach the ovary within the infundibulopelvic ligament and anastomose with terminal branches of the uterine arteries.

The embryologic development and final anatomy of the reproductive system can be confusing initially. Understanding such development requires the construction of a 3-dimensional image of the embryonic structures themselves and their relationship to each other and to those structures they will form in the adult. Such imagining requires time and careful thought but is rewarded in clinical practice when congenital anomalies, such as uterine septation, are encountered and their etiology is then more easily appreciated.

SUGGESTED READINGS

Droegemueller W et al: *Comprehensive Gynecology,* Mosby, 1987.

Moore KL: *The Developing Human: Clinically Oriented Embryology,* 4th ed. Saunders, 1988.

2 | Menstrual Physiology

Lesley R. Levine, MD

Understanding the hormonal mechanisms and endometrial reactions involved in the menstrual cycle provides a basis for many diagnostic and treatment modalities used in gynecology today.

The menstrual cycle and endometrial response occur in preparation for fertilization and pregnancy. The onset of menstruation at puberty is called **menarche.** The cycle begins on the first day of menstruation and lasts until the first day of the next menstruation. The average **cycle length** is 28 days, but a length of 21–40 days is normal if it occurs regularly.

At birth, the newborn ovary contains 2 million potentially viable germ cells. (This amount is considerably less than the peak of 6–7 million, which occurs in the 20-week fetus.) By puberty, only 300,000 follicles are left. Of this entire amount, 400 or so will successfully ovulate. For each ovum thus produced, about 1000 others will grow and fail.

MENSTRUAL CYCLE

Generally, the cycle is divided into 3 phases, **follicular, ovulation**, and **luteal** phases, the entire purpose of which is the selection, development, and support of a single mature, or dominant, follicle.

Follicular Phase
During this phase, a dominant follicle is selected. In approximately 10–14 days, a sequence of hormonal actions on the primordial follicles causes a dominant follicle to appear and many others to become **atretic,** or involuted.

The **primordial follicle** is simply an ovum that was arrested in the prophase stage of meiotic division and is surrounded by a single layer of granulosa cells. These cells are constantly growing, independent of gonadotropin stimulation. They will start to grow at *all* times of the month, even during pregnancy.

Follicle-stimulating hormone (FSH) is secreted by the anterior pituitary in response to declining levels of estrogen and progesterone from the previous cycle. FSH affects the spontaneously growing primordial follicle by increasing FSH receptors and signaling the intracellular production of estrogen by the granulosa cells. The combination of FSH and estrogen in the microenvironment of the follicle stimulates proliferation of the granulosa cells, thus leading to the development of more FSH receptors, the production of more estrogen, and the stimulation of still more granulosa cells. In this locally induced positive feedback system, a dominant follicle is usually established between the fifth and the seventh day. Peripheral levels of **estradiol** (the most significant estrogen) begin to rise on the seventh day (Figure 2–1).

Furthermore, initially low levels of estrogen secreted by the ovary exert a positive feedback signal to the anterior pituitary to release more FSH. This signal is also received in the hypothalamus, which secretes **gonadotropin-releasing hormone (GnRH).** However, as estrogen concentrations reach a critical level, the feedback becomes a negative influence, and the amount of FSH secreted decreases. At this point, the follicle with the most FSH receptors has a significant advantage in continuing on its course of development. Another hormone secreted by the dominant follicle is **inhibin,** which also decreases the amount of FSH secreted.

Follicles not destined to ovulate produce more androgens in the microenvironment because fewer FSH receptors are available and therefore fewer precursors are converted to estrogen. The precursors are instead converted to androgens, which also block aromatization and formation of estrogen. Atresia of these follicles can happen at any time during the cycle. As FSH levels decline, those follicles with fewer FSH receptors produce more androgens, which leads to a "wave" of atresia. Thus, the follicular phase creates a dominant follicle. The dominant follicle ensures its success locally with high levels of estrogen to increase FSH receptors and globally by decreasing the amount of FSH available to the other follicles.

The dominant follicle continues to develop to the preovulatory phase. The proliferation of granulosa cells secrete more and more estrogen into a fluid-filled **antrum** that bathes the germ cell in a protein- and hormone-rich environment. Cells surrounding the granulosa layer, known as **theca cells,** develop a rich vasculature, which may also permit selective delivery of FSH.

In preparation for ovulation, the dominant follicle must develop **luteinizing hormone (LH)** receptors. LH is secreted in small amounts during the follicular phase but has little effect until recep-

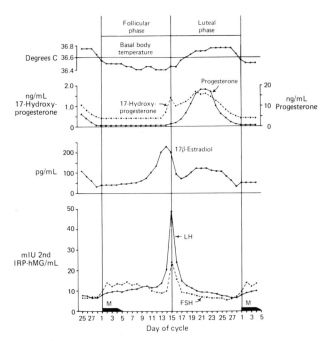

Figure 2-1. Typical basal body temperature and plasma hormone concentration during a normal 28-day human menstrual cycle. M, menstruation; IRP-hMG, international reference standard for gonadotropins. *(Reproduced, with permission, from Midgley AR in:* Human Reproduction. *Hafez ESE, Evans TN [editors]. Harper & Row, 1973.)*

tors are developed on the granulosa cells. In the presence of high levels of estrogen in the follicle, FSH changes its focus from the production of FSH receptors to the development of LH receptors. Peripheral estradiol levels exert a positive feedback effect on the secretion of LH, which increases rapidly toward the end of the follicular phase. LH induces the production of **progesterone** in the granulosa cells. (The granulosa cells become rich in lipids and have a yellow appearance, hence the name luteinizing.)

At this point, the preovulatory environment is marked by the following:

(1) A preovulatory follicle with a thick granulosa layer produces high levels of estrogen and some progesterone, and a richly vascularized theca layer circulates high levels of FSH and LH to the follicle.

(2) Levels of LH increase rapidly in response to high levels of estrogen and some progesterone. Another smaller surge of FSH occurs in response to increasing levels of progesterone. This surge is thought to complete the action of FSH on the dominant follicle and the further atresia of any competing follicles.

(3) The many atretic follicles produce circulating androgens, which may contribute to an increased sex drive at the time of ovulation.

Ovulation

Estradiol levels continue to rise, producing a proportionate increase in LH, known as the **LH surge.** The peak of the LH surge occurs 10–12 hours before ovulation, and knowledge of its timing is an important clinical tool in fertility treatments. The high levels of LH are important because they (1) initiate the resumption of meiosis in the oocyte to complete the reduction division, (2) induce further luteinization of the granulosa cell to produce more progesterone necessary in the luteal phase, and (3) induce production of prostaglandins locally that are responsible for the actual breakdown of the follicle and release of the oocyte. Rising levels of progesterone have a negative feedback effect on LH and contribute to the end of the surge.

Release of the oocyte is due to local effects of prostaglandins, progesterone, and other proteolytic enzymes (collagenase and plasmin) accumulated in the fluid of the follicle. Intrafollicular pressure does not increase; instead, the wall surrounding the follicles degenerates. Inhibition of prostaglandin synthesis may block follicular rupture. Clinically, this effect could be relevant in a patient who is having difficulty with fertility and is taking large amounts of antiprostaglandins (eg, ibuprofen).

The LH surge also causes a large decrease in the amount of peripheral estradiol. This decrease may be due to a downregulation of LH receptors and a corresponding decrease in steroid production.

Ovulation requires not only an LH surge but also a fully prepared and ready-to-respond follicle. This is a remarkably coordinated effort in which the rising estradiol levels signal the readiness of the dominant follicle and precipitate the necessary secretion of LH to release the oocyte for fertilization.

Luteal Phase

After ovulation occurs, the follicle collapses on itself, and the granulosa cells increase in size to become the **corpus luteum** (yellow body). The corpus luteum secretes estrogens, androgens, and most significantly, progesterone. Progesterone reaches its maximum level peripherally about 8 days after the LH surge (Figure 2–1). Locally, in the ovary, progesterone suppresses new follicular growth. As a result, the dominant follicle for the next cycle may be produced in the contralateral ovary.

LH levels slowly decrease during this period. Inhibin, released from the corpus luteum, also decreases gonadotropins. As LH levels decrease, the corpus luteum degenerates. Less estradiol and progesterone are secreted, and lower circulating levels of these hormones initiate a rise in FSH levels for the beginning of the next follicular phase.

The time from the LH surge to the onset of menstruation is 14 days. Cycle length can vary as a result of differing lengths of the follicular phase, but once ovulation has occurred, the corpus luteum degenerates at a fairly rapid and consistent pace. The only way to interrupt the failing corpus luteum is with hormonal support in the form of **human chorionic gonadotropin (hCG)**, a hormone secreted during pregnancy. Like LH, hCG supports the corpus luteum, which, in turn, supplies the progesterone and estradiol necessary to maintain an early gestation.

A healthy corpus luteum results only from a healthy dominant follicle. If the mechanisms of the follicular phase are interrupted such that an unhealthy follicle is produced, an **inadequate luteal phase** occurs in which the corpus luteum is not fully functional and does not produce adequate concentrations of progesterone. This situation may occur in less than 5% of cycles and is occasionally the cause of infertility or recurrent spontaneous abortions.

ENDOMETRIAL CYCLE

If the ovum released during ovulation is fertilized, it must be supported and protected. Endometrial reactions to the hormonal changes of the ovarian cycle are designed to provide a nutrient- and blood-rich compartment to support the early zygote and embryo (Figure 2–2).

Proliferative Phase

The proliferative phase corresponds with the follicular phase of the ovarian cycle. Circulating levels of estradiol directly affect

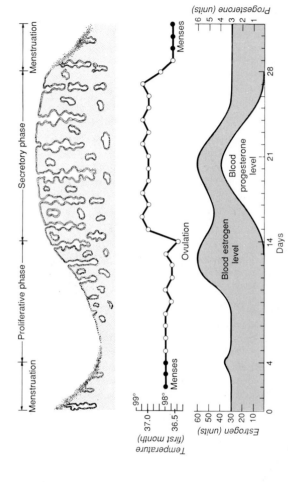

Figure 2-2. Menstrual cycle: hormones, endometrial changes, and basal body temperature. (*Modified and reproduced, with permission, from: Benson RC: Handbook of Obstetrics & Gynecology, 8th ed. Lange, 1983.*)

the structure of the endometrial lining. The endometrium is composed of glands made of epithelial cells, stroma, and other supporting structures, such as arteries.

After menstruation, the entire lining of the uterus is desquamated, and only a thin layer of stroma and epithelial cells remains. Estradiol directly stimulates the reconstruction of the endometrium by means of specific receptors in the epithelial and stromal cells. There is progressive growth of glands and stroma, as evidenced by the numerous mitoses, characteristic of this phase. By the time of ovulation, a continuous, smooth layer of endometrial tissue lines the entire uterine cavity, and this tissue is well vascularized by a large increase in the volume of the spiral arteries.

Secretory Phase

The presence of progesterone, circulating during the luteal phase, stops the continued growth of epithelial and stromal cells. The glands now become tortuous and filled with secretions, which is characteristic of this phase. The spiral arteries continue to grow and coil around the glands, while the stroma becomes more edematous.

All these changes are designed to support an early zygote in the morula stage (2–3 days after fertilization). At this stage, nutrient-rich secretions fill the glands and offer support by simple diffusion. The morula grows unattached in this environment for approximately 6 days, at which time the blastocyst has outgrown the ability to support itself by simple diffusion and begins the process of placentation. This process takes advantage of the intricate vascular plexus developed among the glands, under the epithelial lining.

Menstruation

In the absence of fertilization, the corpus luteum follows its consistent pattern of degeneration, and circulating levels of estradiol and progesterone decrease, leading to a sequence of events, particularly the cessation of growth and vasospasm. Vasospasm causes ischemia, necrosis, and desquamation of the endometrial lining. Prostaglandins (specifically, PGE and $PGF_{2\alpha}$) are released and contribute to the vasospasm.

Normal menstrual flow removes two-thirds of the functional endometrium and involves approximately 40 mL of blood loss. It usually lasts 4–5 days, by which time estradiol from the follicular phase of the ovarian cycle begins to heal and regenerate the endometrial tissue.

CENTRAL REGULATION OF THE MENSTRUAL CYCLE

Regulation of the menstrual cycle is a highly complex phenomenon. The sequence of events presented so far exclude a major but as yet not well understood aspect of regulation: the role of the hypothalamus and GnRH. GnRH is synthesized in the arcuate nucleus of the hypothalamus and released locally into the portal circulation. It is a very short-acting and specific coordinator that plays a permissive, not a controlling, role. Because its half-life is 3–4 minutes, it must be continuously released. Studies have shown that GnRH is secreted in a pulsatile manner and in a critical range. Changing the pulse frequency of GnRH will directly affect the secretion of FSH and LH into the peripheral circulation. Infusing GnRH continuously will stop all FSH and LH release. Clinically, GnRH analogues can be used to decrease FSH and LH cyclicity and to treat estrogen-dependent conditions, such as endometriosis, precocious puberty, and even myomas.

SUGGESTED READINGS

Current role of GnRH agonists in obstetrics and gynecology. (Proceedings from the symposium.) *Obstet Gynecol Surv* 1989;**44**:293.

Guyton AC (editor): *Textbook of Medical Physiology,* 8th ed. Saunders, 1991.

Pernoll ML (editor): *Current Obstetric & Gynecologic Diagnosis & Treatment,* 7th ed. Appleton & Lange, 1991.

Section II:
General Gynecology

Approach to the Patient: Gynecologic History & Pelvic Examination | 3

Jeanette S. Brown, MD

This chapter focuses on obtaining the patient's gynecologic history and performing a pelvic examination. However, a complete medical history, including the patient's age and occupation, family and social history, review of systems, and medications and allergies, should also be obtained at the time of the initial examination.

The gynecologic history and pelvic examination may be an uncomfortable and sometimes embarrassing experience for the patient. When possible, the history should be taken with the patient fully clothed. Before the pelvic examination begins, allow time to discuss any questions the patient may have and to explore any difficulties that she may have encountered in previous examinations. If this is the patient's first pelvic examination, thoroughly review the procedure, including a demonstration of how the speculum is used.

Nonjudgmental and open-ended questions are useful to elicit a comprehensive history. For this reason, the following section on gynecologic history includes sample questions to ask the patient, as well as examples of how this information is recorded in the patient's chart. Also, because clear communication is so important in the approach to the patient, sample explanations are also given in the next section on the pelvic examination.

GYNECOLOGIC HISTORY

Chief Complaint/Present Illness (CC/PI)

The gynecologic history may begin with the following question: Do you have a particular problem or problems that brought you here today? After the patient describes her problem in her own words, the clinician should clarify her specific problem with direct questions that include a review of the severity, timing, location, and length of time the problem has been present. *Example:* CC/PI: Severe cramping at menses, in the mid pelvis, radiating to the lower back, becoming progressively worse over the last 2 yr, and now disrupting her work 2–3 d/mo.*

Pregnancies

It is important to obtain a complete obstetrical history (Chapter 32) and to ask clear, specific questions such as the following: "Have you ever been pregnant? How many times have you been pregnant? What was the outcome of each pregnancy?" The circumstances surrounding each gestation (eg, number of weeks of gestation at loss or termination, additional procedures that were needed) and any complications (eg, hemorrhage, endometritis, perforation) are discussed and noted. The following abbreviations are used to record the response:

- G   Gravidity (number of pregnancies)
- P   Parity (number of term deliveries)
- SAB   Spontaneous abortion
- TAB   Therapeutic abortion
- *Example:* 28 YO accountant G2 P1 TAB1.

Menstrual History

The menstrual history should include details about the patient's menstrual period. Thus, questions such as "What was the date of your last menstrual period?" should be asked. The date of the last normal menstrual period (LMP) should be noted, and, if indicated, the date of the previous menstrual period (PMP) is recorded. When appropriate, the age of menarche or the age of menopause is included. Review the usual cycle length, number of days of flow, and the amount of flow. Although it is difficult to exactly quantify the amount of flow, it can be estimated by the number of pads or tampons used. Abnormal, intermenstrual, or postcoital bleeding is also noted. *Example:* LMP 2/16; every 26–28 days; cycle lasting 3–4 days; using 3–4 tampons/day.

---

*Typical abbreviations used in patient's charts are as follows: YO (years old); d (day), mo (month), yr (year); Dx (diagnosis), Hx (history), Rx (treatment), IUD (intrauterine device); PID (pelvic inflammatory disease); outpt (outpatient); gyn (gynecologic).

Sexual History

The following questions are appropriate for assessing the patient's sexual history: "Have you ever been sexually active? Are you currently sexually active? Are you sexually active with men, women, or both?" The clinician should note the number of current partners and relationship status (eg, single, significantly involved, married). It is also important to ask the patient if she is having any sexual problems she would like to discuss. If there is a problem, the sexual knowledge base of the patient, her orgasmic ability, and whether she experiences dyspareunia should be determined. *Example:* significantly involved and sexually active with one male partner; no sexual problems.

Contraception

The clinician should ascertain what type of contraception is used and how often, for example, by asking the following questions: "What type of contraception do you use? Are you using it consistently?" If the patient is not satisfied with her present birth control method, other methods should be discussed. Any prior complication with a birth control method should be noted. *Example:* diaphragm, inconsistently; Hx IUD with endometritis.

Infections & Sexually Transmitted Diseases

Obtaining the patient's history of infections and sexually transmitted diseases is important and may include the following questions: "Have you ever had a sexually transmitted disease? Have you ever had pelvic inflammatory disease? Have your uterus, tubes, or ovaries ever been infected?" The type of disease is noted, as well as the treatment and whether the treatment was performed on an outpatient or inpatient basis. *Example:* Hx *Chlamydia* with outpt Rx; no Hx PID.

Additional Pertinent Gynecologic History

To provide optimal care, the clinician should obtain information about other gynecologic procedures, such as the results of Papanicolaou (Pap) tests and the treatments the patient received, by asking simple, straightforward questions such as the following: "When was the last time you had a Pap smear done?" The clinician then notes the date of the patient's last Papanicolaou smear, her history of abnormal Papanicolaou smears and follow-up treatments, and any gynecologic or abdominal surgeries. *Example:* benign Pap 6 months prior; no Hx abnormal Pap; no Hx gyn/abdominal surgery.

Summary of Gynecologic History

On conclusion of the interview of the patient's gynecologic history, the information is summarized as follows: CC/PI: Severe cramping at menses, in the mid pelvis, radiating to the lower back, becoming progressively worse over the last 2 yr, and now disrupting her work 2–3 d/mo. Gyn history: 28 YO accountant G2 P1 TAB1; LMP 2/16; every 26–28 days; cycle lasting 3–5 days; using 4 tampons/day; significantly involved and sexually active with one male partner; no sexual problems; diaphragm, inconsistently; Hx IUD with endometritis; Hx *Chlamydia* with outpt Rx; no Hx PID;

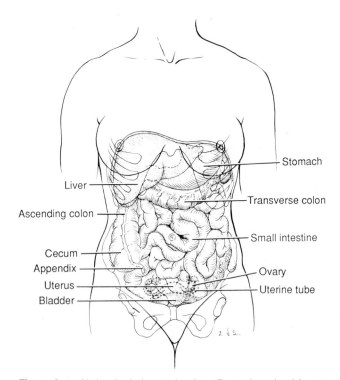

Figure 3-1. Abdominal viscera in situ. *(Reproduced, with permission, from Pernoll ML [editor]:* Current Obstetric & Gynecologic Diagnosis & Treatment, *7th ed. Appleton & Lange, 1991.)*

benign Pap 6 months prior; no Hx abnormal Pap; no Hx gyn/abdominal surgery.

PELVIC EXAMINATION

After the history is completed, the patient changes into an examination gown and waist drape. Blood pressure and weight are measured and recorded. A complete physical examination should be performed. However, for the sake of brevity, only the abdominal and pelvic examinations are discussed below. The breast examination is discussed in Chapter 17.

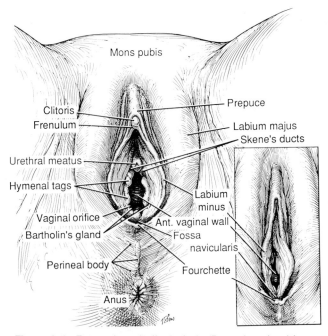

Figure 3-2. External genitalia (vulva). *(Reproduced, with permission, from Cunningham FG, McDonald PC, Gant NF: Williams Obstetrics, 18th ed. Appleton & Lange, 1989.)*

A running commentary is maintained throughout the examination to explain each step of the procedure as well as the physical findings, both normal and abnormal. If the patient has described experiencing pain in a particular area, the examination should begin at a nontender site.

The first part of the pelvic examination is the abdominal examination. This can be a time in which to build trust between the patient and the examiner. For example, it is often reassuring to the patient for the clinician to describe the underlying organ as each quadrant of the abdomen is palpated (Figure 3–1). Rather than use the word "relax" to better palpate an area, it is often more productive to offer a suggestion such as "please soften these muscles here."

After the abdominal examination is complete, the patient is asked to slide her buttocks to the base of the examination table and to place her feet in the stirrups, then the stirrups are adjusted to a comfortable length.

External Genitalia

The examination may begin with the following explanations: "First, I am going to examine the outside of the vagina, which is called the vulva; now I am placing my fingers at the bottom of the lips of the vulva or labia." The clinician then separates the labia at the fourchette to allow for clear inspection of the inner aspects of the labia, clitoris, urethra, Skene's glands, vaginal orifice, and Bartholin's gland opening (Figure 3–2). These areas are inspected for inflammation, ulceration, or lesions. If abnormalities are present on the vulva, they can be shown to the patient with a mirror.

Rarely are the Skene's or Bartholin's glands visible unless they are inflamed. If inflammation of the Skene's gland is suspected, the gland can be "milked" by placing one finger in the anterior vagina and gently pressing along the urethra. If any discharge appears at the gland opening adjacent to the urethra, the Skene's gland is inflamed.

A Bartholin's abscess or cyst can occur when the duct is blocked or inflamed. In the acute stage, the abscess is tender and inflamed. If the abscess does not resolve with sitz baths, treatment consists of incision and drainage. A Word catheter is then placed for 2–3 weeks to allow for epithelization of a new drainage tract. A recurrent abscess can be marsupialized (Figure 3–3).

Speculum Examination

The clinician should choose an appropriate type and size of speculum for the patient (Figure 3–4). The speculum should be

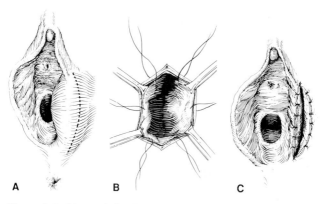

Figure 3–3. Marsupialization of Bartholin's cyst. ***A:*** The cyst or abscess is incised. ***B:*** Interrupted sutures secure the cyst lining to the skin edges. ***C:*** Completed marsupialization. *(Reproduced, with permission, from Benson RC: Handbook of Obstetrics & Gynecology, 8th ed. Lange, 1983.)*

prewarmed on a heating pad or with water. Lubricating jelly should not be used because it may interfere with the Papanicolaou smear. Touching the patient's inner thigh with the speculum not only tests the temperature but also prepares the patient for insertion of the speculum into the vagina.

It is beneficial to explain to the patient what is happening with comments such as "I am going to place the speculum now; you may feel some downward pressure." The shaft screw is tightened, and the speculum is grasped in the palm of the hand with the index and middle fingers around the blades for insertion. The labia are separated at the posterior fourchette, and the blades are inserted in a vertical position in a posterior direction. As the speculum is advanced, it is slowly rotated clockwise so that it is in a horizontal position when at the cervix. Again, it is useful to explain what is happening to the patient with the following statement: "I am opening the speculum now, and you may feel some increased pressure." Then the speculum is opened slowly to the point where the entire cervix can be seen (Figure 3–5).

Papanicolaou Smear

It is useful to address the patient in the following manner before the Papanicolaou smear is obtained: "I am going to do the

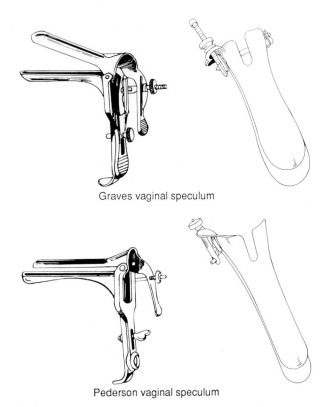

Graves vaginal speculum

Pederson vaginal speculum

Figure 3-4. Two types of specula. Most often, the Graves speculum is chosen for the multiparous patient and the Pederson speculum for the nulliparous patient. *(Reproduced, with permission, from Benson RC:* Handbook of Obstetrics & Gynecology, *8th ed. Lange, 1983.)*

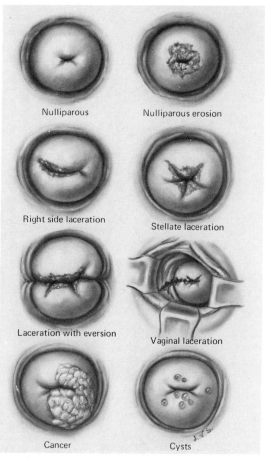

Figure 3-5. The uterine cervix: normal and pathologic appearance. *(Reproduced, with permission, from Pernoll ML [editor]:* Current Obstetric & Gynecologic Diagnosis & Treatment, *7th ed. Appleton & Lange, 1991.)*

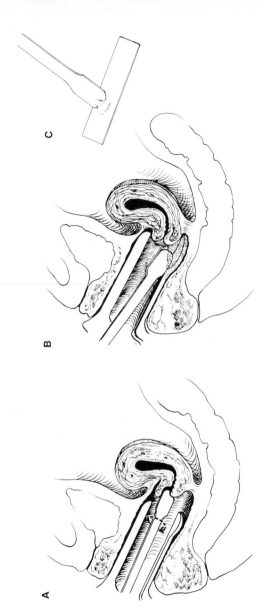

Figure 3–6. Collection of Papanicolaou cytosmear. **A:** Obtain an endocervical sample from the complete squamocolumnar junction with a moistened cotton swab or endocervical brush in the os. An exocervical sample is collected by pressing a cervical spatula against the cervix and rotating it 360 degrees. **B:** Obtain vaginal pool material from the posterior fornix. **C:** All samples are spread evenly on a glass slide and fixed immediately. *(Reproduced, with permission, from Benson RC: Handbook of Obstetrics & Gynecology, 8th ed. Lange, 1983.)*

Pap smear now, and you may or may not feel slight cramping.''
False-negative Papanicolaou results for dysplasia and cancer have
been attributed to poor collection techniques. Proper collection of
an endocervical, exocervical, and vaginal pool is shown in Figure
3–6.

Immediately fix the specimen to ensure that air drying and
cytolysis do not occur. After the Papanicolaou smear is complete,
the speculum is removed by rotating it in a counterclockwise direction. The vaginal walls are inspected as the speculum is removed.

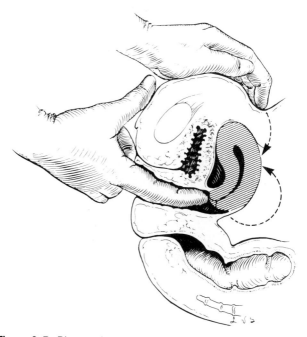

Figure 3–7. Bimanual examination. The two fingers in the vagina are placed under the cervix and used to lift the uterus
toward the adbominal hand. *(Reproduced, with permission,
from Benson RC: Handbook of Obstetrics & Gynecology, 8th
ed. Lange, 1983.)*

Bimanual Examination

Before the bimanual examination begins, it is helpful to out-line the procedure to the patient with a clear explanation, such as the following: "I will be placing 2 fingers in the vagina, and my other hand will be on your lower abdomen to feel the size and shape of your uterus, tubes, and ovaries." During the bimanual examination (Figure 3–7), the position, size, and contour of the uterus are assessed. When the uterus is anteverted, the abdominal hand can easily palpate the fundus (Figure 3–8). When the uterus is retroverted, the fundus can be palpated by the vaginal fingers reaching behind the cervix (Figure 3–9) and by the rectovaginal fingers during the rectovaginal examination. The size of the uterus is noted as compared to the number of weeks of gestation of a gravid uterus (Figure 3–10), and the contour of the uterus (eg,

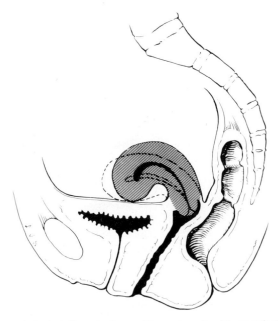

Figure 3-8. Anteflexed uterus. *(Reproduced, with permission, from Benson RC: Handbook of Obstetrics & Gynecology, 8th ed. Lange, 1983.)*

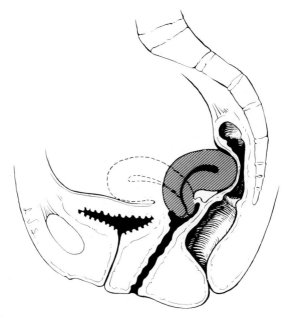

Figure 3-9. Retroflexed uterus. *(Reproduced, with permission, from Benson RC:* Handbook of Obstetrics & Gynecology, *8th ed. Lange, 1983.)*

smooth or irregular) is described, including specific notations of enlarged areas.

After assessing the condition of the uterus, the clinician examines the ovaries. The vaginal fingers are moved from under the cervix to the right side of the vaginal fornix to examine the right ovary. In a sweeping motion, the abdominal hand moves over the ovary toward the vaginal hand, and the size, shape, and contour of the ovary are noted. In particular, any tenderness or enlargement is noted. The left ovary is examined using a similar procedure on the left side of the pelvic area.

The last step of the bimanual examination is the rectovaginal examination. The clinician may again find it useful to offer an explanation such as the following: "I am going to place one finger in the vagina and one finger in the rectum to examine the back of

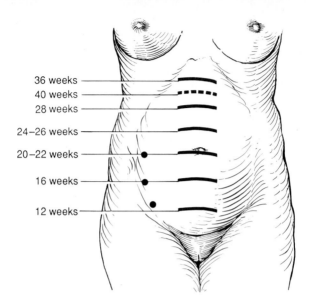

Figure 3-10. Height of the fundus at various times during pregnancy. *(Reproduced, with permission, from Benson RC:* Handbook of Obstetrics & Gynecology, *8th ed. Lange, 1983.)*

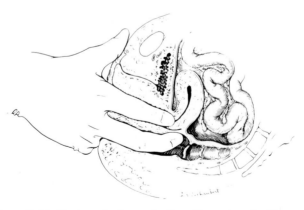

Figure 3-11. Rectovaginal examination. *(Reproduced, with permission, from Pernoll ML [editor]:* Current Obstetric & Gynecologic Diagnosis & Treatment, *7th ed. Appleton & Lange, 1991.)*

the uterus and ovaries.'' ***Note:*** Before the rectal examination begins, the examination glove is changed to prevent infectious agents in the vagina (eg, human papillomavirus) from contaminating the rectum. Then, the rectovaginal area is examined as shown in Figure 3–11, and the findings are noted.

SUGGESTED READINGS

Bates B: *A Guide to Physical Examination and History Taking,* 5th ed. Lippincott, 1991.

Jones HW; Colston WA; Burnett LS: *Novak's Textbook of Gynecology,* 11th ed. Williams & Wilkins, 1988.

Youssef AF: *Atlas of Gynaecological Diagnosis.* Churchill Livingstone, 1984.

4 | Papanicolaou Smear & Cervical Intraepithelial Neoplasia

Elizabeth C. Saviano, RNC, MSN

Since the Papanicolaou (or Pap) smear was introduced in 1943 as a method of cytologic screening for early detection of preinvasive lesions of the uterine cervix, the mortality rate from cervical cancer has been reduced by nearly 50%. The Pap test has enabled clinicians to more readily detect and treat precancerous changes known as **dysplasia**, or **cervical intraepithelial neoplasia (CIN)**.

CERVICAL INTRAEPITHELIAL NEOPLASIA

The prevalence of all grades of CIN in the general population is about 2%, and the average age at onset is 20–25. The onset of CIN is epidemiologically related to a woman's age at the time of first coitus. Because many young women are becoming sexually active at an early age, the incidence of CIN in women 15–19 years old has risen dramatically in recent years. The oncogene that causes CIN is most likely sexually transmitted. In the last 10 years, researchers have clearly established that some types of the sexually transmitted human papillomavirus (HPV) lead to the development of CIN.

CIN is a focal, noninvasive lesion and, as shown in Figure 4–1, is graded according to how deeply the epithelial layer of the cervix is affected: 25% is affected in CIN I (mild dysplasia), 50% in CIN II (moderate), and 75% or more in CIN III (severe). CIN can progress from the mild to the severe form over several years. Severe CIN can develop into carcinoma in situ and finally into invasive carcinoma of the cervix.

PAPANICOLAOU SMEAR SCREENING

The goal of cytologic screening is to identify those who need a diagnostic workup for CIN or cervical cancer based on an abnor-

CERVICAL INTRAEPITHELIAL NEOPLASIA

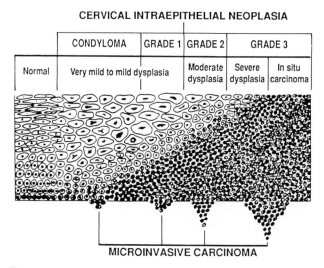

MICROINVASIVE CARCINOMA

Figure 4–1. Intraepithelial precursors to invasive carcinoma of the cervix. *(Slightly modified and reproduced, with permission, from Winkler B, Rickart RM: Human papillomavirus and gynecologic neoplasia.* Curr Probl Obstet Gynecol Fertil *1987;**10**:49.)*

mal Pap smear result. The Pap test is an easy, cost-effective means of screening a large population. However, the false-negative rate can be as high as 20%. These false-negative reports may be due to poor collection technique, air drying of the specimen, or laboratory error.

Frequency of Papanicolaou Tests

Pap screening should begin at age 18 or the age of first coitus, whichever is first. Annual Pap smear tests are recommended for all sexually active women. Women who have been treated for herpes simplex type 2, HPV, CIN, carcinoma in situ, or invasive cancer should be retested every 6–12 months, or more often if indicated.

Women who have late exposure to coitus with one lifetime sexual partner have a minimal risk of developing a cervical abnormality. The risk of cervical cancer in women who have had no exposure to coitus is almost zero. Women who are at low exposure risk for developing cervical carcinoma can be retested at intervals longer than 1 year. Women who have undergone hysterectomy for benign disease should have cytologic screening every 3–5 years.

Women born between 1940 and 1971 who have a known exposure to diethylstilbestrol (DES) in utero are at high risk for developing clear-cell adenocarcinoma of the vagina and cervix. Cytologic evaluation of this group is recommended every 6–12 months beginning at the onset of menstruation, at age 14, or earlier if abnormal bleeding or discharge is exhibited. The Pap smear sample should include cells from all 4 vaginal walls, as well as the endocervix and ectocervix. If annual Pap screening is difficult in this high-risk group, at least one colposcopic examination using Schiller's staining on the vagina and cervix is recommended for women under age 25.

Interpretation of Papanicolaou Test Results

As shown in Table 4–1, several classification systems exist for cytologic description. Currently, cytologists tend to use descriptive interpretation rather than the Papanicolaou numerical classes to report results. The physician and the cytologist must communicate clearly regarding terminology, methodology, and results; therefore, it is useful for the physician to establish a working relationship with the local cytologist, who can be a resource when results are in question.

A. Normal Results: A negative or benign result means that analysis of the Pap smear revealed no abnormalities. Findings such

Table 4–1. Classification systems for Papanicolaou smear results.

Papanicolaou Classes	Descriptive Interpretation	National Cancer Institute
I	Benign; no abnormal cells	Normal
II	Atypia or inflammation	Atypia
III	Mild to moderate dysplasia; CIN[1] I or II	Low-grade SILb[2]
IV	Severe dysplasia; CIN[1] III or CIS[3]	High-grade SIL[2]
V	Squamous carcinoma	Carcinoma

[1] Cervical intraepithelial neoplasia.
[2] Squamous intraepithelial lesions; b category includes cytologic changes of koilocytosis.
[3] Cancer in situ.

as metaplasia, or cellular reactions without atypia, hyperkeratosis, and parakeratosis, although not abnormal, may be very early signs of CIN. In these cases, the Pap test should be repeated in 1 year.

When the Pap smear result is benign but the smear contains no endocervical cells, the sampling is inadequate. In this case, the schedule for repeating the Pap smear is determined by the patient's risk factors.

B. Atypia: Although cytologic atypia is not an indication of the presence of cancer or even precancer, it is not normal. As many as 30% of women with atypical Pap smear results have an underlying CIN.

Inflammatory atypia may suggest the presence of infection with abnormal reparative changes. Vaginitis must be considered, and cervical cultures specifically for gonorrhea and *Chlamydia* are indicated. Appropriate treatment should be completed before the Pap smear is repeated.

As shown in Figure 4–2, the Pap smear should be repeated in

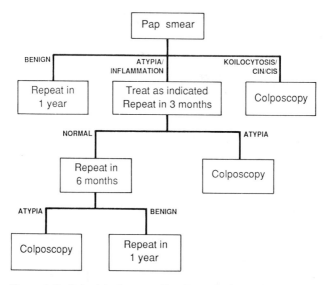

Figure 4-2. Schedule for repeating Papanicolaou smears with atypical findings. CIN, cervical intraepithelial neoplasia; CIS, carcinoma in situ.

3 months in all cases of atypia. If the finding is again atypical, colposcopy is warranted; however, if the repeat Pap smear is normal, a third smear should be taken 6 months later.

C. Koilocytosis: The koilocyte is an epithelial cell with an enlarged hyperchromatic nucleus surrounded by a clear space, or perinuclear "halo." Koilocytic changes on the Pap smear suggest the presence of an HPV infection. The incidence of HPV infection is thought to be about 10% in sexually active women. The presence of koilocytes, with or without atypia, indicates the need for a thorough colposcopic evaluation of the cervix, vagina, vulva, and anus for HPV lesions.

D. Cervical Intraepithelial Neoplasia: Although a lower grade CIN is considered less ominous than a higher grade lesion, the risk of invasion cannot be predicted solely on the Pap smear results. Regardless of the grade of CIN, colposcopic evaluation of the cervix with directed biopsy is necessary to eliminate the possibility of an underlying cancer.

E. Invasive Cancer of the Cervix: A lesion that extends beyond the epithelial layer and invades the cervical stroma is a true carcinoma. The methods for staging and treating invasive cervical cancers are discussed in Chapter 26.

DIAGNOSTIC PROCEDURES

Colposcopy

Colposcopy, the examination of the genital tract with lighted magnification, is indicated for the following cases: (1) abnormal Pap smear results, as defined above; (2) grossly visible lesions, regardless of the Pap smear report; (3) unexplained, abnormal bleeding; or (4) persistent vaginal discharge. The colposcopic examination is used to evaluate the need for directed biopsy. (The accuracy of colposcopically directed biopsy approaches 90%. The accuracy of the colposcopic examination is based on the skill of the colposcopist.)

Magnification enables the clinician to see details of the cervical epithelium, specifically, the area of change on the cervix from squamous to columnar epithelium. This area is called the squamocolumnar junction, also referred to as the **transformation zone** (T-zone). All CIN occurs in the T-zone.

A. Examination Technique: After a repeat Pap smear is obtained, the cervix and vagina are washed with a liberal amount of

3–5% aqueous acetic acid to intensify the appearance of capillary and epithelial abnormalities. The colposcopist then examines the cervix to identify normal landmarks. Colposcopic examinations are considered satisfactory when the distal margins of the T-zone and the full extent of any lesion can be seen. An endocervical speculum can be used to obtain a better view of the cervical canal. The examination is considered unsatisfactory when the above criteria are not met.

B. Abnormal Findings: Areas with varying thicknesses of "white epithelium" and punctate or mosaic patterns of surface capillaries indicate probable CIN. Invasion is suspected when irregular branching with corkscrew and hairpin capillary shapes is noted.

Endocervical Curettage

In the nonpregnant patient, light endocervical curettage is useful for assessing potential involvement of the part of the cervical canal that cannot be seen during colposcopic examination. A positive endocervical curettage result, indicating that CIN or carcinoma in situ is located high in the cervical canal, warrants further evaluation by conization of the cervix.

Colposcopically Directed Punch Biopsy

The most suspicious lesions are biopsied (Figures 4–3 and 4–4). Kevorkian-Younge or Tischler punch forceps allow the clinician to control the sample size without crushing the biopsy specimen. Schiller's iodine solution can be used to further delineate lesions for biopsy. Normal epithelium contains glycogen, which stains a deep brown when painted with Schiller's solution. Abnormal epithelium, such as CIN, does not contain glycogen and therefore does not stain. Multiple biopsy specimens may be obtained with little discomfort to the patient. In the sensitive patient, a paracervical block using 1% lidocaine may be preferred. Immediately on completion of the biopsy, the specimen should be placed in formalin. Bleeding at the biopsy site is usually minimal and can be controlled with an application of 5% silver nitrate or Monsel's paste.

Colposcopy & Biopsy During Pregnancy

When manipulation of the cervix will not put a woman at risk for preterm labor, colposcopy and directed biopsy may be safely performed during pregnancy. The colposcopist should keep in

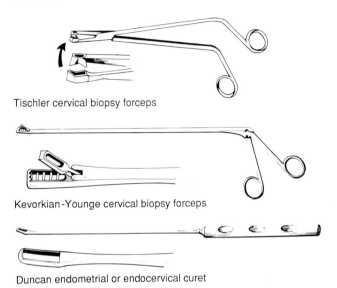

Tischler cervical biopsy forceps

Kevorkian-Younge cervical biopsy forceps

Duncan endometrial or endocervical curet

Figure 4-3. Biopsy instruments. *(Reproduced, with permission, from Pernoll ML [editor]:* Current Obstetric & Gynecologic Diagnosis & Treatment, *7th ed. Appleton & Lange, 1991.)*

mind that, with the increased cervical vascularity during pregnancy, bleeding may be more profuse when a biopsy is preformed. Endocervical curettage is often not appropriate because of the increased risk of rupturing the amniotic membrane. If cervical biopsy shows anything less than invasive carcinoma, treatment for CIN may be postponed until after delivery.

Cone Biopsy

Cold conization of the cervix is indicated when distal margins of a lesion cannot be seen, as in an unsatisfactory colposcopic examination, or when the results of an endocervical curettage are positive. Conization is also indicated when a more advanced PAP smear result is not consistent with colposcopic finding or biopsies. Cone biopsy is performed in the operating room under general or regional anesthesia. During cone biopsy, a portion of the cervix from the squamous junction to the internal os is removed (Figure

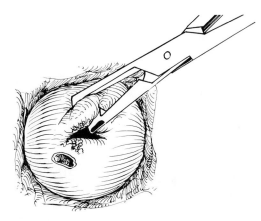

Figure 4-4. Multiple punch biopsy of the cervix with Tischler forceps. *(Reproduced, with permission, from Benson RC:* Handbook of Obstetrics & Gynecology, *8th ed. Lange, 1983.)*

4–5). Cone biopsy is contraindicated in the pregnant patient unless there is a strong suspicion of invasion.

Evaluation of the Vagina, Vulva, & Anus

Colposcopic examination of the vaginal, vulvar, and anal epithelium is always indicated when the Pap smear result is abnormal. Areas of pigmentation or white epithelium, whether flat or papillary, are suspect and should be biopsied.

TREATMENT OF CERVICAL INTRAEPITHELIAL NEOPLASIA

Treatment of the cervical lesions is based on the results of the colposcopic examination and histologic analysis. Figure 4–6 outlines the appropriate interventions.

Cryotherapy

Nitrous oxide freezing for desquamation of abnormal cervical cells is an inexpensive, quick office procedure with few side effects. It is the appropriate therapy for treating lesions that can be seen

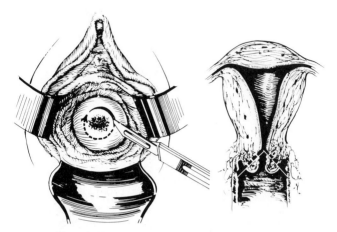

Figure 4-5. Conization of the cervix. *(Reproduced, with permission, from Benson RC:* Handbook of Obstetrics & Gynecology, *8th ed. Lange, 1983.)*

in their entirety during the colposcopic examination. Local anesthesia is not usually necessary, although many women do complain of mild to moderate cramping during the procedure. Prolonged posttherapy discharge is common. Cryotherapy may also change the position of the T-zone, rendering future colposcopic examinations more difficult. Treatment success is 80–90%. Failure is usually the result of treating a lesion that is too large for the cryotherapy probe.

Laser Ablation

CO_2 laser therapy is used to remove lesions that are either too large for cryotherapy or that extend minimally into the internal os. Laser ablation can be performed as an office or an operating room procedure under local anesthesia. Bleeding after laser ablation is the most frequent complication. This treatment is successful in 80–90% of cases.

Treatment Follow-Up

A repeat colposcopic examination and Pap smear test should be performed 3 months after treatment. Waiting 3 months allows

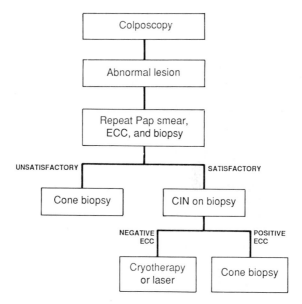

Figure 4-6. Interventions for cervical intraepithelial neoplasia (CIN). ECC, endocervical curettage.

the cervix to heal completely after therapy. If colposcopy reveals that a previously persistent lesion is gone and if the Pap smear is normal, 2 additional Pap smears should be taken at 3-month intervals.

An accurate indication of cure is defined as normal findings on 3 Pap smears within 1 year of therapy. Because women with histories of CIN are considered to be at greater risk for developing cervical carcinoma, they should have Pap smear tests every 6–12 months throughout their lives.

TREATMENT OF HUMAN
PAPILLOMAVIRUS INFECTION

Several studies have demonstrated the presence of HPV-DNA in more than 90% of cervical cancers. Because of the strong link between HPV infection and the development of carcinoma in the genital tract, HPV lesions should be treated.

Vulva

   A. Chemical: The treatment of choice for HPV lesions of the vulva is topical application of 50–85% trichloroacetic acid (TCA). Several weekly applications may be required. A strength of 25–30% Podophyllum resin may also be used topically but carries a greater risk of local and systemic toxicity. Podophyllum resin is contraindicated for use in pregnancy.

   B. Laser: Diffuse, large, or persistent lesions of the vulva may need to be removed by CO_2 laser vaporization.

Vagina

   Well-defined HPV lesions may respond well to careful vaginal application of TCA. Another therapy that is widely used and clinically accepted (but not approved for vaginal use by the US Food and Drug Administration) is the vaginal application of topical 5-fluorouracil. The patient uses half an applicatorful of 5-fluorouracil cream in the vagina for 3–5 nights sequentially. Care must be taken to instruct the patient on how to prevent burns to the vulva and urethra; for example, zinc oxide or a silicone-based ointment is applied to the vulva for protection. The success rate after one treatment course with 5-fluorouracil is about 90%. A second course of 5-fluorouracil therapy resolves lesions in 95% of cases. Because transmission of HPV is through genital contact, all sexual partners of women with HPV lesions should be referred for colposcopic examination. Evaluation and treatment of sexual partners may be the key to further reducing the incidence and recurrence of HPV and possible cervical cancer.

SUGGESTED READINGS

Coppleson M, Pixley E, Reid B: *Colposcopy: A Scientific and Practical Approach to the Cervix, Vagina, and Vulva in Health and Disease,* 3rd ed. Charles C Thomas, 1986.

Ferenczy A: Comparison of 5-fluorouracil and CO_2 laser for treatment of vaginal condylomata. *Obstet Gynecol* 1984;**64:**773.

Nelson JH, Averette HE, Richard RM: Cervical intraepithelial neoplasia and early invasive cervical carcinoma. *CA* 1989;**39:**157.

Genital Tract Infections | 5

Joseph A. Bachicha, MD

A significant component of health care for women involves the diagnosis and treatment of various infections of the upper and lower genital tracts or dealing with their sequelae. This section focuses on common illnesses caused by microbial organisms that infect the genital tract. All treatment recommendations are based on the most recent criteria developed by the Centers for Disease Control (CDC). Appropriate care of women who seek medical assistance for evaluation of genital tract infection includes a detailed history, physical examination, medical and behavioral risk assessment, laboratory tests, curative or palliative therapy, case reporting when required, and appropriate follow-up. The diagnosis of a sexually transmitted infection reflects unprotected sexual activity in which patients with one infection are at risk of acquiring others. Notification and evaluation of the partner might be necessary. Finally, education in risk reduction is essential in every patient encounter.

In Chapter 37, Common Infections During Pregnancy, *Chlamydia,* gonorrhea, herpes simplex virus, and syphilis are discussed in further detail. The reader may find it useful to review Chapter 5 in conjunction with Chapter 37.

VAGINITIS

Vaginitis is suspected when the patient presents with complaints of vaginal itching, burning, or an unusually heavy discharge with a foul vaginal odor (Table 5-1). The causative agent is usually isolated in a wet smear preparation. In these preparations, a specimen of vaginal discharge is divided onto 2 slides, one to be mixed with normal saline and the other with potassium hydroxide (KOH). After 1 or 2 drops of saline are mixed with a specimen of discharge, a cover slip is placed over the slide, and it is viewed under 10 × and 40 × magnification. In the absence of an

47

Table 5-1. Common causes of vaginitis.

	Clinical Appearance	Potassium Hydroxide Slide	Saline Slide	Treatment
Trichomonas	Green or yellow discharge; "strawberry cervix"	***	Motile flagella	Metronidazole[1]
Bacterial vaginosis	Watery, thin, grayish-white, frothy discharge	Positive "whiff" test	Clue cells and white blood cells	Metronidazole[1]
Candida	Thick, white, "cottage cheese," curdy discharge	Hyphae	***	Terconazole or miconazole

[1]Alcohol should not be consumed when taking metronidazole because of associated nausea and vomiting.

obvious organism, increased numbers of white cells on the saline preparation indicate cervicitis, and *Chlamydia,* gonorrhea, or herpes should be suspected. Specific cultures for these organisms should be performed to confirm the diagnosis. Routine vaginal cultures are not helpful because the normal vaginal flora, like the flora of the oral cavity and gut, is extensive.

Trichomoniasis

Trichomonas is usually a sexually transmitted organism. Wet smear preparations will disclose *Trichonomas vaginalis* organisms if they are present. When present, these organisms are often accompanied by numerous white blood cells. *T vaginalis* is pear-shaped and very mobile as a result of its flagella (Figure 5–1).

All patients infected with *T vaginalis* should be treated. The recommended regimen consists of metronidazole, 2 g orally in a single dose. An alternative regimen is metronidazole, 500 mg orally twice daily for 7 days. If failure occurs with either regimen, the patient should be treated again, with metronidazole, 500 mg twice daily for 7 days. If repeated failure occurs, the patient may be treated with a single 2-g dose of metronidazole daily for 3–5 days. Sex partners should be treated with either the single-dose or the 7-day regimen.

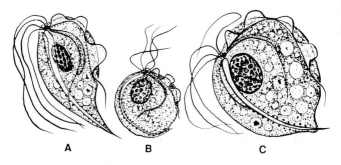

Figure 5–1. *Trichomonas vaginalis* as found in vaginal and prostatic secretions. *A:* Normal trophozoite. *B:* Round form after division. *C:* Common form seen in stained preparation. Cysts not found. *(Reproduced, with permission, from Jawetz E, Meinick JL, Adelberg EA: Review of Medical Microbiology, 16th ed. Lange, 1984.)*

Candidiasis

Candida (yeast) organisms are not considered sexually transmitted, although in rare instances they may be. Yeast infections are common during pregnancy, in diabetic patients, and in women who take oral contraceptives or who take antibiotics for other reasons. Unremitting, recurrent, heavy *Candida* infections may be a sign of infection with the human immunodeficiency virus (HIV). A wet smear is prepared by adding a few drops of 10% KOH on the slide with a specimen sample. The KOH will destroy other organisms, cells, and debris, leaving the spores or hyphae (Figure 5–2).

Many treatment regimens have been proposed, and 3- or 7-day programs are superior to single-dose therapy. Loose-fitting, moisture-absorbent cotton clothing, especially underwear, is encouraged, as is the avoidance of nylon underwear and tight trousers or pantyhose. Highly perfumed toilet paper and soaps, excessive douching (more than once per week), and the heavy use of feminine hygiene sprays are to be avoided. These products can irritate the vulva, may mask signs of infection, and may alter the pH balance of the vagina to promote infection. Wiping front to back will decrease the spread of bacteria from bowel to vagina.

The recommended treatment regimen is as follows: tercona-

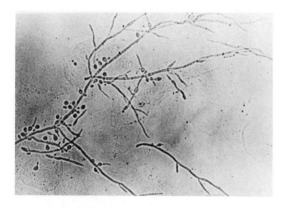

Figure 5–2. KOH preparation showing branched and budding *Candida albicans. (Reproduced, with permission, from Pernoll ML [editor]:* Current Obstetric & Gynecologic Diagnosis & Treatment, *7th ed. Appleton & Lange, 1991.)*

zole, 80-mg suppository of 0.4% cream, or miconazole nitrate, 200-mg suppository, inserted in the vagina at night for 3 nights. Alternative regimens include miconazole nitrate, 100-mg suppository inserted in the vagina at night for 7 nights, or clotrimazole or butoconazole at the same dose and frequency. Sex partners do not need to be treated unless *Candida* infections of the penis or foreskin are present.

Bacterial Vaginosis

Bacterial vaginosis is present when microscopic examination of a wet smear reveals "clue cells," which are epithelial cells covered with bacteria that give the cells a stippled or grainy appearance. This disease, also known as nonspecific vaginitis, is most likely caused by *Gardnerella vaginalis* (formerly called *Corynebacterium* and *Haemophilus vaginalis,* Figure 5–3). On the KOH slide, amines with a characteristic "fishy" odor are released if bacterial vaginosis is present. This is known as a positive "whiff" test and, in the presence of clue cells, confirms the diagnosis. Asymptomatic

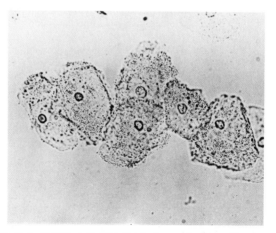

Figure 5–3. Saline wet mount of clue cells from *Gardnerella vaginalis* infection. Note the absence of inflammatory cells. *(Reproduced, with permission, from Pernoll ML [editor]:* Current Obstetric & Gynecologic Diagnosis & Treatment, *7th ed. Appleton & Lange, 1991.)*

infections are common, and treatment is not recommended for such findings.

The treatment regimen consists of metronidazole, 500 mg orally twice daily for 7 days. An alternative regimen is clindamycin, 300 mg orally twice daily for 7 days. The clinical counterpart of bacterial vaginosis has been identified in the male partner, and he can be treated in a similar manner.

CERVICITIS

Cervicitis, an inflammation and infection of the cervix, is suspected when an obvious vaginal pathogen has been excluded. *Chlamydia,* gonorrhea, and herpes are the 3 most common infections of the cervix and may produce a profuse vaginal discharge containing numerous white blood cells. These infections are definitively diagnosed by culture.

Chlamydia

It is estimated that more than 3 million women experience chlamydial infections annually in the USA, and *Chlamydia* has replaced gonorrhea as the most common sexually transmitted infection. It often exists with other infections, especially gonorrhea, and may be either asymptomatic or associated with nonspecific complaints, such as vaginal discharge. In settings in which antigen tests or cultures for *Chlamydia* are not routine or available, treatment is often prescribed on the basis of a clinical diagnosis of cervicitis or in conjunction with treatment for gonorrhea. *Chlamydia* testing may be especially useful in pregnant women, adolescents, women with more than one sexual partner, and women with a history of previous sexually transmitted infections (see Chapter 37). *Note:* Patients who have had sexual contact with an infected partner must be treated.

The recommended regimen for treating a chlamydial infection is as follows: doxycycline, 100 mg orally twice daily for 7 days, or tetracycline, 500 mg orally 4 times daily for 7 days. Alternative regimens consist of the following: erythromycin base, 500 mg orally 4 times daily for 7 days, or erythromycin ethylsuccinate, 800 mg orally 4 times daily for 7 days. If erythromycin is not tolerated, sulfisoxazole, 500 mg orally 4 times daily for 10 days, is appropriate. Because resistance of *C trachomatis* to these regimens has not been documented, a test of cure is not necessary. Sex partners of patients with *Chlamydia* should also be treated.

Gonorrhea

Gonorrhea is a genital infection that rivals *Chlamydia* in prevalence and whose treatment has been complicated by the emergence of strains that are resistant to antibiotic therapy. These strains include penicillinase-producing *Neisseria gonorrhea* (PPNG), tetracycline-resistant *N gonorrhea,* and others with chromosomally mediated resistance to other antibiotics.

All cases of suspected gonorrhea should be confirmed by culture and sensitivity to ensure appropriate antibiotic coverage. Single-dose treatment is a major advance in eliminating uncomplicated urethral, endocervical, or rectal gonorrhea. In some studies, 50% of gonorrhea cases coexist with *Chlamydia*. Therefore, it is recommended that all patients with gonorrhea also be treated with a 7-day course of doxycycline or tetracycline (see Chapter 37).

The recommended regimen is as follows: ceftriaxone, 250 mg intramuscularly once, plus doxycycline, 100 mg orally twice daily for 7 days, or tetracycline, 500 mg orally 4 times daily for 7 days. Alternative regimens include the following options: cefotaxime, 1 g, or ceftizoxime, 500 mg, intramuscularly once; ciprofloxacin, 500 mg, or norfloxacin, 800 mg, orally once; ofloxacin, 400 mg orally once; or spectinomycin, 2 g intramuscularly once, followed by doxycycline or tetracycline, as described above. In confirmed non-PPNG cases, the following regimen is used: amoxicillin, 3 g orally once, with probenecid, 1 g orally once, followed by doxycycline, as described above.

A serologic test for syphilis and counseling and testing for the human immunodeficiency virus (HIV) should be offered to all patients with gonorrhea. *Note:* Any patients that have been exposed to gonorrhea should be examined, cultures should be performed, and treatment should be given. Treatment failure after combined ceftriaxone and doxycycline therapy is rare, and a test of cure is not needed. Patients treated with other regimens should have test of cure cultures taken within one week after completion of therapy.

HERPES SIMPLEX VIRUS

Herpes simplex virus (HSV) infections have had a profound impact on the well being of women in the past decade and are second only to HIV infection in the social disruption they have caused. The actual incidence of HSV infection is unknown, but the number of physician visits for HSV infection increased from

30,000 in 1966 to almost 300,000 in 1981. Infection results from the inoculation of the virus onto a susceptible mucus membrane or through introduction into the skin by close contact with a carrier who may or may not be symptomatic. Most genital infections are caused by HSV type 2, whereas those caused by HSV type 1 reflect orogenital contact (see Chapter 37).

Primary HSV infections tend to be of greater severity and longer duration than the recurrent ones. Patients seeking attention usually complain of numerous vesicular or ulcerated lesions that are extremely painful. The infection can lead to vaginal discharge from cervicitis or urethral discharge from urethritis. Fever, myalgias, and malaise occur in about 40% of patients. The symptoms generally last approximately 2 weeks, and healing requires another 1–2 weeks.

Recurrent HSV infections tend to be milder and of shorter duration than primary infections. Recurrences are more likely due to reactivation of latent virus in the ganglion rather than reinfection. Irritation of the sacral dermatomes may herald a recurrence and is the source of the itching, tingling, or pain sometimes experienced by a patient before the appearance of a lesion. Recurrent herpes tends to occur 5–12 days before the menstrual period and is over in 5–10 days. Aside from neonatal transmission, which can cause several neonatal neurological complications, the primary difficulty with herpes is its psychological burden and subsequent interference with sexual relationships.

Clinical diagnosis is based on the history of genital lesions, which progress from vesicles to ulcers without scarring and are accompanied by pain. Further clinical evidence consists of prodromes and recurrences. Serum antigen tests for herpes are available but have a high false-positive rate. The definitive test is a viral culture.

Patients should be counseled that herpes may be chronic and recurring, with no known cure, but that partial control of the signs and symptoms is possible. Systemic acyclovir treatment accelerates healing but cannot eradicate the infection. Topical acyclovir is less effective than the oral form. For the first clinical episode, the recommended regimen is acyclovir, 200 mg orally 5 times daily for 7–10 days or until clinical resolution. For patients with severe disease or complications requiring hospitalization, the recommended regimen is acyclovir, 5 mg/kg body weight intravenously every 8 hours for 5–7 days or until clinical resolution.

Most episodes of recurrent herpes are unaffected by acyclovir. In severe, recurrent cases, some patients who begin therapy at the start of the prodrome may experience some relief. Dosage regimen for recurrent herpes is as follows: acyclovir, 200 mg orally 5 times daily for 5 days or 800 mg orally 2 times daily for 5 days.

Daily suppressive therapy can reduce recurrences by at least 75% in patients with more than 6 episodes per year. After a year of suppressive therapy, acyclovir should be discontinued to reassess the patient's recurrence rate. Daily suppressive therapy consists of acyclovir, 200 mg orally 2–5 times daily or 400 mg orally twice a day.

Patients with herpes should be advised to refrain from sexual activity when lesions are present. If this not possible, condom use should be strongly recommended. Herpes and other ulcerating infections have been associated with an increased risk of acquiring HIV infection, and condom use should be recommended for all sexual exposure if the partnership is not mutually monogamous.

SYPHILIS

About 1% of women with gonorrhea also have syphilis. The disease has little impact on the genital tract itself and may be asymptomatic. If left untreated, it may have a great impact on the central nervous and cardiac systems. The incidence of syphilis has increased recently, largely in troubling association with rising HIV infection rates in women. The causative agent is *Treponema pallidum,* which is transmitted through direct contact with a syphilis lesion when the spirochetes pass through mucus membranes or broken skin (see Chapter 37).

In **primary syphilis,** the incubation period is 10–90 days, and the first clinical sign is the chancre, which is a firm, indurated, painless lesion with a raised and firm border (Figure 5–4). There may be painless local lymphadenopathy. The chancre may persist for 3–6 weeks and heal spontaneously. Diagnosis at this stage is made by identification of spirochetes with darkfield microscopy. Serologic tests, such as the VDRL or rapid plasma reagin tests, are usually nonreactive when the chancre appears but become reactive in 1–4 weeks.

Secondary syphilis, which lasts 2–20 weeks after infection, exhibits various physical manifestations. Copper-colored, maculopapular lesions may appear on the palms and soles, and moist, highly contagious lesions may be seen around the rectum, vagina, or in the oral cavity. Generalized lymphadenopathy may occur, and the eyelashes and lateral third of the eyebrows may be lost. Untreated secondary syphilis resolves in 4–12 weeks.

PRIMARY SYPHILIS

Spirochetes penetrate the skin, usually of the penis, vulva, or cervix or occasionally elsewhere.

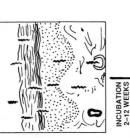

Lymphocytes and plasma cells proliferate; hard chancre forms at site of entry; local lymph nodes enlarge.

INCUBATION 2–12 WEEKS

Diagnosis. Fresh smear. Dark-field illumination reveals live (moving) organisms.

3–6 WEEKS

SECONDARY SYPHILIS (2–20 weeks)

Organisms disseminate
- Skin rash (with lymphocytic infiltration)
- Mucosal ulcer
- Fever

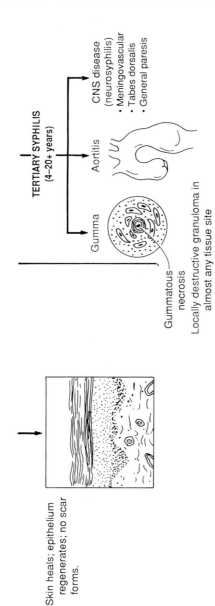

Skin heals; epithelium regenerates; no scar forms.

TERTIARY SYPHILIS
(4–20+ years)

Gumma

Aortitis

CNS disease (neurosyphilis)
• Meningovascular
• Tabes dorsalis
• General paresis

Gummatous necrosis

Locally destructive granuloma in almost any tissue site

Figure 5–4. Course and pathologic features of syphilis. *(Reproduced, with permission, from Chandrasoma P, Taylor CR: Concise Pathology, Appleton & Lange, 1991.)*

During **latent syphilis** there are no signs or symptoms of disease. Latency may last a lifetime or may be followed by **tertiary syphilis.** Manifestations of tertiary syphilis include gumma, which is benign, aortitis, and neurosyphilis.

Any patient exposed to a sexually transmitted disease should have a screening test performed, often the VDRL test. Laboratories report a positive result as the highest dilution of the serum that yields a positive result. VDRL titers of 1:8 or less indicate false-positive serologic reactions; the VDRL test should be repeated to eliminate laboratory error. If the second result is positive, the VDRL result should be confirmed with a more specific test, the fluorescent treponemal antibody absorption (FTA-ABS) test. A positive FTA-ABS result confirms the diagnosis, and a negative test result means the VDRL result was false positive. An attempt should be made to determine the duration of infection because the treatment protocols vary depending on the stage of the disease.

Treatment of primary and secondary syphilis and latent syphilis of less than 1 year's duration is benzathine penicillin G, 2.4 million units intramuscularly once. An alternative regimen for nonpregnant patients allergic to penicillin consists of tetracycline, 500 mg orally 4 times daily for 14 days, or doxycycline, 100 mg orally twice daily for 14 days. A spinal tap followed by examination of the cerebrospinal fluid is recommended if there are neurologic signs or symptoms; evidence of active disease, such as aortitis, gumma, or iritis; planned treatment with a nonpenicillin agent; or a serum nontreponemal antibody titer ratio of 1:32 or greater.

Because of its chronic course and long asymptomatic periods, follow-up of syphilis is important. Physical examinations and serological tests should be performed at 3 and 6 months. If signs or symptoms indicate persistent disease or if nontreponemal antibody tests do not show a decrease after treatment, the cerebrospinal fluid should be evaluated and the patient retreated as necessary. For patients with primary syphilis, all partners for the past 3–6 months should be evaluated, and for patients with secondary syphilis, all partners within 12 months should be evaluated.

PELVIC INFLAMMATORY DISEASE

Pelvic inflammatory disease (PID) is a nonspecific term for a variety of findings in the upper female genital tract characterized by inflammation and infection. Endometritis, salpingitis, peritonitis, and tubo-ovarian abscess are included under the PID category. The most common organisms causing PID are *Chlamydia* and gonorrhea, although anaerobes, gram-negative rods, and mycoplasmas may be involved. Nearly 1 million new cases of PID are diagnosed yearly in the USA, and about 1 woman in 7 is thought to have already had at least one episode. PID can result in significant morbidity, especially infertility and ectopic pregnancy as a result of tubal damage and adhesions. Sexually active teenage women are the highest risk group. Women who are 15–19 years old have about a 1 in 8 risk of developing PID. About 300,000 women are hospitalized annually with PID, and there are more than 2.5 million outpatient visits for the disease.

Risk factors for the development of PID include the following: (1) more than one sex partner, (2) young age at first intercourse, (3) a high frequency of intercourse, and (4) a new partner within the 30 days before the diagnosis of PID. Associated risk factors include the use of the intrauterine device, especially within the first 3 months after insertion, and vaginal douching. Low education, low income, and race are also associated factors. Nonwhite women are 2.5 times more likely to be hospitalized for PID than white women.

Diagnosis

Accurate diagnosis of pelvic inflammatory disease may be difficult. The differential diagnosis includes ectopic pregnancy, appendicitis, ruptured ovarian cyst, ovarian torsion, or spontaneous abortion. Laparoscopic evaluation is the gold standard of diagnosis. Edema and erythema of the fallopian tubes, often accompanied by purulent exudate, are the hallmark findings. Laparoscopy is useful as a diagnostic tool, but it is expensive and carries with it operative and anesthetic risks.

Widely applicable, inexpensive, noninvasive, easy-to-perform methods have been developed to diagnose PID with some measure of accuracy. Abdominal pain, cervical motion tenderness, or uterine and adnexal tenderness, together with at least one nonspecific indicator (fever ≥ 38 °C, white blood count above 10,000) are the most accepted clinical criteria. Presence of an adnexal mass suggests the presence of a tubo-ovarian abscess (Figure 5–5). Upper abdominal pain may indicate Fitz-Hugh–Curtis syndrome, an inflammation of the liver capsule that results in adhesions from the liver to the abdominal wall or viscera. Ultrasonography is often used to exclude intrauterine or ectopic pregnancy or to document

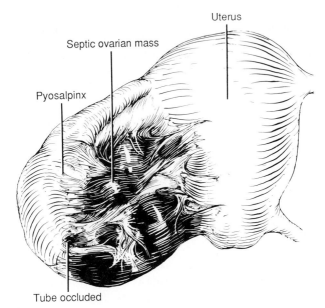

Figure 5-5. Tubo-ovarian abscess. *(Reproduced, with permission, from Benson RC:* Handbook of Obstetrics & Gynecology, *8th ed. Lange, 1983.)*

the presence of an adnexal mass. Some studies suggest that vaginal ultrasonography and endometrial biopsy together may be an alternative to laparoscopic diagnosis.

Note that not all PID episodes produce symptoms. "Silent" PID may produce tubal damage as severe as PID that produces pain and may account for a significant proportion of infertility problems and ectopic pregnancies.

Treatment

Elimination of signs and symptoms and preservation of fertility are the twin goals of treatment. Because of its presumed polymicrobial etiology, the treatment of PID requires broad-spectrum antibiotics. Outpatient management is the norm, but hospitalization is recommended if any of the following are present: unclear diagnosis, pelvic abscess, poor patient compliance, severe illness, or failed response to ambulatory treatment. Formerly, aggressive surgery in the form of total abdominal hysterectomy with bilateral salpingo-oophorectomy was advocated as the treatment of choice for tubo-ovarian abscess. It is now recognized that medical therapy with intravenous antibiotics is the mainstay of abscess treatment, with surgery reserved for the most recalcitrant cases.

For ambulatory management of PID, the recommended regimen is cefoxitin, 2 g intramuscularly once, plus probenecid, 1 g orally, or ceftriaxone, 250 mg intramuscularly once, plus doxycycline, 100 mg orally twice daily for 10–14 days, or tetracycline, 500 mg orally 4 times daily for 10–14 days. An alternative regimen for patients unable to tolerate doxycycline or tetracycline consists of erythromycin, 500 mg orally 4 times daily for 10–14 days.

Inpatient treatment includes the following and is continued for 48 hours after clinical improvement: cefoxitin, 2 g intravenously every 6 hours, or cefotetan, 2 g intravenously every 12 hours, plus doxycycline, 100 mg orally or intravenously twice daily. After the patient is discharged, treatment continues with doxycycline, 100 mg orally twice daily for 10–14 days, or tetracycline, 500 mg orally 4 times daily for 10–14 days. The alternative regimen is as follows: clindamycin, 900 mg intravenously every 8 hours, plus gentamicin, loading dose intravenously or intramuscularly (2 mg/kg of body weight) followed by a maintenance dose (1.5 mg/kg) every 8 hours, continued for 48 hours after clinical improvement.

After the patient is discharged, treatment continues with doxycycline or tetracycline, as noted above. Continuation of clindamycin, 450 mg orally 5 times daily for 10–14 days, is an alternative, although doxycycline is the treatment of choice for suspected chlamydial infection.

PREGNANCY CONSIDERATIONS

Infections during pregnancy are discussed extensively in Chapter 37. Additional relevant considerations include the following.

Trichomonas: Metronidazole is contraindicated in the first trimester because of the risk of congenital malformations. Its use in the remainder of pregnancy is controversial; some physicians recommend its use in severe infections. An alternative, although less efficacious, treatment is clotrimazole, 100 mg inserted in the vagina nightly for 7 days.

Candida: Terconazole is not recommended for use during pregnancy. Clinical experience with clotrimazole, nystatin, and miconazole is greater, although these medications may be less effective. They remain the cornerstones of treatment of yeast infections during pregnancy.

SUGGESTED READINGS

Benson MD, Brown E, Keith L: Sexually transmitted diseases. In: *Current Problems in Obstetrics and Gynecology and Fertility,* Vol 8 (December), Year Book, 1985.

Centers for Disease Control: CDC guideline for treatment of sexually transmitted diseases. *MMWR* 1989;**38**:1.

Glass RH: *Office Gynecology.* Williams & Wilkins, 1981.

Contraception, Sterilization, & Abortion | 6

Dilys M. Walker, MD

In 1987, 92% of sexually active couples exposed to unwanted pregnancy were using some form of birth control. Overall, the most frequently used method of contraception is sterilization (22% female and 16% male) followed closely by oral contraceptive pills (32%) then condoms (16%).

In discussions of contraception, the terms **method effectiveness** and **use effectiveness** are frequently used. Method effectiveness describes the failure rates observed when the method is used correctly 100% of the time and is estimated by lowest observed failure rates (pregnancy). Use effectiveness is a more practical measure and reflects actual usage, which is often not correct 100% of the time and is estimated by typical user failure rates. These rates are expressed as pregnancies per 100 woman-years, which is defined as the number of pregnancies that occur during the first year after 100 women begin using a particular method. In addition to the inherent efficacy of each particular method of birth control, typical failure rates are influenced by a couple's motivation, their inherent potential to conceive, and their frequency of intercourse. In the following discussion, typical failure rates are used to approximate use effectiveness.

BARRIER METHODS

Barrier methods of contraception prevent pregnancy by blocking passage of sperm into the cervical canal. These are all temporally related to coitus and are therefore only used at, or around, the time of intercourse.

Condom

Condoms have become increasingly popular over the past 10 years. Among sexually active 17–19 year olds, there has been a particularly striking increase in condom usage from 25% in 1978 to 58% in 1988. This dramatic increase has been attributed to the ability of condoms to prevent transmission of acquired immune deficiency syndrome (AIDS) and other sexually transmitted diseases as well as their effectiveness as a form of contraception. In addition, aggressive marketing strategies and increased public display of condoms have heightened public awareness. Advertising campaigns are now directed at women as well as men, which has helped increase the proportion of condoms purchased by women to 50%.

A. Effectiveness and Mechanism of Action: In general, condoms used alone have typical failure rates of 10–15%. These rates are lower if the condom is used together with a spermicidal agent, either jelly, cream, or foam. Spermicidal condoms are also available and contain an inner and outer coating of the spermicide nonoxynol-9. For optimal effectiveness, the condom must be placed on the erect penis before genital contact and removed immediately after intercourse. The condom acts as a barrier to the passage of sperm into the vagina and cervical canal.

B. Benefits: Condoms offer the following benefits:

(1) Condoms may be the single most effective means of protection against HIV.

(2) Condoms decrease transmission of gonorrhea, *Chlamydia*, syphilis, condyloma, and herpes.

(3) By helping to prevent transmission of these sexually transmitted diseases, condoms decrease both the risk of infertility, caused by pelvic inflammatory disease, and cervical intraepithelial neoplasia, caused by condyloma.

(4) Condoms are relatively inexpensive to use and have become increasingly accessible over the counter in drug stores and are available in some public bathroom dispensers.

C. Risks and Contraindications: There are no serious medical risks or side effects associated with condom use. Some men or women may experience an allergic reaction to the rubber or spermicide. In this situation, the clinician could recommend using natural fiber condoms, usually lambskin, which are effective in preventing pregnancy but do not protect against sexually transmitted diseases because of their porous nature.

Recently, a "female condom" has been developed that is made of latex and worn like a G-string with a pouch that unrolls into the vagina with penetration. These have generally not been widely accepted.

Diaphragm

A. Effectiveness and Mechanism of Action: A couple must be highly motivated to successfully use a diaphragm for contraception because its effectiveness is directly related to correct and consistent use. Typical first-year failure rates are 10–15%.

The diaphragm is a dome-shaped rubber cap that is filled with approximately 15 mL (1 tbsp) of spermicide and then placed in the posterior vagina just behind the pubic bone and covering the cervix (Figure 6–1). It acts as a barrier by blocking and inactivating sperm before they can enter the cervix. The diaphragm may be placed up to 2–3 hours before intercourse and must be in place before genital contact. After intercourse, it must remain in the vagina for 6–8 hours. If intercourse is resumed before 6 hours, additional spermicide must be placed in the vagina without removing the diaphragm.

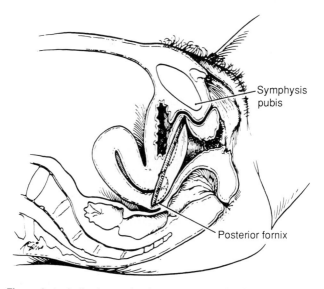

Symphysis pubis

Posterior fornix

Figure 6–1. A diaphragm in place creates a physical barrier between the vagina and cervix and importantly provides for intimate contact between the contraceptive jelly or cream and the cervix. (The woman is lying supine.) *(Reproduced, with permission, from Cunningham FG, McDonald PC, Gant NF:* Williams Obstetrics, *18th ed. Appleton & Lange, 1989.)*

Diaphragms are available in various sizes and must be individually fit by a health care provider.

   B. Benefits: The benefits provided by diaphragms are as follows:

(1) The diaphragm is useful for women who have infrequent intercourse or are highly motivated and committed to its use.
(2) As with condoms, the diaphragm is associated with a decreased transmission of sexually transmitted diseases, although it is not effective in preventing transmission of HIV.
(3) Decreased rates of cervical intraepithelial neoplasia have been noted in diaphragm users.
(4) The diaphragm is an appropriate alternative for women with medical contraindications to the use of hormonal methods of contraception.

   C. Risks and Contraindications: As with condoms, there are no serious side effects to using the diaphragm. The following is a list of relative contraindications:

(1) Allergy to rubber, spermicidal jelly, or cream.
(2) Recurrent cystitis (after diaphragm has been refit).
(3) Anatomy that does not allow a satisfactory placement or fit.
(4) History of toxic shock syndrome.
(5) Prior pregnancy while using the diaphragm.

Cervical Cap
   Like the diaphragm, the cervical cap is made of rubber but is a much smaller dome that fits snugly over the cervix. The cap is filled with spermicide before it is placed in the posterior vagina so that it covers the cervix. Unlike the diaphragm, the cervical cap may remain in place for up to 24 hours. Cervical caps are available in 4 different sizes and must be specially fit by a trained professional. The woman must feel comfortable checking the placement each time it is used to ensure that the cervix is covered. The failure rates are similar to those for the diaphragm and are highly dependent on motivation.

Vaginal Sponge
   The contraceptive sponge is a circular sponge 6 cm in diameter and 2 cm thick that contains 1 g of the spermicide nonoxynol-9. Placed in the posterior vagina so that it covers the cervix, the vaginal sponge not only inactivates sperm but also provides a mechanical barrier to sperm. The sponge may be placed immediately be-

fore intercourse and is left in place for 6 hours after intercourse. It can provide up to 24 hours of continuous contraception. The sponge is available over the counter in one size only. Its effectiveness, benefits, and contraindications are similar to those for the diaphragm.

Intrauterine Device

The intrauterine device (IUD) is a foreign object that is placed into the uterine cavity to prevent pregnancy. Since their introduction, IUDs have been made of various materials and in numerous shapes. The IUDs most widely used 20 years ago (ie, the Copper 7, Lippes Loop, and Dalkon Shield) are no longer available in the USA because of associated complications, including pelvic infections and septic abortions. Today in the USA new IUDs are being studied in clinical trials; however, only 2 IUDs are approved by the US Food and Drug Administration: TCu 380A and Progestasert. Both devices are T-shaped and have been shown to be safe and effective (Figure 6–2).

A. Effectiveness and Mechanism of Action: IUDs are considered highly effective with typical first-year failure rates of only 3%. These pregnancies are most often the result of an undetected IUD expulsion. The exact mechanism by which the IUD prevents pregnancy is not fully understood. The following mechanisms have been suggested and supported:

(1) Implantation is inhibited as a result of the local inflammatory reaction to the IUD as a foreign body.
(2) Alterations in tubal motility affect transport of both oocyte and sperm.
(3) Progesterone-containing IUDs have the additional effects of producing an atrophic endometrium and thickening the cervical mucus.

The TCu 380A is a T-shaped device made of polyethylene wound with a copper wire. This device is currently approved for 8 years of continuous use. The Progestasert is also T-shaped and contains progesterone in a silicone oil base, which is slowly released into the system. This device is approved for 1 year of continuous contraception. IUDs are usually placed at the time of the menses and are immediately effective.

B. Benefits: The IUD is a highly effective method of contraception that provides continuous protection. After the patient has undergone the initial insertion procedure, she can feel confident

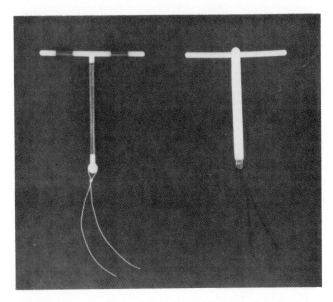

Figure 6-2. Intrauterine contraceptive devices available in 1989. At left is a Copper T 380A *(Courtesy of GynoPharma, Inc., Somerville, New Jersey)* and to the right a Progestasert *(Courtesy of ALZA Corp., Palo Alto, California).*

that she is adequately protected from unwanted pregnancy. No further action or motivation is required other than monthly checks for the IUD strings.

    C. Side Effects: The following are the most frequently observed side effects and complications related to the IUD:

(1) Menorrhagia (10–15%).
(2) Dysmenorrhea (10–15%).
(3) Expulsion (2–20%).
(4) Pelvic inflammatory disease. The IUD provides no protection against HIV or other sexually transmitted diseases. If a woman develops a pelvic infection with an IUD in place, she must be treated aggressively with antibiotics and have the IUD removed.
(5) Uterine perforation (< 1%).

If a woman becomes pregnant with an IUD in place, the risk of spontaneous abortion is 50%. If the IUD is removed in the first trimester, the risk of spontaneous abortion decreases to 25%. Of all women with IUDs who become pregnant, 5% have ectopic pregnancies, compared with an overall ectopic pregnancy rate of about 1%.

D. Contraindications: The IUD is not an appropriate contraceptive choice in many situations. For example, in the younger woman at high risk for exposure to sexually transmitted diseases, the potential for developing pelvic inflammatory disease with an IUD and its associated sequelae of infertility and chronic pain may far outweigh the contraceptive benefits. This potential risk underscores the need for open dialogue between the patient and her health care provider to determine the most appropriate and effective method of contraception. The generally accepted contraindications to using an IUD are summarized in Table 6–1.

ORAL HORMONAL CONTRACEPTIVES

Currently, more than 20 different types of oral contraceptive pills are on the market. Most of these are combined pills; that is, they consist of various combinations and types of estrogen and progestin (see Table 6–2 for a list of commonly prescribed low-dose oral contraceptive pills). Combined pills are available as 21-day regimens or 28-day regimens with the last 7 days as placebos or iron supplements.

Table 6-1. Contraindications to using intrauterine devices (IUDs).

Absolute contraindications
Active pelvic infection.
Pregnancy.
Relative contraindications
Purulent cervicitis.
Postpartum endometritis.
Impaired response to infection.
Recurrent sexually transmitted diseases.
Multiple sexual partners.
History of ectopic pregnancy.
History of pelvic inflammatory disease.
Impaired coagulation.
Anatomic uterine anomaly.

Table 6-2. Commonly used low-dose oral contraceptives.[1]

Name	Type	Progestin	Estrogen (Ethinyl Estradiol)
Lo/Ovral	Combination	0.3 mg dl-norgestrel	30 μg
Nordette and Levlen	Combination	0.15 mg levonorgestrel	30 μg
Norinyl 1/35 and Ortho-Novum 1/35	Combination	1 mg norethindrone	35 μg
Loestrin 1.5/30	Combination	1.5 mg norethindrone acetate	30 μg
Demulen 1/35	Combination	1 mg ethynodiol diacetate	35 μg
Brevicon and Modicon	Combination	0.5 mg norethindrone	35 μg
Ovcon 35	Combination	0.4 mg norethindrone	35 μg
Ortho-novum 10/11	Biphasic	0.5 mg norethindrone (days 1–10) 1 mg norethindrone (days 11–21)	35 μg
Ortho-novum 777	Triphasic	0.5 mg norethindrone (days 1–7) 0.75 mg norethindrone (days 8–14) 1 mg norethindrone (days 15–21)	35 μg
Tri-Norinyl	Triphasic	0.5 mg norethindrone (days 1–7) 1 mg norethindrone (days 8–16) 0.5 mg norethindrone (days 17–21)	35 μg
Triphasil and Tri-Levlen	Triphasic	0.05 mg levonorgestrel (days 1–6) 0.075 mg levonorgestrel (days 7–11) 0.125 mg levonorgestrel (days 12–21)	30 μg 40 μg 30 μg
Micronor and Nor-QD	Progestin-only mini-pill	0.35 mg norethindrone to be taken continuously	
Ovrette	Progestin-only mini-pill	0.075 mg dl-norgestrel to be taken continuously	

[1] Reproduced, with permission, from Schroeder SA et al: *Current Medical Diagnosis & Treatment*, 30th ed. Appleton & Lange, 1991.

Triphasic and biphasic pills also contain a combination of estrogen and progestin, except that the progestin level varies over the 21-day period. These pills are intended to more closely approximate the hormonal pattern that occurs during a normal menstrual cycle.

The "sequential" regimen is no longer used in the USA. In this regimen, the first 15–16 pills contained only estrogen, and the remaining 5 pills contained a combination of estrogen and progestin. These pills are no longer used in the USA because of their association with increased rates of endometrial cancer.

Oral contraceptives were approved by the US Food and Drug Administration in 1960. Since then, the dosages of both estrogen and progestin have decreased dramatically. Most pills now contain only 0.035 mg of estrogen and less than 1 mg of progestin (compared with 0.15 mg of estrogen and 10 mg of progestin in the 1960s).

Daily progestin tablets, known as the minipill, contain only progestin and are slightly less effective than the combined pills. These pills are useful for women who are older or who have a medical contraindication to an estrogen-containing pill. Progestin-only pills are less likely to be associated with headaches, elevated blood pressure, or alterations in carbohydrate metabolism.

Mechanism of Action

Combined oral contraceptive pills prevent pregnancy primarily by suppressing ovulation by altering the cyclical hypothalamic-pituitary-ovarian secretion of follicle-stimulating hormone (FSH) and luteinizing hormone (LH). The normal midcycle LH surge that triggers ovulation is inhibited by the exogenous estrogen and progestin in the pill. The progestin-only pill can also alter the midcycle LH surge and inhibit ovulation, although less reliably than the combined pill. Therefore, the effectiveness of the progestin-only pill depends more on the mechanisms listed below, which are important for both types of pills:

(1) Alteration of cervical mucus to hamper movement of sperm.
(2) Change in the character of the endometrial lining to inhibit implantation.
(3) Alteration of ovum transport.

Effectiveness

The typical first-year failure rate for oral contraceptives is 3%. When some medications are used concurrently with oral contraceptives, they decrease the effectiveness of the pill through their effects on liver enzymes and metabolism. The most common of these medications include phenytoin, carbamazepine, and antico-agulants. When these medications are taken concurrently with oral contraceptives, a backup method of contraception should be used (eg, condoms, diaphragm, or vaginal sponge).

Benefits

The following list outlines some of the known health benefits for oral contraceptive pill users:

(1) Regulation of menses, useful for young women with irregular periods or menorrhagia.
(2) Protection from ovarian and endometrial cancer.
(3) Treatment of functional ovarian cysts.
(4) Decrease in the incidence of benign breast masses, fibrocystic disease, and fibroadenomas.
(5) Decrease in incidence of pelvic inflammatory disease due to changes of cervical mucus.

Note that, even though oral contraceptives can help reduce the in-cidence of pelvic inflammatory disease, they provide no protection against HIV.

Side Effects

Many women experience no side effects while taking oral con-traceptives. However, there is a long list of potential side effects that women experience to varying degrees. These side effects can often be diminished or eliminated by changing to a different type of pill and selecting the combination of estrogen and progestin that is least associated with the given side effect. The following is a list of the most common side effects:

(1) Bleeding irregularities, including missed periods, scanty bleed-ing, spotting, or breakthrough bleeding.
(2) Weight gain.
(3) Skin changes, acne, and chloasma.
(4) Breast tenderness or fullness.
(5) Increased incidence of benign liver tumors (adenomas).
(6) Depression or mood changes.

Some of the more serious but less common side effects include:

(1) Hypertension (less than 5%).
(2) Stroke (less than 0.05%).

(3) Thrombotic disease.

Contraindications

Table 6–3 lists the absolute and relative contraindications to using oral contraceptives. These contraindications must be considered when deciding whether or not to recommend oral contraceptives.

POSTCOITAL OR "MORNING-AFTER" PILL

The so-called morning-after pill is a hormone regimen that is effective in preventing pregnancy if taken within 72 hours of unprotected intercourse. The regimen prescribed most often is as follows: 2 Ovral tablets (each table contains 0.050 mg of ethinyl estradiol and 0.5 mg of norgestrel) are taken initially, followed by another 2 tablets 12 hours later. High doses of diethylstilbestrol (DES) may also be given in a 5-day course. These hormonal regimens are thought to prevent pregnancy by suppressing ovulation or altering transport of the ovum through the fallopian tube. Studies have indicated failure rates of 1–2%.

IMPLANTS & INJECTABLES

Implants

In this method of contraception, capsules that contain the progestational hormone levonorgestrel are implanted subdermally

Table 6–3. Contraindications to using oral contraceptives.

Absolute contraindications
  Thromboembolic disease or history of thrombophlebitis.
  Cerebrovascular accident.
  Ischemic heart disease.
  Breast cancer.
  Estrogen-dependent neoplasm.
  Vaginal bleeding of unknown cause.
  Pregnancy.
  Liver tumor or impaired liver function.
  Pregnancy-related cholestasis.
Relative contraindications
  Migraine headaches.
  Hypertension.
  More than 35 years of age and a smoker.
  Diabetes.
  Sickle cell disease.

in the upper arm. The levonorgestrel is released slowly over months to years. Currently, Norplant is the only implant approved for use in the USA by the Food and Drug Administration. It consists of 6 silicone implants, each containing the progestin levonorgestrel. These implants are placed subdermally in a fan shape in the upper inner arm. Each capsule is 3.5 cm long and 2.5 mm in diameter. The slow release of levonorgestrel is effective in preventing pregnancy for up to 5 years. The typical first-year failure rate is 0.04%, giving a method effectiveness of greater than 99%. Norplant is a reversible, highly effective method of long-term contraception that is unrelated to intercourse.

Norplant is thought to prevent pregnancy by inhibiting ovulation, thickening cervical mucus, and altering the endometrial lining. The most common side effects are as follows: irregular bleeding and spotting, acne, mood changes, and complications at the insertion or removal site. The few contraindications to its use include active liver disease, unexplained vaginal bleeding, pregnancy, thrombophlebitis, and cerebrovascular disease.

Capronor is a similar levonorgestrel implant system that is currently being used in clinical trials and has not yet been approved by the US Food and Drug Administration. The capsules are biodegradable and are effective for 18 months of continuous protection.

Injections

Another means of providing contraception is to inject hormones intramuscularly to create a depot from which the contraceptive agent is gradually released. Medroxyprogesterone acetate (Depo-Provera) is the hormone used most often in these injections. This progestin has a mechanism of action that is similar to that of Norplant; however, this single injection provides only 3 months of continuous contraception. Although Depo-Provera is used widely throughout the world, it is not approved by the US Food and Drug Administration as a contraceptive because early studies performed on beagles showed an increased risk for breast cancer. These results have been widely disputed and are generally disregarded because similar studies in humans have not supported these findings.

FERTILITY AWARENESS

Fertility awareness, an extension of the **rhythm method,** involves daily charting of basal body temperatures and evaluation of cervical mucus to accurately predict ovulation. Once a woman has learned to predict when she is ovulating, she can then calculate her fertile period, which generally lasts from 7 days before ovulation to 3 days after ovulation. She can then either abstain or use another method of birth control during that time. The method effectiveness rate is 80%, significantly lower than for most other methods. This method has no side effects or contraindications and is useful for women who, for religious or other reasons, are unable to use other forms of contraception. Learning to accurately chart menstrual cycles and predict ovulation is also helpful for couples who are actively trying to conceive. This method provides no protection against HIV or other sexually transmitted diseases.

COITUS INTERRUPTUS

Coitus interruptus, sometimes called "withdrawal," is when the man withdraws his penis from the vagina just before ejaculation. This method is generally about 80% effective. One reason for the high failure rate is that preejaculatory fluid contains sperm that may lead to pregnancy. As with fertility awareness, this method provides no protection against HIV or other sexually transmitted diseases.

STERILIZATION

Throughout the world, sterilization is the most widely accepted form of contraception. This procedure is considered permanent and therefore is recommended only for couples who are not interested in future childbearing. This aspect must be emphasized when counseling couples who are inquiring about sterilization because some couples believe that this procedure is easily "reversed." Reversal of tubal ligation or vasectomy requires microsurgical techniques and results in future pregnancy in only one-third of the cases. Although male sterilization is generally associated with fewer complications, women undergo the procedure more often than men. For both men and women, the procedure can be performed on an outpatient basis with either local or general anesthesia.

Female Sterilization

Fallopian tube ligation is the most common method of female sterilization. Tubal ligation may be performed immediately after vaginal delivery, in conjunction with a cesarean section, or as an elective outpatient procedure. There are many approaches to tubal ligation, ranging from the most common laparoscopic procedures to laparotomy, minilaparotomy, culdoscopy, or a transvaginal approach.

A. Laparoscopic Procedures: Laparoscopic tubal ligation is a widely accepted procedure and may be performed either under general anesthesia or with local anesthesia and intravenous sedation. The procedure can be completed in only 10–15 minutes. The techniques used most often are as follows: (1) occlusion of the oviducts using metal clips or silastic rubber rings (with a failure rate of 0.2–0.5%) and (2) bipolar electrocautery of the ampullary section of the tube bilaterally (with a failure rate of 0.1–2.0%).

B. Procedures Requiring an Abdominal Incision: The primary abdominal approaches to tubal sterilization are summarized in Figure 6–3.

C. Complications Associated with Tubal Ligation: The complications that occur with tubal ligations are primarily those associated with any surgery and are as follows:

(1) Failure (0.2–0.4%). If a woman becomes pregnant after a tubal ligation, she has up to a 50% chance of having an ectopic pregnancy.
(2) Infection. The risk of infection is similar to that for other surgical procedures.
(3) Bleeding. Occasionally, broad ligament hematomas may form.
(4) Anesthesia. The risks related to the anesthetic during tubal ligation are the same as in other surgical procedures that require anesthesia.

Male Sterilization

Vasectomy, or ligation of the vas deferens, results in male sterilization by blocking the passage of sperm from the testes. The procedure is done on an outpatient basis through a small incision in the scrotum under local anesthesia and requires only 20 minutes to perform. Compared with female sterilization, vasectomy is less expensive to perform and is associated with lower mortality and morbidity.

Before sterility can be ensured, sperm counts must be checked until 2 consecutive counts are zero. This may take several weeks to months and depends on frequency of ejaculation.

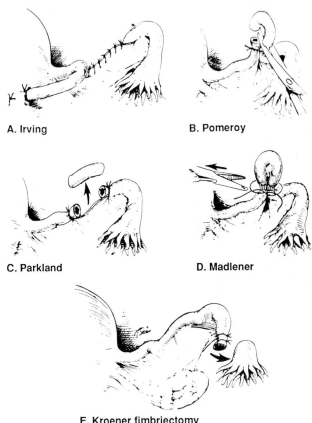

A. Irving

B. Pomeroy

C. Parkland

D. Madlener

E. Kroener fimbriectomy

Figure 6–3. Various techniques for tubal sterilization. **A.** Irving procedure: The medial cut end of the oviduct is buried in the myometrium posteriorly and the distal cut end is buried in the mesosalpinx. **B.** Pomeroy procedure: A loop of oviduct is ligated, and the knuckle of the tube above the ligature is excised. **C.** Parkland procedure: A midsegment of tube is separated from the mesosalpinx at an avascular site; the separated tubal segment is ligated proximally and distally and then excised. **D.** Madlener procedure: A knuckle of oviduct is crushed and ligated without resection. **E.** Kroener procedure: The tube is ligated across the ampulla, and the distal portion of the ampulla, including all of the fimbriae, is resected. *(Reproduced, with permission, from Cunningham FG, McDonald PC, and Gant NF: Williams Obstetrics, 18th ed. Appleton & Lange, 1989.)*

ELECTIVE ABORTION

Abortion is the general term referring to the loss of any previable pregnancy. Approximately 15–20% of all pregnancies end in spontaneous abortion, irrespective of medical intervention. An **elective abortion** is a surgical intervention in which the fetus and placental tissues are evacuated from the uterus at a previable stage. This is also known as a **therapeutic abortion.** A **first-trimester abortion** is evacuation of the products of conception during the first 13 weeks of gestation as determined by the last menstrual period (LMP). A **second-trimester,** or **midtrimester, abortion** is evacuation of the uterus from 14–24 weeks of gestation as determined by LMP.

Legal Issues

Abortion is legal in many countries, often with specific guidelines and restrictions. Laws governing abortion practices vary, with some countries having highly permissive laws that allow unrestricted access to abortion and other countries having rigorous restrictions on abortion. Today in the USA, abortion is again a highly charged and controversial issue. Its legal status is being redefined by US government officials as they begin to reconsider the landmark Supreme Court Roe versus Wade decision.

In 1973 the US Supreme Court ruled in *Roe versus Wade* that women have the right to terminate their pregnancy in the first trimester. Beyond the first trimester, individual states have laws that provide guidelines and limitations for abortion procedures.

Evaluation

Extensive counseling must be provided for all women seeking an abortion. All options should be discussed, including adoption and motherhood in addition to abortion. Social services and professional counselors should be available to aid the woman in making this difficult decision and to support her through the process. Once a woman has made the decision to proceed with an abortion, she should be supported in that choice.

The following are generally accepted indications for performing an abortion.

A. Medical Indications: In general, any condition in which pregnancy will seriously jeopardize the mother's health.

(1) Severe diabetes mellitus.
(2) Renal insufficiency.

(3) Heart disease (eg, class III or greater functional impairment, Eisenmenger complex, Fallot's tetralogy, myocarditis).

(4) Pulmonary disease (eg, cystic fibrosis, pulmonary hypertension).

(5) Cancer (eg, invasive cervical cancer, Hodgkin's disease).

(6) Hematologic disorders (eg, thromboembolic disease, hemaglobinopathies, clotting defects).

(7) Gastrointestinal tract disorders (eg, severe ulcerative colitis, cholestatic jaundice of pregnancy).

(8) Specific medical disorders (eg, serious cases of systemic lupus erythematosus, rheumatoid arthritis, adrenal insufficiency, acute hepatitis, and AIDS).

B. Obstetric Indications:

(1) Intrauterine infections that may result in fetal anomaly (eg, rubella).

(2) Ingestion of medication early in pregnancy known to cause fetal anomalies.

(3) Uterine anomalies or injury (eg, prior ruptured uterus or extensive myomas).

(4) Isoimmunization, particularly in the case of a prior infant with hydrops fetalis.

(5) Congenital factors, which can lead to fetal deformities or genetic anomalies (eg, Marfan syndrome, Down syndrome).

C. Social Indications:

(1) The patient does not desire the pregnancy or is unable to care for her children because of poverty, family size, or lack of support from her partner.

(2) The pregnancy is the result of rape or incest.

(3) The patient suffers from a severe mental disorder (eg, schizophrenia or depression).

D. Preabortion Work-Up: A preabortion work-up should include the following:

(1) **Complete history and physical examination** with evaluation for possible exposure to sexually transmitted diseases.

(2) **Accurate dating of the pregnancy** by last menstrual period and confirmation with uterine sizing. Ultrasonography should be used when a discrepancy exists between uterine size and gestational age based on dates.

(3) **Laboratory data,** especially hematocrit and Rh status. If the patient is Rh-negative, she must receive Rh (D) immunoglobu-

lin (RhoGAM) after the procedure to prevent RH sensitization that could affect future pregnancies.

(4) **Contraceptive counseling.** Plans should be made for postabortion contraception.

Anesthesia

Elective abortions are usually performed under local anesthesia, although general anesthesia is often used in later gestations. Studies have shown that overall mortality rates are lowest when abortions are performed under local anesthesia by paracervical block with 15 mL of 1% chloroprocaine or lidocaine and intravenous sedation with a narcotic agent such as fentanyl, 50 μg. Not only is local anesthesia associated with fewer risks, it is also far less expensive than general anesthesia. Moreover, having the patient awake during the procedure is useful because she is able to communicate any discomfort directly to the physician performing the procedure.

Procedures

All abortion procedures should be preceded by cervical dilation, which can be done safely and successfully using osmotic dilators. *Laminaria* tents or synthetic dilators (Lamicel or Dilapan) are narrow cylinders that are placed into the cervical canal and slowly expand by absorbing the surrounding water. These dilators are generally placed in the cervix 6–24 hours before the procedure and significantly reduce the incidence of cervical lacerations and uterine perforation that can be caused by mechanical dilation at the time of the procedure.

A. First-Trimester Abortion Procedures:

1. Vacuum curettage–Vacuum curettage is considered the standard procedure for first-trimester abortions. After the cervix is dilated either with osmotic dilators before or mechanical dilators at the time of the procedure, a suction cannula is passed into the intrauterine cavity. The cannula is connected to a vacuum pump that creates negative pressures of 50–60 mm Hg, and the uterine contents are evacuated. Finally, a sharp curette is used to confirm that the uterus is empty. This procedure has an average blood loss of less than 100 mL and requires about 3 minutes to perform.

2. Dilatation and curettage–This procedure is similar to vacuum curettage, except that the uterus is evacuated by sharp curettage alone. This method is recommended for first-trimester abortions only when suction equipment is unavailable. Compared with vacuum curettage, it is associated with a higher incidence of complications and takes longer to perform.

3. RU486–RU486 has received extensive publicity as the "abortion drug." Although not currently available in the USA, RU486 has been used extensively in France, where it was developed. RU486 is a competitive antagonist to progesterone and has been shown to be safe and effective in European studies. Given orally within the first few weeks after a missed period, it causes complete sloughing of the endometrial lining, which either prevents implantation or removes an implanted zygote. It is unclear when or if this agent will become available for general use in the USA.

B. Second-Trimester Abortion Procedures:

1. Dilatation and evacuation–Dilatation and evacuation is probably the most common abortion procedure for second-trimester abortion and is similar to the dilatation and curettage method described above for first-trimester abortions. After the cervix is dilated, the uterine contents are evacuated with grasping forceps and manual curettage. Ultrasonographic guidance during this procedure is useful to ensure that the uterus is completely emptied. Ultrasonography is also helpful in later abortions to accurately estimate gestational age.

2. Prostaglandins–Two prostaglandins, PGE_2 and PGF_2, are now being used to induce labor, particularly for second-trimester abortions. These agents are useful for cervical dilatation and expulsion of the fetus but may require adjuvant curettage to remove retained placental tissue. The prostaglandin E_2 is placed in the vagina in the form of a suppository or gel and often requires more than 12 hours to be effective. Prostaglandins are associated with the unpleasant side effects of fever, nausea, and diarrhea. This method may be more traumatic than dilatation and evacuation for the patient, although it requires less expertise on the part of the surgeon.

3. Intra-amniotic saline–Intra-amniotic injection of hypertonic saline was a common second-trimester abortion procedure before dilatation and evacuation and prostaglandin use became the favored procedures. When hypertonic saline is injected directly into the amniotic sac, it induces labor.

This method has been associated with the following serious side effects: (1) disseminated intravascular coagulation, (2) hypernatremia, (3) hypervolemia and heart failure, (4) myometrial necrosis, and (5) retained products of conception. Because of these complications, hypertonic urea is now used instead of saline and is associated with fewer harmful side effects.

4. Hysterectomy and hysterotomy–Hysterectomy is rarely indicated as a method of abortion primarily because of the increased risks associated with this procedure, in particular, the risk of excessive blood loss when performing a hysterectomy on a pregnant uterus. This procedure may be considered when a woman desires an abortion and sterilization and has large uterine fibroids.

Hysterotomy requires a laparotomy to make an incision in the uterus and then remove the fetus and placental tissues. This procedure is rarely indicated and has the disadvantages of possibly delivering a live fetus as well as compromising future child-bearing potential.

Complications

Interestingly, the risks associated with first-trimester abortion are lower than if the pregnancy were carried to term. In general, the morbidity rate associated with first-trimester abortions is 5%, whereas the morbidity rate associated with second-trimester abortions is 15–25%. The main risks and complications are as follows:

(1) **Bleeding.** May be caused by failure of the uterus to contract after aspiration. Can be treated with intramuscular injections of ergonovine maleate or prostaglandin or intravenous injections of oxytocin.
(2) **Infection.** Should be suspected in any patient with fever, pelvic pain, or purulent discharge.
(3) **Retained products of conception.** Should be suspected in cases with immediate or delayed vaginal bleeding. Requires reaspiration.
(4) **Injury to the cervix or uterus** (cervical lacerations or uterine perforations). Can occur with dilatation of the cervix. Occasionally, hysterectomy must be performed to control bleeding caused by a ruptured uterus.

No significant long-term complications have been documented for single first-trimester abortions. Some data suggest repeated abortions may be associated with Asherman's syndrome or recurrent miscarriages.

SUGGESTED READINGS

Hatcher RA et al: *Contraceptive Technology 1990–1992,* 15th ed. Irvington, 1990.

Speroff L, Glass RH, Kase NG: *Clinical Gynecologic Endocrinology and Infertility,* 4th ed. Williams & Wilkins, 1989.

Tietze C. In: *Fertility Regulation and the Public Health: Selected Papers of Christopher Tietze.* Tietze SL, Lincoln R (editors). Springer-Verlag, 1987.

Ultrasonography in Obstetrics & Gynecology | 7

Ruth B. Goldstein, MD

Because of its excellent diagnostic accuracy, patient safety, and relative low cost, ultrasonography has become a nearly indispensable tool in evaluating obstetric and gynecologic pathology. Sophisticated ultrasound equipment is widely available in the USA today, and most of it is portable, so critically ill patients can be examined at the bedside or in the operating room.

High-resolution, real-time ultrasonography has dramatically improved fetal assessment. No other diagnostic test for suspected abnormalities in a fetus (eg, computed tomography, tomography, magnetic resonance imaging, fetoscopy) approaches the accuracy and safety of ultrasonography. Ultrasonographic examination of the fetus may be the most thorough physical examination possible. This chapter discusses some of the more important uses of ultrasonography in the general practice of obstetrics and gynecology.

STANDARD SONOGRAM

Non-ionizing sound waves of a frequency just greater than audible sound are emitted by an ultrasound transducer (crystal). Between transmissions, the transducer is changed to act like an echo receiver. The sound waves reflect and scatter within tissues and at organ boundaries, resulting in returning echoes of different amplitudes. The time elapsed between the origin and return of the ultrasound waves is translated into depth information, and this information, in combination with the amplitude of the returning echo, is electronically converted into a 2-dimensional gray-scale image (sonogram) by a computer. The computer operates fast enough to project onto the monitor a real-time, moving picture of the area being examined.

Two basic types of ultrasonography are most often used in obstetrics and gynecology: **transabdominal sonography** (TAS) and

endovaginal sonography (EVS), also known as **transvaginal sonography.** As the name implies, TAS involves transmitting the sound waves through the surface of the abdomen to examine the pelvic organs. Developed more recently, the EVS technique involves inserting a probe into the vagina so that sound is transmitted transvaginally. Because the probe is placed nearer the pelvic organs and because higher frequency transducers are used, images of higher resolution can be obtained with this technique.

ULTRASONOGRAPHY IN OBSTETRICS

Currently, routine use of obstetric ultrasonography is not recommended in the USA. However, because most authorities believe that it is safe and useful, indications for its use are relatively liberal. Obstetric ultrasonography is most commonly indicated to

(1) Confirm fetal life.
(2) Date the pregnancy.
(3) Evaluate the fetal growth and the amniotic fluid volume.
(4) Resolve size and date discrepancy (includes multiple gestations).
(5) Evaluate the fetus for anomalies.
(6) Ascertain the position of the placenta (eg, to exclude placenta previa).

Two "levels" of sonograms are recommended. The first, the Level I Sonogram or the standard obstetric sonogram, includes an assessment of fetal life and number, the position of the fetus and the placenta, an estimation of the amniotic fluid volume, and fetal biometry (fetal measurements) performed to determine fetal size and gestational age. The cerebral ventricles and spine, fluid-filled stomach, umbilical cord insertion into the abdominal wall, and bladder and kidney regions are also documented during this examination to exclude major fetal anomalies. A more detailed examination of fetal morphology, or Level II Sonogram, is indicated if the fetus is known to be at increased risk for an anomaly. This fetal survey, targeted to search for specific anomalies, should be performed by experienced examiners, usually at a prenatal diagnostic center.

Estimating Gestational Age in the First Trimester

Ultrasonography is now the most widely used method for determining gestational age. Sonologists, like obstetricians, date the pregnancy from the first day of the last normal menstrual period, and the gestational age is reported in menstrual weeks.

In the first trimester, gestational age is sonographically estimated by measuring the size of the embryo or gestational sac. In a normally progressing pregnancy, a gestational sac is first detectable on TAS when the mean sac diameter (MSD) is approximately 5–6 mm (Table 7-1), which is equivalent to a 5-week gestation. As gestation progresses to 6 weeks, the yolk sac becomes visible (MSD is approximately 15 mm). Next, the embryo becomes sonographically visible, at which point the long axis of the embryo, or the crown-rump length (CRL), can be measured (Figure 7-1) to determine gestational age (CRL equals about 5 mm or 6.5 weeks of gestation). Between 6.5 and 12 weeks, the CRL is accurate in estimating gestational age to within plus or minus 7 days; after about 12 weeks, the CRL measurement is a less accurate parameter for estimating age because of the extension and flexion of the fetus.

Estimating Gestational Age in the Second & Third Trimesters

By the beginning of the second trimester, the details of fetal anatomy can be seen more clearly on the ultrasonogram, and the size of the head, the abdomen, and the long bones can be measured to estimate fetal age. The biparietal diameter, head circumference, abdominal circumference, and femoral length (Figure 7-2) are used to estimate fetal size and age. In the first 20 weeks of gestation, this age estimate is quite accurate (± 1 week). However, in the latter half of gestation, more biologic variations occur, and other factors have greater influence on fetal growth; thus, sonographic estimation of age becomes less accurate (± 2–4 weeks) as gestation progresses. For this reason, it is recommended that sonograms for dating be obtained in the first 20 weeks of gestation.

Table 7-1. Transabdominal sonography: estimation of gestational age.

Gestational Age	Accuracy	Parameters[1]
5–6.5 weeks	± 7 days	MSD
7–13 weeks	± 5–7 days	CRL
14–20 weeks	± 7–10 days	BPD, HC, AC, FL
20–40 weeks	± 2–4 weeks	BPD, HC, AC, FL

[1]MSD, mean sac diameter; CRL, crown-rump length; BPD, biparietal diameter; HC, head circumference; AC, abdominal circumference; FL, femur length.

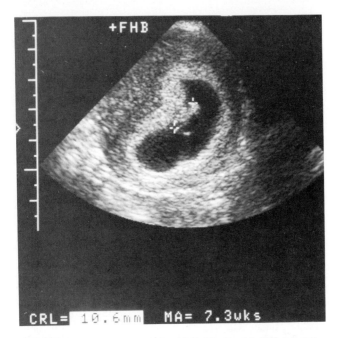

Figure 7-1. Crown-rump length (CRL). The length of the embryo is measured and, in this case, corresponds to 7.3 menstrual weeks (MA). Cardiac pulsations were observed with real-time imaging.

Further, many more fetal anomalies can be (incidentally) observed on a sonogram obtained at 18 weeks compared with one obtained at 8 or 10 weeks. For example, anencephaly, an unequivocally lethal anomaly, can be missed on a routine sonographic examination performed at 11 weeks. Similarly, myelomeningoceles and other neural tube defects, gastrointestinal defects, and even renal agenesis can go undetected on an early first-trimester sonogram. Therefore, it is recommended that, *if only one sonogram for dating is obtained, it should be obtained at approximately 18 weeks.*

In the second and third trimesters, the ultrasonographic report should include the sonographic estimate of both fetal age and weight. The fetal weight, calculated from the sonographic measurements, is reported in grams and as a percentile according to the expected weight based on the date of the last menstrual period (LMP). When the gestational age and weight based on the sonogram disagree with those based on the LMP, it is important to determine whether the LMP date is incorrect or whether the fetus is either too large or too small. If the patient is first scanned before 20 weeks, the sonographic age estimate is usually reliable, and it is likely that a 4-week discrepancy in size reflects an incorrect LMP date. However, in the "late entry" patient first scanned in the third trimester, a small fetus may indicate a truly growth-retarded fetus. Changing dates in this setting would result in overlooking a growth-retarded fetus. Therefore, after 20 weeks, the menstrual dates should be changed only with the greatest caution and with very good reason. It is for this reason that the sonologist does not change dates based *solely* on the sonogram in the second half of gestation.

Threatened Abortion & Ectopic Pregnancy

It is common for women to experience vaginal bleeding in the first trimester of pregnancy (about 25% of clinically recognized pregnancies), and as many as 50% of these women will spontaneously abort. However, more than 90% of these pregnancies will remain viable when vaginal bleeding occurs but a living embryo (ie, heart motion) is detected after 8 weeks on the sonogram. Thus, the observation of fetal heart motion dramatically changes the prognosis from a loss rate of 50% to less than 10%. In contrast, a well-formed embryo or fetus observed on the TAS without detectable heart motion is unequivocal evidence of a fetal demise.

In the first trimester, the source of bleeding is often never uncovered. Later, in the second and third trimesters, vaginal bleeding may be caused by a placental abruption or placenta previa. A subchorionic clot can be seen in about 5–20% of women evaluated for vaginal bleeding. This clot is usually secondary to a partial placental abruption, which can also be seen on the sonogram. The more serious retroplacental hematomas are much more difficult to see on sonograms (because of the similar echotexture of clot and placenta). In the third trimester, placenta previa is diagnosed accurately with ultrasound. In the first half of gestation, many false-positive diagnoses of placental previa occur (usually a marginal or partial previa) because the placenta appears dangerously close to the cervix. However, as the lower uterine segment lengthens during gestation, the distance between the edge of the placenta and the

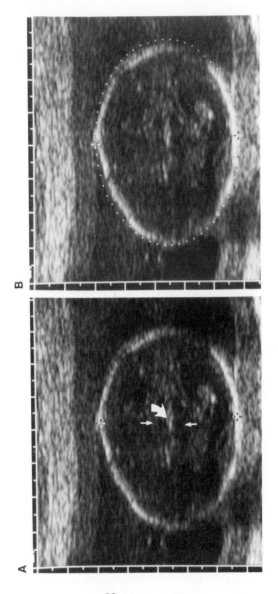

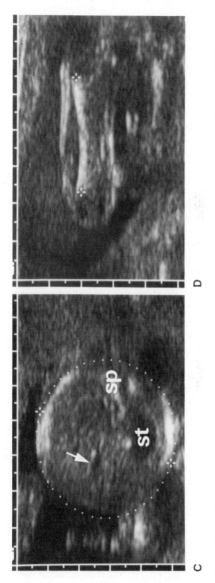

Figure 7-2. Biometric measurements in a fetus at 18 menstrual weeks. *A:* The biparietal diameter (BPD) is measured on an axial image through the fetal head at the level of the hypoechoic thalamus (*straight arrows*) and the echogenic line indicating the third ventricle (*curved arrow*). *B:* Head circumference is measured on the same plane of imaging as the BPD. *C:* Abdominal circumference is measured in a transverse plane through the abdomen at the level of the stomach (st) and right portal vein of the liver (*arrow*); spine (sp). *D:* The length of the diaphysis of the femur is also measured.

cervix increases, and the placental position can be more accurately estimated.

If the patient presents with vaginal bleeding or pelvic pain very early during pregnancy, it may be more difficult to confirm or negate the presence of embryonic life because, even though the gestational sac is visible on the sonogram, the embryo is not. In this case, the diagnostic possibilities include the following:

(1) A pregnancy too early for the embryo to be detectable by ultrasonography (< 7 weeks using TAS).

(2) A very early embryonic demise that has resulted in expulsion of part of the sac and embryo, degeneration of the embryo, or arrest in development at an early stage of embryonic life (ie, an "empty" sac).

(3) A pseudogestational sac associated with an ectopic pregnancy.

Sonographic observations of the early gestational sac in conjunction with quantitative human chorionic gonadotropin (β-hCG) can be useful for distinguishing among these diagnostic considerations.

Threshold (discriminatory) sac sizes have been established, after which embryonic structures should be detectable using TAS. A yolk sac should be detectable in all normal pregnancies when the MSD is 20 mm or more (> 7 weeks), and an embryo should be detectable when the MSD is 25 mm or more (roughly after 7–8 weeks) (Table 7–2). In many cases, the embryonic structures will be detectable well before the sac has achieved these sizes, but these threshold sizes are chosen as conservative limits so that all normal pregnancies will fall within these guidelines.

Threshold sac size criteria have also been established for EVS.

Table 7–2. β-hCG and size threshold for detecting gestational sacs or embryonic structures using transabdominal and endovaginal sonography.

	TAS	EVS
Gestational sac (β-hCG)	1800 mIU/mL[1]	1000 mIU/mL[1]
Yolk sac (diameter)	≥ 20 mm	≥ 8 mm[2]
Embryo (diameter)	≥ 25 mm	≥ 16 mm[3]

[1] Second International Standard.
[2] Some use more conservative criterion of 13 mm in diameter.
[3] Some use more conservative criterion of 18 mm in diameter.

In fact, EVS can confirm a normally developing gestation about 1 week earlier than TAS because of its higher resolution. As listed in Table 7-2, with EVS, a yolk sac is visible in all normal pregnancies when the MSD is 8 mm (about 5.5 weeks), and an embryo is detectable when the MSD is 16 mm (about 6.5 weeks).

The utility of these threshold MSD dimensions is illustrated in the following examples:

(1) A woman presents with vaginal spotting. According to her LMP, she is 8 weeks pregnant. She and her doctor are concerned that the pregnancy is nonviable. On the transabdominal sonogram, an intrauterine sac is observed, and the MSD measures 32 mm. No yolk sac or embryo is detected. Because we know that in all normal pregnancies both the yolk sac and the embryo should be detectable when the MSD is 25 mm or more, we can be certain that this measurement represents an abnormal gestation, usually an embryonic demise or a blighted ovum, and the uterus can be evacuated.

(2) Similarly, if menstrual dates are uncertain and a very small sac is observed (eg, MSD = 6 mm), the absence of a detectable yolk sac or embryo may be completely normal and may merely reflect a gestational age that is earlier than expected. Serial scans or β-hCG titers would be the most appropriate analytic tools in this situation.

Another parameter that is useful in diagnosing the causes of vaginal bleeding or pelvic pain is the titer of the serum β-hCG, which increases proportionately with gestational age (logarithmically) until approximately 8 menstrual weeks. In a normal pregnancy an intrauterine gestational sac is detectable using TAS at a β-hCG level of 1800 mIU/mL.* With the greater resolution of EVS, an intrauterine gestational sac is detectable at a β-hCG level of 1000 mIU/mL.* EVS and β-hCG levels can be used jointly when a woman presents with vaginal bleeding or pelvic pain and a positive pregnancy test, but she is unsure of the date of her last normal menstrual period. If the β-hCG level is 1000 mIU/mL or more and if the sonogram does *not* reveal an intrauterine gestational sac, an ectopic pregnancy is a likely possibility. However, if the β-hCG level is low ($\leq$ 1000 mIU/mL), the absence of an intrauterine gestational sac is less meaningful.

Several key sonographic observations can be dramatic aids in di-

---

*Second International Standard; for a specific definition, see the section titled Chorionic Gonadotropin Tests in Chapter 8. Laboratory reference standards of these titers may vary from one institution to another, so numeric values are not necessarily transferable from one laboratory to another. It is extremely important to know which reference the laboratory uses to estimate β-hCG.

agnosing ectopic pregnancy. According to recent information (Callen, 1988), of all women referred to the ultrasound laboratory for potential ectopic pregnancies, approximately 18% do have ectopic pregnancies. However, when no intrauterine pregnancy is detected by ultrasonography, the percentage of women with ectopic pregnancies increases to 43%; furthermore, when an adnexal mass or cul-de-sac fluid is also detected, approximately 71% have ectopic pregnancies. Approximately 100% of the women have ectopic pregnancies when both a mass and fluid are detected but no intrauterine gestation is found. Note, however, that the sonogram may be completely normal in up to 20% of women with ectopic pregnancies. Therefore, the diagnosis of ectopic pregnancy is essentially one of *exclusion*. Any pregnant woman presenting with pelvic pain and vaginal bleeding in whom an intrauterine gestation cannot be identified with ultrasonography is strongly suspected of having an ectopic pregnancy.

The observation of an intrauterine sac alone is not sufficient evidence for the diagnosis of an intrauterine pregnancy. In 10–20% of ectopic gestations, a saclike structure, or pseudogestational sac, is observed within the central uterine cavity. This structure reflects a combination of thickened endometrium (decidua) and blood. In many cases, a true gestational sac can be distinguished from a pseudogestational sac by the characteristic appearance of the double decidual line ("double decidual sac" sign) that is present only in a true gestational sac (Figure 7–3). The decidua capsularis (the decidua lifted by the developing embryo and chorionic fluid) forms the inner echogenic line and the decidua vera or parietalis (the decidualized endometrium on the opposite side of the implanted embryo) forms the outer echogenic line. Unless an embryo has implanted within the uterus, the decidua capsularis will not form and therefore the double decidual morphology will not be present. Because the interpretation of this sonographic observation may be subjective, this observation is not as definitive sonographic evidence of an intrauterine pregnancy as the presence of a yolk sac or embryo. More important, if any doubt remains about the nature of an intrauterine sac, the scan should be repeated in 3–4 days when the yolk sac and the embryo should be detectable.

ULTRASONOGRAPHY IN GYNECOLOGY

Normal Pelvis

During transabdominal sonography, the filled urinary bladder acts as an acoustic window through which the ultrasound waves can pass. To expedite the examination, the patient is asked to drink 3 or 4 glasses of water 1 hour before the examination. After the TAS, if the examiner concludes that a better evaluation might be achieved with EVS, the patient's bladder is emptied, and EVS is performed. Because mobile pelvic masses and intra-abdominal fluid collections may be missed using only EVS, EVS is nearly always used in conjunction with TAS.

Uterus

The normal postpubertal uterus has a smooth contour and measures approximately 7 × 4 × 5 cm. Multiparity may increase the size by 1–2 cm in all directions. The prepubertal uterus is smaller (3 × 1 × 1 cm) and proportioned differently than in the menstruating woman, with the cervix accounting for two-thirds of the uterine length. After menopause, the uterus atrophies to approximately 1–2 cm thick and 3–7 cm long. The size, position, echotexture, contour, and endometrial cavity of the uterus and cervix can be easily evaluated with ultrasonography.

On sonograms the myometrium is homogeneous low- to moderate-level echotexture. Focal areas of decreased echotexture and contour irregularities are most often due to leiomyomas (fibroids). Occasionally, calcification can be detected in conjunction with fibroids.

A thin echogenic line defines the central uterine cavity and represents the interface of the opposed endometrial surfaces. Changes in the thickness of the endometrium are not detectable on sonograms. In the postmenopausal woman, the endometrium becomes thinner; a thick endometrial layer (> 5 mm) on a sonogram is considered pathologic and warrants further evaluation.

An abnormally thick endometrium may also occur in association with endometrial hyperplasia, polyps, carcinoma, or adenomyosis. Similarly, the endometrial echo complex may be focally distorted by submucosal myomas, endometrial polyps, or endometrial cancer. The appearance of an endometrial abnormality is often nonspecific, and a tissue diagnosis (ie, biopsy) becomes necessary. In patients with adenomyosis (a condition in which there is abnormal growth of the glandular basal endometrium into the myometrium), usually the only sonographic finding is a diffuse and smooth enlargement of the uterus.

Scars or tumors in the cervix may obstruct the endometrial cavity, resulting in hydrometra, pyometra, or hematometra. In these cases, the echo complex for normal endometrium is replaced by one that indicates the presence of fluid.

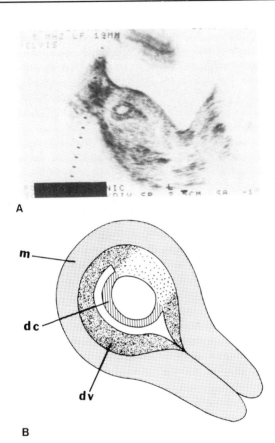

A

B

Figure 7-3. Sonographic depiction of decidua in early intrauter-ine and extrauterine pregnancies. *A:* Longitudinal real-time son-ogram of early (4-week) intrauterine pregnancy before sono-graphic depiction of an embryo. Two layers of decidua surround the developing gestational sac. *B:* Diagram of the 2 decidual layers that can be seen in early intrauterine pregnancy. The in-nermost ring of decidua surrounds the developing gestational sac and represents the decidual capsularis (dc). The thickened endometrium forms the decidua vera (dv) (m, myometrium). (*continued*)

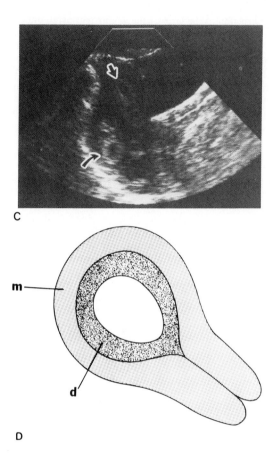

Figure 7-3 (cont). *C:* Longitudinal real-time sonogram of a ruptured ectopic pregnancy (***curved arrow***) associated with a decidual cast (***arrow***) in the uterus. The decidual cast is composed of only one layer. *D:* Diagram of the decidual cast that is associated with an ectopic pregnancy (d, decidua; m, myometrium). *(Reproduced, with permission, from Sanders RC, James AE, Jr: The Principles and Practice of Ultrasonography in Obstetrics and Gynecology, 3rd ed. Appleton-Century-Crofts, 1985.)*

Obstruction at the level of the vagina (eg, by an imperforate hymen, vaginal septum obstructing a duplicated uterus, or vaginal atresia) causes fluid to collect in both the uterus and vagina (hydrometrocolpus). Since most of these fluid collections produce at least low-level echoes (ie, not "simple" fluid echoes), the blood, pus, and mucous often cannot be distinguished by the sonographic appearance. Bright reflectors within the fluid suggest air and should raise suspicion of infection if the patient has not been instrumented (ie, if air has not been introduced during a dilatation and curettage).

Uterine malformations such as didelphia, bicornuate uterus, or uterus subseptus can be sonographically detected by the presence of 2 endometrial echo complexes. However, more precise anatomic delineation of these anomalies is achieved with magnetic resonance imaging (MRI).

Adnexa

The adnexa include ovaries, fallopian tubes, and the ligaments of the ovaries (mesovarium of the broad ligament). The ligaments and fallopian tubes are not evident on sonograms unless they are abnormal. When the fallopian tubes become distended by blood (hematosalpinx), pus (pyosalpinx), or fluid (hydrosalpinx), they appear as fluid-filled tubular structures adjacent to the uterus in the posterior or posterolateral cul-de-sac. Normally, a small amount of fluid is noted in the cul-de-sac of women of childbearing age.

The ovary appears as an oval solid mass with small peripheral (follicular) cysts. Ovarian size changes with age and stage of the menstrual cycle. In the child the ovary is small ($1 \times 1 \times 1$ cm) with a volume of 1 mL or less. The size increases until puberty, when the normal ovarian size is approximately $2 \times 2 \times 3$ cm with a volume of 10–12 mL. After menopause, the ovarian volume decreases to 2.5 mL or less.

Ovarian Masses

Most ovarian masses and neoplasms are cystic. Fortunately, the majority of ovarian cysts detected by ultrasound are both benign and nonneoplastic. While sonography cannot always distinguish a benign cyst from a malignant one, sonographic observations of simple "anechoic" fluid, a smooth indiscernible wall, and the absence of septations or irregularity suggest a benign cyst. In contrast, mural nodularity, thick septations, and associated ascites suggest malignancy.

The management of an adnexal cyst depends on the age of the patient, the size of the cyst, and the appearance of the cyst on the sonogram (see Chapter 10, The Pelvic Mass). Any ovarian cyst larger than 2.5 cm in diameter is considered abnormal (for comparison, the average mature follicle diameter is 20–22 mm).

The differential diagnosis of a cystic adnexal mass includes functional cyst (follicular, corpus luteum, theca lutein, and ovarian remnant), paraovarian cyst (wolffian duct remnant), endometrioma, tubo-ovarian abscess, hydrosalpinx, ectopic pregnancy, or neoplasm. In women of childbearing age, functional cysts are most common. Small unilocular cysts (ie, < 6 cm in diameter) are usually functional cysts (follicular or corpus luteul, not neoplasm). Because functioning cysts are so common, most small to moderately sized ovarian cysts (< 5–6 cm in diameter) in ovulatory women are not true neoplasms and often resolve without surgery. If the cyst is more than 6 cm in diameter, the likelihood of spontaneous resolution is diminished. However, even if a cyst is greater than 6 cm in diameter but is sonographically anechoic and unilocular, it is very unlikely to be malignant. Although the cyst may be a neoplasm and require surgical removal, most are benign neoplasms and can be monitored with serial sonograms for at least 4–6 weeks without significantly increasing the risk to the patient.

The sonographic appearance of an ovarian mass should be interpreted in the context of the clinical setting. For example, in a febrile patient, a thick-walled mass containing echogenic fluid is likely to be an abscess. If the patient is 8 weeks pregnant and the cyst is unilocular, it is most likely a corpus luteum cyst. If the patient is postmenopausal and the wall is nodular with thick septations, it is more likely to be malignant. Since the advent of higher resolution endovaginal transducers, not only are all types of cysts being detected earlier (ie, when they are smaller), but also finer details of the internal structure are now visible.

Dermoid cysts (cystic teratomas) tend to have a characteristic sonographic appearance: echogenic fluid and focal, high-amplitude reflectors with acoustic shadowing (caused by the presence of teeth or hair). Unfortunately, these high-amplitude reflectors may simulate bowel gas; therefore, these lesions may be camouflaged, and in rare cases, even large lesions can go undetected on sonograms, an important fact to recall if the physical examination discloses a large, definite adnexal mass but the sonogram fails to reveal one.

Small, solid tumors (ie, < 3 cm in diameter) are extremely difficult to detect on sonograms because they are similar in echotexture to the normal ovary. Solid tumors of the ovary (metastases, endometrioid tumors, dysgerminomas, and sex cord-stromal tumors) are rare, especially in women of childbearing age. If a solid lesion is observed in the adnexa of a premenopausal woman, it is more likely to be an exophytic leiomyoma than a solid ovarian neoplasm. The characteristic appearance of a leiomyoma may also be confirmed with magnetic resonance imaging if suspicion for a solid ovarian mass persists.

SUGGESTED READINGS

Callen PW: *Ultrasonography in Obstetrics and Gynecology,* 2nd ed. Saunders, 1988.

Fleischer AC et al (editors): *The Principles and Practice of Ultrasonography in Obstetrics and Gynecology,* 4th ed. Appleton & Lange, 1991.

Ectopic Pregnancy | 8

Audrey S. Koh, MD

An ectopic pregnancy occurs when a fertilized egg implants outside the uterine cavity and begins to grow (Figure 8–1). Both the prevalence and the incidence rates of ectopic pregnancy are increasing. In 1987, 1.7%, or 1 in 59, of the pregnancies reported to the Centers for Disease Control were ectopic. Despite a decreasing mortality rate for ectopic pregnancy, it is one of the leading causes of maternal death in the USA, accounting for 12% of maternal deaths in 1987.

Most ectopic pregnancies (97.7%) occur in the fallopian tube; less frequently, they occur in the abdomen (1.4%), in the cervix (0.2%), or in an ovary (0.2%). Among tubal gestations, 41% of implantations are in the distal third (ampullatory portion) of the tube, 38% in the middle third, 12% in the isthmus, 5% in the fimbria, and 1.4% in the interstitium. Combined intrauterine and ectopic pregnancies are extremely rare, as are multiple ectopic pregnancies.

PATHOGENESIS

The abnormally located implantation site is usually unable to withstand the distention and intrusive vascularization of the pregnancy and thus ruptures. In a tubal gestation, this rupture is from the tubal lumen into the connective tissue between the endosalpinx and the tubal serosa. As this hematoma expands, blood seeps distally out of the space between the fimbrial tissue and the serosa. Ultimately, the serosa itself ruptures, resulting in either abortion with regression of the ectopic gestation or secondary reimplantation at another site.

The uterine lining responds to the hormonal changes of pregnancy with a decidual reaction. When the ectopic embryo dies, the decidua is sloughed, resulting in vaginal bleeding.

The risk factors for the majority of ectopic pregnancies are related to tubal dysfunction or damage (Table 8–1).

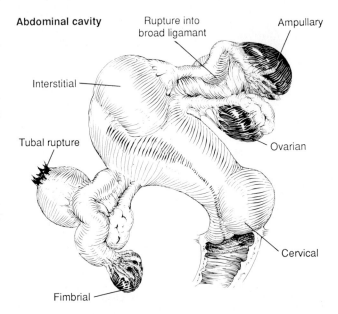

Figure 8-1. Sites of ectopic pregnancies. *(Reproduced, with permission, from Benson RC:* Handbook of Obstetrics & Gynecology, *8th ed. Lange, 1983.)*

Table 8-1. Risk factors for ectopic pregnancy.

Major risk factors
Use of intrauterine device
Prior tubal surgery
Prior pelvic inflammatory disease
Infertility
Minor risk factors
Prior abdominal or pelvic surgery
Prior appendicitis
Salpingitis isthmica nodosa
In utero diethylstilbestrol (DES) exposure
In vitro fertilization and embryo transfer (IVF-ET)

Table 8-2. Symptoms of ectopic pregnancy.

Symptoms	Percentage of Cases
Abdominal pain	90
Vaginal bleeding	80
Amenorrhea	75
Dizziness, fainting	25
Normal pregnancy symptoms	15

CLINICAL FINDINGS

The common symptoms of ectopic pregnancy are listed in Table 8-2. Abdominal or pelvic pain, ranging from low-grade soreness to a colicky cramping, is generally present even before tubal rupture. With acute rupture, the pain is often sharp and becomes diffuse. Shoulder pain may result from diaphragmatic irritation by a hemoperitoneum. However, there is no specific pain pattern for ectopic pregnancy.

Frequently, patients report normal menstrual cycles, but when questioned further, they often report abnormal timing or flow of "menses." Characteristically, the bleeding is light and results from uterine decidual slough.

The presenting signs of ectopic pregnancy are listed in Table 8-3. The so-called classic triad of ectopic pregnancy, that is, **pelvic or abdominal pain, abnormal vaginal bleeding, and an adnexal mass,** occurs in only one-third of patients. Note that of the 50% of patients with an adnexal mass, one-fifth of those masses are on the side opposite the ectopic pregnancy and usually represent a corpus luteum cyst. Although the uterus may be enlarged as a result of hormonal stimulation, it is not as large as expected for the duration of amenorrhea.

Table 8-3. Signs of ectopic pregnancy.

Signs	Percentage of Cases
Abdominal tenderness	90
Adnexal tenderness	85
Adnexal mass	50
Uterine enlargement	25
Orthostatic changes	10
Fever	5–10

Table 8-4. Differential diagnosis of ectopic pregnancy.[1]

	Ectopic Pregnancy	Appendicitis	Salpingitis	Ruptured Corpus Luteum Cyst	Uterine Abortion
Pain	Unilateral cramps and tenderness before rupture.	Epigastric, periumbilical, then right lower quadrant pain; tenderness localizing at McBurney's point. Rebound tenderness.	Usually in both lower quadrants, with or without rebound. Dysuria sometimes present.	Unilateral, becoming in general with progressive bleeding.	Midline cramps.
Nausea and vomiting	Occasionally before, frequently after rupture.	Usual. Precedes shift of pain to right lower quadrant.	Infrequent.	Rare. No symptoms or signs of pregnancy.	Almost never.
Vaginal bleeding	Some aberration; missed period, spotting.	Unrelated to menses.	Hypermenorrhea or metrorrhagia, or both.	Period delayed, then bleeding, often with pain.	Longer amenorrhea, then spotting, then brisk bleeding.
Temperature and pulse	37.2–37.8 °C (99–100 °F). Pulse variable: normal before, rapid after rupture.	37.2–37.8 °C (99–100 °F). Pulse rapid: 99–100.	37.2–40 °C (99–104 °F). Pulse elevated in proportion to fever.	Not over 37.2 °C (99 °F). Pulse normal unless blood loss marked, then rapid.	To 37.2 °C (99 °F) if spontaneous; to 40 °C (104 °F) if infected.

Pelvic examination	Unilateral tenderness, especially on movement of cervix. Crepitant mass on one side or in cul-de-sac.	No masses. Rectal tenderness high on right side.	Bilateral tenderness on movement of cervix. Masses only when pyosalpinx or tubo-ovarian abscess is present.	Tenderness over affected ovary. No masses. Uterus firm and not enlarged.	Cervix slightly patulous. Uterus slightly enlarged, irregularly softened. Tender only with infection.
Culdocentesis	Nonclotting blood.	Rarely purulent.	Purulent.	Bloody fluid.	Negative.
β-hCG	Positive.	Negative.	Negative.	Positive or negative.[2]	Positive.
Laboratory findings	White cell count of 15,000/μL. Red cell count strikingly low if blood loss large. Sedimentation rate slightly elevated.	White cell count 10,000–18,000/μL (rarely normal). Red cell count normal. Sedimentation rate slightly elevated.	White cell count 15,000–30,000/μL. Red cell count normal. Sedimentation rate markedly elevated.	White cell count normal to 10,000/μL. Red cell count normal. Sedimentation rate normal.	White cell count 15,000/μL if spontaneous; to 30,000/μL if infection. Red cell count normal. Sedimentation rate slightly to moderately elevated.

[1] Modified and reproduced, with permission, from Pernoll ML (editor): Current Obstetric & Gynecologic Diagnosis & Treatment, 7th ed. Appleton & Lange, 1991.
[2] When there is a concomitant pregnancy.

DIFFERENTIAL DIAGNOSIS

The signs and symptoms of ectopic pregnancy are frequently similar to those of other pathologic conditions. The most common of these conditions are characterized in Table 8-4. Less common conditions include torsion of adnexa, endometriosis, dysfunctional uterine bleeding, and degenerating myoma. Spontaneous abortions are included in the differential diagnosis of the patient with a positive pregnancy test. The types of spontaneous abortions are as follows:

(1) Complete: the entire products of conception are passed vaginally and the uterus is empty.

(2) Incomplete: the pregnancy has partially aborted and the remainder is still in utero.

(3) Threatened: the pregnancy is maintained in utero despite symptoms suggestive of aborting.

(4) Missed: the gestation is nonviable but has not been aborted.

DIAGNOSIS

Ectopic pregnancies can be diagnosed using human chorionic gonadotropin (hCG) tests, ultrasound imaging, dilatation and curettage (D&C), culdocentesis, and laparoscopy.

General Approach

A general approach to diagnosing ectopic pregnancy is summarized in Figure 8-2. In the clinically stable patient, the hCG level should be measured. Because a normal intrauterine pregnancy is discernible by transabdominal ultrasonography at an hCG level of 1800 mIU/mL (and at lower hCG levels [1000 mIU/mL] with endovaginal ultrasonography), sonography should be performed on patients with hCG levels above this threshold (see Chapter 7).

When the hCG level is under 1800 mIU/mL, serial titers should be checked. Falling hCG titers or titers with subnormal doubling times most likely indicate an ectopic pregnancy or an aborting intrauterine pregnancy. A normal intrauterine pregnancy should demonstrate normal hCG doubling times; when these titers reach 1800 mIU/mL, the diagnosis can be confirmed by sonography.

Human Chorionic Gonadotropin Tests

Ectopic pregnancies usually produce less hCG than normal pregnancies. The normal hCG doubling time is approximately 48 hours. Thus, an ectopic pregnancy should be suspected if the hCG titers do not double in 48 hours.

hCG is composed of alpha (α) and beta (β) subunits; the β-hCG radioimmunoassays are most specific for pregnancy. *Note:* Different laboratories use different standards; serial β-hCG titers must be compared using a consistent laboratory standard. Use the following equation as an approximate guideline:

1 ng/mL = 5 mIU/mL 2nd IS (Second International Standard)
= 10 mIU/mL IRP (First International Standard or International Reference Preparation)
= 10 mIU/mL 3rd IS-WHO (Third International Standard, World Health Organization)

In this chapter, hCG levels refer to Second International Standard β-hCG assays. Sensitive urine assays can detect hCG levels as low as 25 mIU/mL. With these sensitive urine pregnancy assays, a negative test excludes 95.5% of ectopic pregnancies.

Ultrasonography

Ultrasonography is a useful diagnostic tool for patients at risk for ectopic pregnancies. The improved detection capability of endovaginal ultrasonography compared with that of transabdominal ultrasonography results in the ability to diagnose ectopic pregnancy earlier. Chapter 7 provides more details concerning the use of ultrasound in the diagnosis of ectopic pregnancy.

Dilatation & Curettage (D&C)

D&C can be used to exclude intrauterine pregnancy when pregnancy is either not desired or unsalvageable. The histologic identification of chorionic villi confirms an intrauterine pregnancy. Identification of a decidual reaction (in 30% of ectopic gestations) or Arias-Stella reaction (a hypersecretory response of the endometrium found in 50% of ectopic gestations) strongly suggests the possibility of an ectopic pregnancy.

Culdocentesis

Culdocentesis is useful in diagnosing hemoperitoneum, which occurs in ruptured as well as unruptured ectopic gestations. A

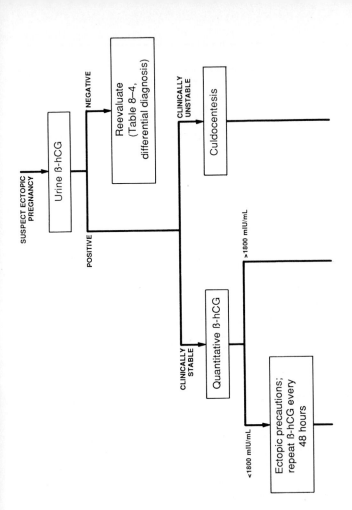

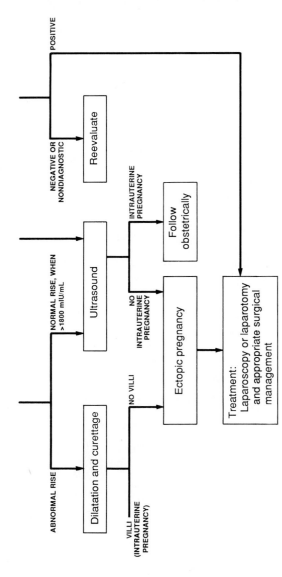

Figure 8-2. Evaluation of possible ectopic pregnancy.

needle is placed transvaginally into the cul-de-sac, and the area is aspirated (Figure 8–3). When no fluid is obtained, the test is **nondiagnostic** and carries no clinical weight. When clear or yellow peritoneal fluid is obtained, the test is **negative** and eliminates the diagnosis of hemoperitoneum. However, this test has a 11–14% false-negative rate as a result of nonhemorrhagic ectopic pregnancies. The test is **positive** when nonclotting blood is obtained during aspiration, as is the case in 80–95% of ectopic pregnancies. False-positive test results can occur with ruptured cysts (commonly, corpus luteum cysts), retrograde menstruation, and incomplete abortions.

Laparoscopy

Laparoscopy provides direct visualization of the pelvic structures; it has both a false-positive and false-negative rate of approximately 4%. It is increasingly being used for both the diagnosis and treatment of ectopic pregnancy.

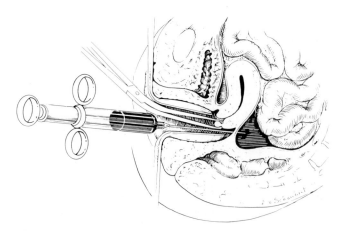

Figure 8–3. Culdocentesis. *(Reproduced, with permission, from Pernoll ML [editor]:* Current Obstetric & Gynecologic Diagnosis & Treatment, *7th ed. Appleton & Lange, 1991.)*

TREATMENT

The treatment of ectopic pregnancy is primarily surgical. The surgical approach used depends on the clinical status of the patient, the location of the pregnancy, and the capabilities of the surgeon, both in terms of training and available instrumentation.

Salpingostomy is the usual treatment for unruptured tubal pregnancies, and for ruptured ectopic gestation without extensive tubal damage (Figure 8–4). This procedure is performed by making an incision over the antimenteric portion of the tubal pregnancy. The products of conception can then be gently removed. Bleeding can be controlled with electro- or laser-coagulation. Hemostasis can also be achieved by injection of vasopressin into, cauterization of, or ligation of the underlying mesenteric vessels. Once hemostasis is achieved, the incision is allowed to heal by secondary intention. If bleeding is not easily controlled, the incision can be closed with fine suture. This procedure can be performed through a laparotomy incision or, in many circumstances, laparoscopically.

A patient presenting in shock with a history consistent with ectopic pregnancy requires immediate surgical exploration. In cases in which future fertility is of no concern or in which tubal rupture has caused extensive damage, salpingectomy (removal of the uterine tube) is the appropriate procedure.

Fimbrial pregnancies that are already in the process of being distally extruded can be gently expressed out of the tube. This approach is not appropriate for most tubal gestations because it can cause dissection of the trophoblastic tissue into the muscularis, resulting in persistent ectopic pregnancies and increased tubal damage.

Interstitial, or cornual, pregnancies can be treated by segmental resection with or without tubal reimplantation. However, because of poor pregnancy rates and the potential for weakened myometrium after tubal reimplantation, salpingectomy may be the appropriate procedure.

Abdominal pregnancy is treated by removing the fetus with ligation of the umbilical cord. The temptation to partially resect the placenta should be resisted because of the significant risk of uncontrollable hemorrhage.

While most ectopic pregnancies are treated surgically, interest in nonsurgical therapies is increasing. On the basis of strict selection criteria, some early ectopic pregnancies in clinically stable patients can be closely observed for resorption or spontaneous abortion. Additionally, methotrexate, a folinic acid antagonist, is being

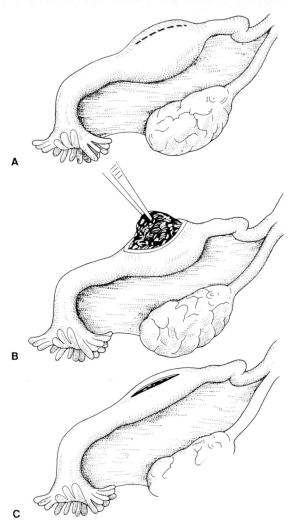

Figure 8–4. Linear salpingostomy. **A:** an incision is made on the antimesenteric aspect of the affected tubal portion. **B:** The conceptus is shelled out. **C:** The incision is not sutured. *(Modified and reproduced, with permission, from Pernoll ML [editor]:* Current Obstetric & Gynecologic Diagnosis & Treatment, *7th ed. Appleton & Lange, 1991.)*

Table 8-5. Prognostic factors for future intrauterine pregnancy.

Factors	Good Prognosis	Poor Prognosis
Fertility history	Normal	Infertility
Pelvic findings	Normal	Abnormal (adhesions)
Affected salpinx	Unruptured	Ruptured
Contralateral salpinx	Normal	Abnormal
Future intrauterine pregnancy rate (%)	80–85	55–65

used systemically to treat early ectopic pregnancies or those that persist after surgical therapy.

PROGNOSIS

The prognosis for a viable pregnancy after an ectopic pregnancy depends on the continuing presence of factors that predisposed the ectopic gestation, the presence or absence of other infertility factors, and the surgical procedure performed (Table 8-5). Overall, after salpingostomy, there is a 55–85% viable pregnancy rate and a 12–15% repeat ectopic rate. For patients with a history of 2 or more ectopic pregnancies that were treated conservatively, there is a 29% rate of repeat ectopic pregnancies among those who conceive.

SUGGESTED READINGS

Bateman BG et al: Vaginal sonography findings and hCG dynamics of early intrauterine and tubal pregnancies. *Obstet Gynecol* 1990;**75**:421.

Leach RE, Ory SJ: Modern management of ectopic pregnancy. *J Reprod Med* 1989;**34**:324.

Nager CW, Murphy AA: Ectopic pregnancy. *Clin Obstet Gynecol* 1991; **34**:403.

Stabile I, Grudzinskas JG: Ectopic pregnancy: A review of incidence, etiology and diagnostic aspects. *Obstet Gynecol Surv* 1990;**45**:335.

9 | Pelvic Pain & Dysmenorrhea

Joseph A. Bachicha, MD

Pelvic pain is a presenting complaint of nearly one-third of all gynecology patients. In fact, it is estimated that at least 50% of menstruating women suffer from **dysmenorrhea,** or painful menstruation, and that these symptoms interfere with normal activities in about 10%. This chapter describes an approach to the most common pain syndromes: **primary** and **secondary dysmenorrhea,** which includes **endometriosis,** and **chronic pelvic pain** (Table 9–1).

PRIMARY DYSMENORRHEA

Primary dysmenorrhea is defined as menstrual pain that is not caused by an organic disease. Research has shown that in women with primary dysmenorrhea the secretory endometrium produces excess prostaglandins F_2 and E_2. Prostaglandins stimulate uterine contractions, sensitize pain nerve endings, and decrease uterine blood flow, leading to relative ischemia.

Symptoms

Classically, primary dysmenorrhea presents 6 months to 2 years after menarche when ovulatory cycles are established. Pain is located in the lower abdomen, is colicky, and may radiate to the low back, labia majora, or inner thighs. Headache, fatigue, nausea, and nervousness may accompany the pain. Symptoms usually begin within a few hours of the onset of menses and last 1–2 days; sometimes, symptoms precede the flow. *Note:* Any woman presenting with pelvic pain must be investigated for organic gynecologic conditions that may contribute to the pain (Table 9–1).

Treatment

When contraception is not needed, prostaglandin synthetase inhibitors are the treatment of choice because they are required for only the duration of symptoms. They have a high rate of effective-

Table 9-1. Causes of pelvic pain.

Gynecologic	Nongynecologic
Primary dysmenorrhea	Urinary tract infection
Secondary dysmenorrhea	Inflammatory bowel disease
Endometriosis	Constipation
Adenomyosis	Appendicitis
Leiomyomata	Trauma
Congenital anomalies	
Hematocolpos	
Imperforate hymen	
Absent vagina	
Cervical abnormalities	
Pelvic inflammatory disease	
Postoperative adhesions	
Intrauterine device	
Ovarian source	
Cyst	
Torsion	
Chronic pelvic pain	
Pregnancy-related causes	
Ectopic pregnancy	
Intrauterine pregnancy	

ness and a low incidence of side effects. Fenamate derivatives (mefenamic acid) and arylpropionic formulations (ibuprofen, naproxen) are appropriate choices. They should be started at the onset of bleeding and continued for the duration of symptoms. Alternatively, for those who cramp before menses begin, these medications can be started at the onset of symptoms. Dosage or formulations may be adjusted to obtain satisfactory relief (Table 9–2).

If these medications are ineffective or if contraception is a consideration, ovulation suppression with oral contraceptives is the treatment of choice. The 90% effectiveness of oral contraceptives in relieving primary dysmenorrhea can be explained in 2 ways. First, they decrease menstrual fluid volume, and second, they prevent the formation of the secretory endometrium, which produces the excess prostaglandins. Sometimes, combined oral contraceptive–prostaglandin synthetase inhibitor therapy is needed for complete relief.

SECONDARY DYSMENORRHEA

Secondary dysmenorrhea is menstrual pain that has an organic cause. This type of dysmenorrhea usually begins after what

Table 9-2. Prostaglandin synthetase inhibitors.

Drug	Strength (mg/tablet)	Dosage
Ibuprofen	200, 400, 600, 800	200–400 mg orally every 4–6 hours
Naproxen sodium	275	550 mg immediately, then 275 mg orally every 6–8 hours
Diflusinal	250, 500	1000 mg immediately, then 500 mg orally twice daily
Fenoprofen calcium	200, 300, 600	200 mg orally every 4–6 hours
Orphenadrine	100	100 mg orally twice daily
Mefenamic acid	250	500 mg immediately, then 250 mg orally every 6 hours
Ketoprofen	25, 50, 75	25–50 mg orally every 6–8 hours

may be years of relatively comfortable menstruation. Endometriosis is the primary cause of secondary dysmenorrhea. Other causes include pelvic inflammatory disease (PID), ovarian cysts, or the presence of an intrauterine device.

Endometriosis

Endometriosis is a condition in which abnormal growth of tissue, histologically resembling endometrial tissue, occurs outside the uterus, including the surfaces of the bowel, bladder, or abdominal wall (Figure 9–1). Rectal pain during defecation, rare in other gynecologic conditions, is common when cul-de-sac involvement with endometriosis is present. Estimates of the prevalence of endometriosis vary, but one study revealed a prevalence of 18% in asymptomatic patients at tubal ligation. The onset of endometriosis is rare in women younger than age 15, but it may occur at any time during the reproductive years.

A. Pathogenesis: The most common suggested causes of endometriosis are as follows: **retrograde menstruation** through the fallopian tubes, **vascular** or **lymphatic dissemination,** or **coelomic metaplasia.** Patients with endometriosis have been noted to have more endometrial tissue in the peritoneal cavity than control patients. Risk factors for the disease include long menstrual periods and lower immunity to endometrial antigens. Endometriosis commonly occurs at the tubal openings, and gravity is a major determi-

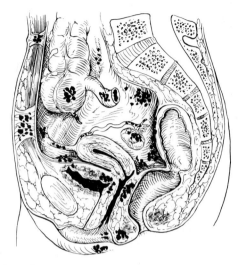

Figure 9–1. Common sites of endometrial implants (endome-triosis). *(Reproduced, with permission, from Way LW [editor]:* Current Surgical Diagnosis & Treatment, *7th ed. Lange, 1985.)*

nant of endometrial implant locations. Mobile organs, such as the fallopian tubes themselves or the squamous epithelium of the va-gina and cervix, are relatively resistant to endometriosis.

A growing body of evidence suggests that women with endo-metriosis have altered immune responses. IgG and IgA antibodies for endometrial and ovarian tissue have been found in the serum, cervix, and peritoneal fluid of women with endometriosis. How-ever, the role of these antibodies in the pathogenesis of the disease is unclear because they are sometimes found when other conditions are present, such as pelvic inflammatory disease.

B. Diagnosis: Endometriosis may be suspected on clinical grounds, but its diagnosis *must* be confirmed by laparoscopy. Re-cent research has identified 3 distinct types: nodular lesions, vesi-cles, and plaque lesions. Nodular lesions, which are usually black but can be any color, may be older and less active than other le-sions. Vesicles, which are 1–3 mm in diameter and are red, yellow, or clear, may indicate endometriosis but may also represent inclu-sion cysts or vascular anomalies. Plaque lesions are white when visible but may be visible only by scanning electron microscopy; these lesions may represent hidden, active disease. Biopsies of suspicious lesions are recommended to confirm the diagnosis. Lysis of adhesions, associated with endometriosis, may be performed at the time of laparoscopy. These adhesions can be a significant factor in causing pelvic pain by causing traction on the bowel.

C. Treatment: The aim of therapy is to relieve symptoms and preserve fertility. In symptomatic women with only a few superficial implants, treatments of choice are electrocauterization or laser vaporization of the implants at the time of diagnostic laparoscopy. With more extensive disease, hormonal therapy may be required as an adjunct to surgical treatment. Asymptomatic patients with mild disease may require no therapy unless infertility is an issue.

Danazol has been the preferred treatment for endometriosis. Danazol is a testosterone derivative that suppresses estrogen production and thus inhibits growth of the estrogen-responsive endometrial implants. Side effects that may occur include weight gain, fluid retention, mood swings, vaginal dryness, and hot flushes. Masculinization is very rare. Recently, GnRH analogues have been used successfully to treat endometriosis and in some centers are now the principal treatment modality.

Endometriosis recurs in 30–40% of patients within 3 years after danazol is discontinued. Similar figures for GnRH agonists are not yet available. Long-term management of patients who do not wish to conceive includes the use of oral contraceptives, antiprostaglandins, or progesterone therapy alone (Table 9–3).

Other Causes

Adenomyosis, the presence of endometrial glands within the uterine wall, and leiomyomas are common causes of secondary dysmenorrhea and are discussed in detail in Chapter 11. Other considerations in the differential diagnosis of secondary dysmenorrhea include congenital anomalies in the younger woman, pelvic inflammatory disease, postoperative adhesions, the presence of an intrauterine device (IUD), and ovarian cysts. Nongynecologic causes of pain, such as constipation, urinary tract infection, or inflammatory bowel disease, should be considered.

A. Congenital Anomalies: Congenital anomalies are rare but should be considered when evaluating the adolescent who presents with dysmenorrhea or chronic pelvic pain. Malformations that obstruct menstrual flow can cause pelvic pain, as well as vaginal pain, abnormal bleeding patterns, or purulent vaginal discharge. When congenital anomalies are a factor in pelvic pain, the physical exam-

Table 9-3. Drug therapy for endometriosis.

Drug	Strength	Dosage
Danazol	200-mg capsule	800 mg daily in divided doses for 6 months
Nafarelin	200 μg/spray	One spray in 1 nostril twice daily for 6 months
Leuprolide	5 mg/mL/syringe	0.5 mg subcutaneously daily for 6 months or 3.75 intramuscularly monthly for 6 months
Depomedroxy progesterone acetate[1]	150 mg	150 mg intramuscularly every 3 months
Medroxyprogesterone acetate	10-mg tablet	10–30 mg orally daily for 90 days

[1] After this medication is discontinued, ovulation may be delayed for more than 1 year.

ination usually reveals a pelvic or vaginal mass and also a bulging imperforate hymen, an absent vagina, or cervical abnormalities. Because various anatomic defects can cause these anomalies, an extensive workup involving pelvic and renal ultrasonography and hysterosalpingography may be required. Appropriate surgery is performed to maximize sexual and reproductive function.

B. Pelvic Inflammatory Disease: Acute and chronic pelvic inflammatory disease is sometimes encountered in pelvic pain states, probably associated with the high levels of prostaglandins released in the inflammatory reaction. Diagnosis and treatment of this condition are covered in Chapter 5. Briefly, history, physical examination, and cultures, especially for gonorrhea and *Chlamydia,* are useful.

C. Postoperative Adhesions: Postoperative adhesions may occur as a result of pelvic surgery, appendicitis, or any abdominal surgery. Generally, adhesions are associated with tenderness to palpation of the adherent structures. Often, however, the association between the presence of adhesions and pelvic pain is not clear. Lysis of adhesions may be useful.

D. Intrauterine Device: It is usually obvious when an IUD is the cause of dysmenorrhea. Pain is probably mediated through production of prostaglandins induced by the IUD itself or by associated subacute endometritis. Removal of the IUD is recommended for intense discomfort, but in the absence of infection, treatment with prostaglandin synthetase inhibitors may be attempted.

E. Ovarian Cysts: On occasion, pelvic pain is caused by intermittent ovarian torsion resulting from a persistent cyst or by rapid distention of a functional ovarian cyst. Such cysts are usually detected during the physical examination and are confirmed using ultrasonography or laparoscopy. Appropriate therapy is administered (see Chapter 10).

CHRONIC PELVIC PAIN

Some women experience chronic or recurring pelvic pain for which no explanation can be found. Because this type of pain has no precise etiology, it is frustrating to both the physician and the patient and is sometimes dismissed as psychologic and untreatable.

Patients with chronic pelvic pain experience constant pain or repeated episodes of pain that interfere with their lives. Often, analgesics are ineffective, the patient's work and sleep suffer, and social supports are strained and diminished. Needs for care and dependence are met (often unconsciously) more easily when the patient is in the role of a sick person.

Management of patients with chronic pelvic pain is challenging and requires considerable skill in assessment. Chronic pelvic pain is a multifactorial condition, and the health care provider is advised to abandon the familiar desire to find a single cause with a single cure or to try multiple medications in a series. A more productive approach is to combine the information obtained from the patient's history, physical examination, and psychological assessment to develop an optimal treatment plan.

The pain history should include a careful chronology of pain development and a description of how the pain spreads to other sites. These details must be matched with an account of the impact of the pain on the patient's work, social, sexual, and home life to understand the meaning of pain in her life. A careful physical examination should also be performed.

Because chronic pelvic pain is a multifactorial condition, the treatment approach needs to be multifaceted. The treatments are not unusual, but when used in combination and with a reassuring, gentle, confident delivery, they are often effective where previous therapies failed. These treatments include high-fiber diets or vegetable laxatives and exercise for constipation, flexion exercises for low back pain, antibiotic therapy for pelvic infections, biofeedback or relaxation training for muscle discomforts, as well as appropriate surgery and analgesics. In addition, psychotherapy is often useful.

Although the cause of chronic pelvic pain may remain a mystery and its symptoms may not be totally eradicated, a thorough search for organic causes, recognition of underlying psychiatric problems, and appropriate medical and surgical therapy can significantly enhance the quality of the patient's life.

SUGGESTED READINGS

Hopkins M et al: Chronic pelvic pain. *Am J Gynecol Health* 1989;**III(1).**
Munsick R: Superficial dyspareunia. In: *Gynecology and Obstetrics.* Sciarra JJ (editor). Harper & Row, 1988.
Steege J: The evaluation and treatment of women with pelvic pain. In: *Gynecology and Obstetrics.* Sciarra JJ (editor). Harper & Row, 1988.

10 | The Pelvic Mass

David Chelmow, MD

Pelvic masses are important at any time during a woman's life because of the symptoms they can cause, including pain, bloating, and fullness, but also because they can represent cancerous or precancerous tumors. The pelvic examination is the primary means of detecting pelvic masses and is an essential part of the routine physical examinations of all women. During gynecologic examinations, health care providers should be attentive to detecting adnexal and pelvic masses, even in the absence of symptoms. However, when symptoms are present, clinicians should be especially careful in diagnosing the source. Ultrasonography, both endovaginal and transabdominal, is useful in visualizing and characterizing a pelvic mass detected during a physical examination. Ultrasonography is also indicated when a woman with symptoms cannot be adequately examined because of pain or body habitus.

This chapter concentrates on the various benign gynecologic sources of a pelvic mass. (Gynecologic oncology is discussed in Chapters 25 through 29.) Differential diagnosis of the pelvic mass can be long and complicated. In addition to ovarian neoplasms, pelvic masses may arise from the uterus, cervix, urinary system, gastrointestinal system, and other anatomic sites (Table 10–1). Because both the differential diagnosis and the significance of a pelvic mass change drastically with each stage of the patient's reproductive life and because the evaluation and treatment vary concomitantly, this chapter is divided accordingly.

PREMENARCHE

Although pelvic masses are uncommon in children, they do occur, and ovarian cancers constitute 1% of malignant tumors in children. An ovarian mass should be considered in evaluating a child that presents with chronic abdominal pain, bloating, or fullness. Because the child's pelvis is small and narrow, adnexal masses

Table 10-1. Nongynecologic sources of pelvic masses.

Stool	Mesenteric cysts
Distended bladder	Colon cancer
Pelvic kidney	Metastatic cancer
Omental cysts	Retroperitoneal mass

tend to rise into the abdomen and are palpable as abdominal masses. It is not uncommon for an adnexal mass to be detected at the time of laparotomy for suspected appendicitis, volvulus, or intussusception.

Examining children presents special difficulties, and extreme gentleness and patience are required during the pelvic examinations. Because the vagina is short and small, rectal examinations are helpful in assessing pelvic masses. In many instances, it may be necessary to perform the examinations under anesthesia. Ultrasonography and computerized tomography (CT) scans also provide much additional information.

The differential diagnosis of a pelvic mass, even in children and young adolescents, is broad. Table 10–2 lists the most common causes of pelvic masses in the premenarchal female. **Functional cysts** are very unusual before menarche; thus, ovarian neoplasm must be carefully considered. The exception is in neonates, in whom it is not uncommon to find functional cysts resulting from stimulation by maternal gonadotropins. These cysts should be observed and should regress spontaneously and rapidly. Similarly, adolescents may have functional cysts around the time of menarche. All types of ovarian tumors have been identified in children, but **germ cell tumors** are the *most* common by far.

Table 10-2. Common causes of pelvic masses in premenarchal females.

Nongynecologic sources (Table 10–1).
Functional cysts (neonates and perimenarchal females).
Benign cysts, especially mature teratomas (dermoid cysts).
Malignant tumors.
   Germ cell tumors (most common types).
   Dysgerminomas, embryonal sinus tumors, immature teratomas.
   Stromal and epithelial tumors.
Adrenal tumors.
   Neuroblastoma.
   Wilms' tumor.

Because functional ovarian tissue is necessary for completion of menarche and because the preservation of fertility is tremendously important, the treatment of an adnexal mass should be as conservative as possible. However, the desire for conservative therapy (cystectomy or oophorectomy only) must be balanced against the risk of disease progression.

REPRODUCTIVE AGE

Functional Cysts

Functional, or physiologic, cysts are the most common source of adnexal masses in women of reproductive age. The 2 main types of functional cysts, **follicle** and **corpus luteum cysts,** are benign and are derived from either an unruptured follicle or the cystic degeneration of a corpus luteum, respectively. Some functional cysts are asymptomatic but are important because they must be differentiated from malignant growths and because they can cause fullness, bloating, and pain. Spontaneous rupture or torsion of the cyst can cause symptoms of an acute abdomen. Hemorrhage from a ruptured corpus luteum cyst can be severe enough to be mistaken for a ruptured ectopic pregnancy and can require surgical intervention.

Because functional cysts have characteristic benign properties and resolve as the menstrual cycle progresses, surgery is usually avoidable. Typically, these cysts are unilateral and are less than 6 cm in diameter, and during pelvic examinations, they feel smooth and cystic. If the results of the physical examination suggest a pelvic mass but are inconclusive, ultrasonography may clarify the type of mass or cyst. On sonograms, the cysts appear unilocular and fluid filled, without evidence of solid components or excrescences. Cysts meeting these criteria should be observed, and the patient should be reexamined after the next menstrual cycle. By definition, both the follicular and corpus luteum cysts resolve by the next cycle, and only cysts that persist more than 3 months may need exploratory surgery and removal. However, pain from these cysts can be severe, and adequate analgesia should be provided during the observation period. An oral contraceptive containing 35 μg of estrogen is often used to suppress the formation of other physiologic cysts that might cause confusion during the observation period. The additional observation time adds negligible risk to the patient with a neoplasm and spares the majority of reproductive-aged women from invasive procedures.

Table 10.3 Benign ovarian neoplasms.

Mature teratoma (dermoid cyst)
Serous and mucinous cystadenoma
Fibroma
Thecoma
Brenner tumor
Endometrioma

Multicystic masses and masses with solid components or excrescences should be considered malignant until proved otherwise. The majority of these masses are benign neoplasms, principally **mature teratomas** and benign and mucinous **cystadenomas.** However, given the dire consequences of not intervening as early as possible when a malignant mass occurs, surgical exploration is necessary. All types of ovarian cancers may occur in this age group (see Chapter 28).

Benign Neoplasms of the Ovary

Table 10–3 lists the most frequently encountered benign ovarian neoplasms. In general, they are unilateral, mobile, smooth, capsuled masses that appear multicystic on ultrasound examination. They are important because they can cause symptoms through torsion, pressure, or rupture and because they must be differentiated from malignant masses (Table 10–4).

Mature teratomas, also known as **dermoid cysts,** occur commonly in women of reproductive age. They contain elements of mature adult structures derived from all 3 embryonic layers: endoderm, mesoderm, and principally ectoderm. These structures include hair, teeth, bone, and skin and, because of the calcified components, are often detectable with routine x-ray studies.

Table 10-4. Characteristics of benign and malignant pelvic masses.

Benign	Malignant
Unilocular	Multilocular
Smooth walled	Irregular
Mobile	Fixed
Unilateral	Bilateral
Cystic	Solid
< 6 cm in diameter	> 6 cm in diameter
	Excrescent

Serous and mucinous cystadenomas are also common. Mucinous tumors are usually multilocular and can become large, whereas serous tumors are usually unilocular. Cystadenomas are commonly encountered during operations to remove their suspected malignant counterparts, the cystadenocarcinomas. Rupture of a mucinous tumor can lead to diffuse intraperitoneal spread, a syndrome called **pseudomyxoma peritonei.**

Fibromas and thecomas are solid benign tumors found in pre- and postmenopausal women. They are rarely associated with ascites and pleural effusions, a situation called **Meigs' syndrome. Brenner tumors** are another type of benign solid tumor often discovered incidentally during surgery. There are rare reports of malignant Brenner tumors.

Endometrioma is another common benign cyst. These cysts are also called "chocolate cysts" because they are filled with a dark fluid and are often associated with endometriosis, pelvic pain, and infertility (see Chapter 9).

These masses should be surgically removed, but because they are benign and usually occur in women of reproductive age, surgery should be as conservative as possible. Dermoids and endometriomas are usually excised. Cystadenomas, fibromas, thecomas, and Brenner tumors are usually treated with unilateral salpingo-oophorectomy. The tumors can be bilateral, so careful examination of the contralateral ovary is important. If the contralateral ovary has a normal appearance, biopsy is usually not performed.

Borderline Tumors

Between the benign cystadenomas and their malignant counterparts, the cystadenocarcinomas, lies an intermediate class of epithelial ovarian tumors—the borderline tumors, or tumors of low malignant potential. These tumors are intermediate in both their histology and prognosis. They can metastasize, but even with advanced spread, survival is appreciable. Overall, 5-year survival is 95%. Recurrence as late as 20 years after the initial diagnosis is possible.

These tumors tend to occur in women of reproductive age, so conservative therapy is desirable and usually possible. Surgery is the treatment of choice. Staging, including preoperative evaluation, exploratory laparotomy, and peritoneal cytology, is performed as for any suspected ovarian cancer (see Chapter 28). The contralateral ovary should be carefully inspected and biopsied if suspicious. Stage IA tumors (confined to a single ovary) can be effectively treated with unilateral salpingo-oophorectomy. For more advanced tumors, surgical resection of all macroscopic disease is the most important therapy. Five-year survival after this therapy alone exceeds 90%. Careful pathologic examination of all specimens is essential to exclude foci of higher grade malignant tumors. Both radiation and chemotherapy are used in more advanced disease.

Other Pelvic Masses

Nonneoplastic conditions must also be considered (Table 10-5) and can often be differentiated from neoplasm without surgery. *Pregnancy must be excluded* when evaluating a pelvic mass. An **ectopic pregnancy** can resemble an adnexal mass and can be life threatening. In the hirsute, obese patient with a history of irregular or absent menses and bilateral enlarged ovaries, the diagnosis of **polycystic ovarian syndrome** should be entertained. Patients with pelvic inflammatory disease may have palpable **tubo-ovarian complexes. Uterine myomas** (see Chapter 11) are common in this age group, and pedunculated and broad ligament myomas can easily be confused with adnexal masses. Ultrasonography is useful in differentiating myomas from other pelvic masses. However, magnetic resonance imaging (MRI) is indicated when ultrasonography cannot differentiate the origin of a pelvic mass.

POSTMENOPAUSE

The risk of ovarian cancer rises sharply after menopause, particularly in women 45–60 years old. Annual pelvic examinations are essential in this age group to detect ovarian cancer early, while it is potentially curable. Functional cysts do not occur in postmenopausal women; thus, *observation is contraindicated* in a postmenopausal woman with a pelvic mass.

Table 10-5. Nonneoplastic pelvic masses in women of reproductive age.

Nongynecologic sources (Table 10-1).
Ectopic pregnancy
Polycystic ovarian syndrome
Tubo-ovarian abscess and hydrosalpinx
Leiomyoma
Paraovarian cyst

Women with ovarian cancer can present with nonspecific symptoms of bloating, abdominal pain, or fullness. Women presenting with such symptoms should undergo thorough pelvic examinations, and ultrasonography should be used if adequate pelvic examinations cannot be performed. The diagnosis of ovarian cancer should be entertained in any postmenopausal woman with unexplained gastrointestinal symptoms.

A normal postmenopausal ovary involutes as the follicles and corpora lutea degenerate; thus, an ovary should *not* be palpable in a postmenopausal woman. For this reason, a palpable ovary in this age group is considered to be cancer until proved otherwise and requires *immediate evaluation*.

SUGGESTED READINGS

Emans SJH, Goldstein DP (editors): Ovarian masses. In: *Pediatric and Adolescent Gynecology.* Little, Brown, 1990.

DiSaia PJ, Creasman WT: The adnexal mass and early ovarian cancer: Borderline malignant epithelial ovarian neoplasms. In: *Clinical Gynecologic Oncology,* 3rd ed. Mosby, 1989.

Droegemueller W et al: Significant signs and symptoms in different age groups: Pelvic and lower abdominal masses, and benign gynecologic lesions: Ovary. In: *Comprehensive Gynecology.* Mosby, 1987.

Soper DE: Pelvic masses. In: *Postreproductive Gynecology.* Shingleton HM (editor). Churchill Livingstone, 1990.

Weingold AB: Pelvic mass. In: *Principles and Practice of Clinical Gynecology,* 2nd ed. Kase NG, Weingold AB, Gershenson DM (editors). Churchill Livingstone, 1990.

Uterine Myomas & Adenomyosis | 11

Abner P. Korn, MD

UTERINE MYOMAS

Uterine myomas, sometimes called fibroids, are very common, occurring in approximately 20% of women over the age of 30. Although they are the most frequent type of solid pelvic tumors that occur in women, they are asymptomatic in many. Clinical presentation ranges from an asymptomatic pelvic mass to abnormal uterine bleeding or to an acute abdomen during pregnancy. A large proportion of gynecologic surgery is performed in therapy of uterine myomas.

Classification

Most myomas begin growth within the myometrium, proliferating from a single smooth muscle cell and incorporating connective tissue elements secondarily. Tumors that remain within myometrium are called **intramural,** whereas tumors that protrude into the endometrial cavity or the peritoneal cavity are called **submucous** or **subserous,** respectively. Occasionally, these tumors occur in the cervix or extend into the broad ligament. A parasitic myoma is one that has developed a blood supply from another intraperitoneal structure, most often the omentum (Figure 11–1).

Pathology

Microscopic examination of myomas reveals long, thin muscle cells with rodlike nuclei configured in a whorled pattern. These tumors may secondarily undergo several of the following types of benign degeneration:

- **Hyalinization:** nuclei vanish often in the central portion of the tumor.

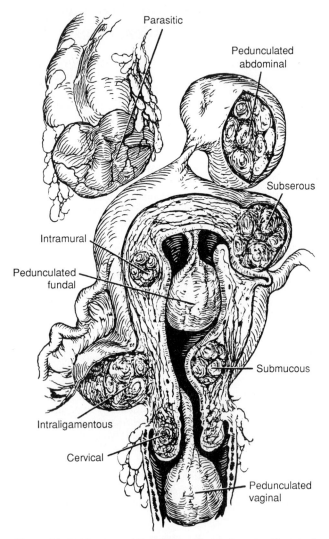

Figure 11-1. Myomas of the uterus. *(Reproduced, with permission, from Benson RC:* Handbook of Obstetrics & Gynecology, *8th ed. Lange, 1983.)*

- **Cystic degeneration:** after hyalinization, the tumor further degenerates until its center is liquid.
- **Calcification:** calcium deposits usually appear in layers and are often visible on radiographs.
- **Necrosis or carneous (red) degeneration:** the tumor outgrows its blood supply and can cause acute abdominal pain (most often seen during pregnancy, possible due to high progesterone levels).

For unknown reasons, myomas occur 3–9 times more frequently among black than white women. Other risk factors for the growth of these tumors are similar to those for endometrial cancer, both conditions stimulated by an estrogen-dominant environment, including nulliparity and obesity. Myomas often differ from normal myometrium in that they contain higher quantities of cytoplasmic estradiol receptors. Growth of myomas may also be stimulated by epidermal growth factor, insulin-like growth factors, and fibroblast growth factor.

The incidence of cancer in what clinically appears to be a myoma is probably less than 1 in 500. Whether sarcoma, a malignant smooth muscle tumor, occurs in preexisting myomas is unknown.

A myoma-like tumor is likely to be a sarcoma if it occurs in a postmenopausal patient or if the tumor exhibits rapid growth. The cut appearance of "raw pork" classically attributed to sarcoma may also be noted in benign lesions. Even the microscopic differentiation of benign and malignant lesions can be difficult. Sarcomas may differ from benign tumors only in the number of mitoses noted, or they may be clearly invasive.

Clinical Findings

A myoma can exhibit various clinical patterns, most commonly perhaps as a pelvic mass or as a pregnant uterus that is unexpectedly larger than the gestational age of the pregnancy. In some cases, it is difficult to differentiate a solitary myoma from an ovarian tumor, although frequently myomas are multiple. Still myomas can be coincident with pathologic adnexa.

Abnormal uterine bleeding is frequently noted either as menorrhagia or metrorrhagia. This bleeding may be due to disruption of the endometrial cavity by a submucous myoma or by dilation of the venous system within the uterus by an intramural myoma.

Pelvic pain resulting from myomas is most often a sensation of pressure in the pelvic area or it is evident as dysmenorrhea (painful menses). Often, urinary frequency results from the enlarged uterus compressing the bladder. Less commonly, severe pelvic pain may occur, generally in the pregnant patient with a myoma undergoing carneous (red) degeneration. Occasionally, a submucous myoma becomes pedunculated and prolapses through the cervical os. Distortion of the endometrial cavity or its blood supply may explain recurrent second-trimester fetal losses in a patient with a uterine myoma. Infertility may result if a submucous myoma interferes with implantation; however, myomas are probably a rare cause of infertility.

Myomas in the pregnant patient may lead to abdominal pain, preterm labor, obstruction of labor, malpresentation, and postpartum hemorrhage. The incidence of degeneration and preterm labor is about 15–20%. Placental abruption occurs in about 50% of patients in whom the myoma lies directly under the placental attachment site. All these complications are more frequent when the myomas are more than 3 cm in diameter.

Laboratory & Radiologic Findings

Anemia frequently occurs in patients with menorrhagia secondary to a uterine myoma. Rarely, polycythemia has been reported and attributed to erythropoietin production by myomas.

The finding of an irregular, enlarged uterus suggests the diagnosis of multiple myomas. Pelvic ultrasonography may provide further evidence as may other imaging techniques, such as magnetic resonance imaging (MRI) and computerized tomography (CT). However, because of their varying appearances, myomas can be confused with ovarian neoplasms. In some cases laparoscopy or laparotomy may be required to reach a firm diagnosis. Hysterosalpingography will reveal an abnormality in many but not all patients with submucous tumors. Hysteroscopy is a more sensitive means of making this diagnosis.

Differential Diagnosis

During pelvic examinations, ovarian tumors, pelvic abscesses, pelvic kidneys, adenomyosis, and uterine sarcomas may resemble myomas in their various forms. The abnormal bleeding caused by submucous myomas can be mistaken for the abnormal bleeding caused by endometrial polyps, hyperplasias, and cancers. *Note:* Patients more than 35 years old who present with abnormal uterine bleeding should undergo endometrial biopsies to exclude an endometrial abnormality.

Treatment

Observation during regular pelvic examinations is sufficient treatment for many patients, generally those without symptoms and with smaller masses. This treatment is especially recommended for patients nearing menopause in whom cessation of tumor growth is anticipated. The choice of treatment for patients with uterine myomas depends on their desire for future pregnancies. The traditional treatment for patients who have completed their childbearing is hysterectomy, which is generally indicated when the tumors are symptomatic, when they have grown rapidly, or when they are large (ie, larger than a pregnant uterus of 12–14 weeks of gestation).

If a hysterectomy is performed, the patient and physician should discuss what will be done if the ovaries are normal. Factors to consider include the risk of future surgery for benign or malignant ovarian tumors versus the need for hormone replacement to avoid menopausal symptoms. In cases in which there has been ovarian disease in the patient or her family, it may be wise to remove the ovaries at an earlier age. However, for the majority of patients, the ovaries should not be removed if they are still functional.

Myomectomy, the removal of the individual tumors with repair of the uterus, is indicated in the symptomatic patient who desires future fertility (Figure 11–2). In some cases of infertility, myomectomy may be indicated. In general, this procedure is used only with patients that desire fertility or that have a strong desire to conserve the uterus. Myomectomy has a high incidence of complications, including transfusion in nearly 20%, febrile morbidity in nearly 30%, and formation of postoperative pelvic adhesions in many patients. These complications are more likely to occur with removal of many large myomas. *The option of observation should always be kept in mind for the asymptomatic patient.* Removing uterine myomas may challenge the operative skills of the gynecologist because of their distortion of pelvic anatomy or because of coexistent disease. Alternatives to myomectomy are (1) electrosurgical resection or laser vaporization of submucous myomas via the hysteroscope, which eliminates abdominal and myometrial incisions, and (2) operative laparoscopic resection of myomas with the removal of the tumors by morcellation or by colpotomy. The potential advantages of these alternatives over an open myomectomy are less incidence of postoperative adhesions, smaller abdominal incisions, and often faster patient recovery.

Medical therapy with continuous administration of gonadotropin-releasing hormone (GnRH) analogues leads to suppression of pituitary gonadotropin release and subsequently to hypoestrogenism. This treatment temporarily reduces the size of myomas (to

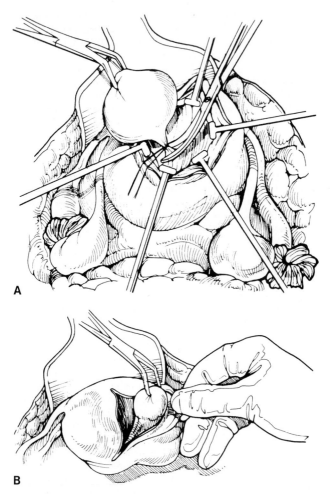

A

B

Figure 11–2. Myomectomy: **A:** The myoma is raised from its defect, and the base is suture ligated. The fibroid is then removed. **B:** Surrounding tissue is palpated to locate other tumors that can be extracted through the same incision. *(Reproduced, with permission, from Stangel JJ [editor]:* Infertility Surgery: A Multimethod Approach to Female Reproductive Surgery, *Appleton & Lange, 1990.)*

about half of pretreatment size). Side effects include hot flushes, and less often, mood changes and vaginal dryness. Long-term use of GnRH analogues usually leads to osteoporosis. When GnRH agonist therapy ceases, the myomas regrow. These factors limit the consideration of use of agonists to perimenopausal patients in whom the tumors are suppressed until natural menopause occurs. The agonist may be useful perioperatively when a smaller uterus may be more easily removed (eg, through the vagina or a smaller abdominal incision). However, use of agonists before myomectomy remains controversial.

Prognosis

Patients who undergo hysterectomy are cured of their disease. After myomectomy, about 20% will require future hysterectomy primarily due to regrowth of tumors. Recurrence is most likely if multiple rather than solitary tumors are removed. Myomectomy to relieve menorrhagia is successful in 80% of patients. Forty percent of infertile patients have conceived after myomectomy, and the rate of spontaneous abortion decreased from 41% to 19% in patients who underwent myomectomy for recurrent miscarriage.

ADENOMYOSIS

Adenomyosis is characterized by growth of endometrial glands into the myometrium. When specimens are carefully analyzed, adenomyosis is found in up to 60% of hysterectomies. The peak incidence occurs in women more than 40 years old. This growth may be present throughout the uterus or only in a focal area. The uterosacral ligaments are also frequent sites of adenomyosis. Adenomyosis is generally responsive to estrogen stimulation and less so to progesterone.

The classic clinical findings are mild uterine enlargement and dysmenorrhea. Menorrhagia may also be present, but frequently, adenomyosis is an incidental finding on pathologic examination of a uterus removed for other reasons. Because the glands involved in adenomyosis are direct invasions of those lining the endometrium, a hysterosalpingogram can sometimes reveal this disorder. Most often, the diagnosis is made on clinical grounds and is treated by hysterectomy. Even if the adenomyosis is localized, excision with uterine preservation can be difficult because of the lack of a clear plane separating the adenomyosis from the surrounding myometrium. Adenomyosis may be considered as a variant of endometriosis that is internal to the uterus instead of external. It is associated with "external" (ovarian or peritoneal) endometriosis in many cases (15–40%).

SUGGESTED READINGS

Buttram VC Jr, Reiter RC: Uterine leiomyomata: Etiology, symptomatology, and management. *Fertil Steril* 1981;**36:**433.

Rice JP, Kay HH, Mahony BS: The clinical significance of uterine leiomyomas in pregnancy. *Am J Obstet Gynecol* 1989;**160:**1212.

Vollenhoven BJ, Lawrence AS, Healy DL: Uterine fibroids: A clinical review. *Br J Obstet Gynecol* 1990;**97:**285.

Dysfunctional Uterine Bleeding | 12

Jeanette S. Brown, MD

Dysfunctional uterine bleeding is abnormal uterine bleeding with no pathologic cause. Most commonly, dysfunctional bleeding is due to anovulation (absence of ovulation). It occurs frequently during puberty, before maturation of ovarian function, and in the perimenopausal period, as ovarian function declines.

Without ovulation and the subsequent production of progesterone from the corpus luteum, the endometrium is stimulated by unopposed estrogen and continues to proliferate. Anovulatory cycles lack the synchronized estrogen and progesterone secretion necessary for stabilization and regular shedding of the endometrium. Therefore, a patient with anovulation often presents with irregular, prolonged bleeding.

EVALUATION & DIAGNOSIS

Evaluation

The evaluation of a patient with abnormal uterine bleeding involves a complete history. The patient's pattern of menstrual bleeding is documented, including cycle length and regularity, duration and amount of flow, midcycle bleeding, and associated symptoms. Normal values for menstruation are as follows:

- Cycle length: 28 days; range 21–35 days.
- Duration: 3–4 days of flow; range of 2–8 days.
- Amount: 35 mL; range 25–80 mL.

Patients with bleeding patterns outside this range are considered to have abnormal bleeding. Descriptive terminology for abnormal bleeding include the following:

- **Menorrhagia:** prolonged, heavy bleeding at regular intervals.
- **Metrorrhagia:** bleeding at irregular intervals.

- **Menometrorrhagia:** prolonged, heavy bleeding at irregular intervals.
- **Polymenorrhea:** frequent regular bleeding at intervals of less than 22 days.

Diagnosis

A complete physical examination is performed, including a Papanicolaou smear and speculum, bimanual, and rectovaginal examinations. Laboratory evaluation routinely includes hematocrit and hemoglobin tests to assess the degree of bleeding and a β-hCG pregnancy test for the sexually active patient. Depending on the clinical situation, additional tests include thyroid function tests, coagulation studies, and liver function tests. After the evaluation is complete, a diagnosis of dysfunctional uterine bleeding can be established if all pathologic causes have been excluded (Table 12–1).

TREATMENT

Young Women

Coagulation studies are indicated for young women (under 35 years old) with severe menorrhagia (Hgb < 10), who require hos-

Table 12–1. Common causes of abnormal uterine bleeding.

Genital sources	Endocrine disorders
Vulva or vaginal carcinoma	Hypothyroidism
Cervical polyp	Hyperthyroidism
Cervical neoplasia	Pituitary adenoma
Endometrial polyp	**Coagulation disorders**
Leiomyoma	von Willebrand's disease
Adenomyosis	Thrombocytopenia
Endometrial hyperplasia	Leukemia
Endometrial carcinoma	**Medications**
Intrauterine pregnancy	Estrogen-containing medications
Threatened abortion	Oral contraceptives
Ectopic pregnancy	Aspirin
Gestational trophoblastic disease	
Gastrointestinal sources	
Hemorrhoids	
Rectal Carcinoma	
Colon Carcinoma	

pital admission or a transfusion. About 20% of these patients have a coagulation defect. A bleeding time, prothrombin time, partial thromboplastic time, and platelet count are sufficient to diagnose a possible coagulation disorder.

Management of dysfunctional uterine bleeding in the adolescent requires stabilization of the endometrium and subsequent cessation of bleeding. The likelihood of endometrial carcinoma is low; therefore, medical management is appropriate. Various treatment regimes have been advocated, including a low-dose combination contraceptive pill (< 35 μg of estrogen). One pill is taken 4 times a day for 5 days. At the completion of the treatment, synchronized withdrawal bleeding occurs. This bleeding is often termed a medical dilatation and curettage (D&C) because a similar result would be accomplished with a surgical D&C.

For the next 6–12 months, the patient is given either oral contraceptives for the sexually active patient or medroxyprogesterone acetate (MPA), 10 mg for 10 days each month. Although treatment does not correct the cause of anovulation, it allows time for maturation of the ovulatory process. When indicated, an iron supplement is also given.

Adult Women

After age 35, endometrial sampling becomes an important part of the evaluation of the patient with abnormal bleeding. The sampling is both diagnostic to rule out endometrial carcinoma and therapeutic to remove the endometrial lining. Patients with risk factors for endometrial carcinoma, such as obesity, chronic anovulation, and nulliparity, should also be considered for endometrial sampling even if they are under 35 years of age.

An office sampling procedure with a suction aspirator is as accurate as a formal D&C (Figure 12–1). A paracervical block is given and dilatation is not required when a cannula 3–4 mm in diameter is used. When an office procedure cannot be performed because of cervical stenosis or patient intolerance, then a D&C in the operating room is indicated (Figures 12–2 and 12–3). Additional indications for a formal D&C are insufficient tissue from the office procedure for diagnosis, atypical hyperplasia, or continued bleeding despite treatment.

Once endometrial pathology has been eliminated, the patient's bleeding pattern can be observed. If the patient has continued abnormal bleeding, MPA, 10 mg for 10–14 days per month is indicated. Alternatively, for women under the age of 45 without contraindications, a low-dose oral contraceptive can be prescribed.

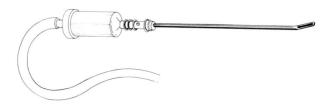

Figure 12-1. Vabra aspirator. *(Reproduced, with permission, from Pernoll ML [editor]:* Current Obstetric & Gynecologic Diagnosis & Treatment, *7th ed. Appleton & Lange, 1991.)*

Acute Excessive Bleeding

For the patient with severe bleeding who continues to bleed despite a D&C, intravenous conjugated estrogens (Premarin), 25 mg every 4–6 hours, can be given until bleeding abates. Treatment is continued with oral conjugated estrogens (2.5 mg 4 times a day for 3–4 weeks). Before the estrogen therapy is complete, MPA, 10 mg for 7–10 days, is added. After withdrawal bleeding occurs, the patient is cycled as outlined above.

For the patient with uncontrollable hemorrhage, who desires future fertility, transcatheter arterial embolization can be considered. It is performed under local anesthesia using pelvic angiography to identify the bleeding site. Selective embolization is achieved with placement of absorbable gelatin sponge (Gelfoam) or wire coil.

Recurrent Dysfunctional Uterine Bleeding

Recurrent abnormal bleeding warrants further investigation or surgery. Hysteroscopy may identify an endometrial polyp or submucosal myoma not previously appreciated. Patients who have completed childbearing are offered a hysterectomy when dysfunctional uterine bleeding is unresponsive to all other treatment modalities.

In those patients with medical contraindications to surgery or who desire to retain their uterus, endometrial ablation under hysteroscopic guidance is indicated. Electrocoagulation or laser ablation is used.

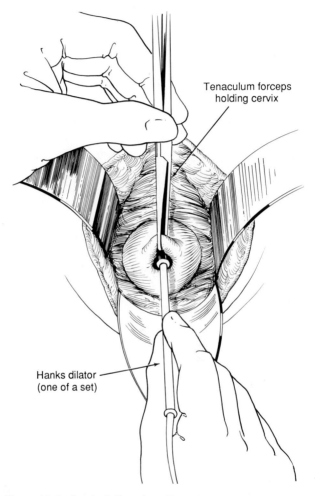

Figure 12-2. Cervical dilatation. *(Reproduced, with permission, from Benson RC:* Handbook of Obstetrics & Gynecology, *8th ed. Lange, 1983.)*

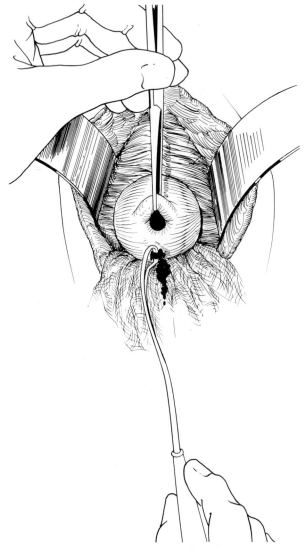

Figure 12-3. Curettage. *(Reproduced, with permission, from Benson RC:* Handbook of Obstetrics & Gynecology, *8th ed. Lange, 1983.)*

SUGGESTED READINGS

Claessens, EA: Acute adolescent menorrhagia. *Am J Obstet Gynecol* 1981;**139**:227.

Dehaeck CM: Transcatheter embolization of pelvic vessels to stop intractable hemorrhage. *Gynecol Oncol* 1986;**24**:9.

Zimmerman C: Dysfunctional uterine bleeding. *Obstet Gynecol Clin North Am* (March) 1988;**15**:107.

13 | Menopause

Jonathan S. Friedes, MD

Colloquially, the term menopause has come to mean the period during and after which a woman ceases to menstruate. More rigorously, this period is known as the climacteric, whereas menopause refers to the actual cessation of menses. The climacteric is due to the loss of functional ovarian follicles. Menopause is perhaps the most apparent result of this process, but the consequent hormonal changes induce various physiologic and psychologic changes. These changes are not pathologic in that they occur in the normal course of life. Nevertheless, they can cause considerable morbidity and mortality, which can be reduced through medical intervention.

The mean age at menopause is 51 years. The age at menopause is not related to age at menarche, reproductive history, nutrition, or socioeconomic status. Smoking does appear to hasten menopause.

MENOPAUSE PHYSIOLOGY

At menarche, the ovaries contain approximately 400,000 follicles. During each ovulatory cycle, approximately 1000 follicles are lost through atresia and ovulation. Even during periods of anovulation, atresia occurs. By a woman's mid-to-late 30s, those follicles remaining are less responsive to gonadatropins, and fewer are capable of maturing into normal ova. Progressively higher levels of follicle-stimulating hormone (FSH) are necessary before ovarian estradiol production exerts its negative feedback on the pituitary. Ovulation and menstruation become less regular and, ultimately, cease.

Although follicular production of estradiol ceases, the stroma of the postmenopausal ovary produces the androgens androstenedione and testosterone. The predominant estrogen in postmenopausal women is estrone, which is produced by the aromatization of ovarian and adrenal androgens in adipose tissue. Ovarian anatomy changes along with ovarian function; postmenopausal ovaries contain a dense stroma, along with rare, scattered follicles.

SECONDARY EFFECTS OF ESTROGEN DEPRIVATION

Urogenital Effects

The tissues of the female reproductive tract, the bladder trigone, and the urethra are all estrogen responsive. In the absence of estrogen, the uterus and cervix become smaller, and the endometrium becomes thin and atrophic. The vaginal and urethral mucosa become atrophic, and vaginal lubrication decreases. Additionally, the tissues surrounding the vagina and urethra lose elasticity.

Osteoporosis

Osteoporosis is the loss of bone density. Most commonly, women suffer asymptomatic compression fractures of vertebral bodies, and the only overt finding is a loss of height. More important clinically are hip fractures, which have a mortality rate of 15% in the first year, as a result of complications.

There are 2 types of osteoporosis. Type I affects mainly trabecular bone, which constitutes most of a vertebral body, and occurs primarily in postmenopausal women. Type II affects cortical and trabecular bone alike and accompanies aging in both sexes. Type II is largely responsible for hip fractures, but the two types have an additive effect.

The exact mechanism of postmenopausal osteoporosis is unknown, but it appears that, in the absence of estrogen, the rate of bone resorption increases, while that of bone formation remains unchanged. Administration of at least 0.625 mg of conjugated estrogens daily halts, and may even reverse, bone loss in both trabecular and cortical bone. Estrogen replacement decreases the incidence of vertebral fractures, but has not been demonstrated to reduce the incidence of hip fractures, probably because these fractures occur later in life and data are not yet available to substantiate such a conclusion.

Various factors affect a woman's risk for osteoporosis. White and Asian women are more prone to developing osteoporosis than black women, and osteoporosis tends to run in families. Factors that increase the risk of osteoporosis include early surgical or spontaneous menopause; smoking; high intake of caffeine, alcohol, or protein; and low intake of vitamin D or calcium. Small, slender women are predisposed toward osteoporosis. Systemic diseases, such as Cushing's syndrome, hyperthyroidism, hyperparathyroidism, and multiple myeloma, can cause or exacerbate osteoporosis, and exogenous glucocorticoids are an important iatrogenic cause.

Vasomotor Effects

The most common symptom of menopause is the hot "flush" or "flash." This symptom is a sudden feeling of warmth in the face, often spreading to the chest and accompanied by nausea, dizziness, palpitations, or diaphoresis. Hot flushes typically last from 30 seconds to 5 minutes. Frequently, they occur at night and are associated with insomnia and night sweats. Most women experience hot flushes for only 2 or 3 years, but during that time, they can be extremely disruptive.

The cause of hot flushes appears to be related to the withdrawal of estrogens. If exogenous estrogens are administered, hot flushes cease. Although hot flushes in normal women are associated with luteinizing hormone (LH) surges, they also occur in women who have undergone hypophysectomy, suggesting that a change in hypothalamic function may account for both phenomena.

Central Nervous System & Behavioral Effects

Postmenopausal women may complain of insomnia, irritability, loss of memory, and inability to concentrate. It is not clear whether these symptoms are a direct effect of estrogen deficiency or a result of disruption of sleep patterns caused by nocturnal hot flushes.

Effects on the Cardiovascular System & Lipid Metabolism

Premenopausal women are less prone to cardiovascular disease than their male counterparts. Within 10 years of menopause, this advantage disappears. A major reason for this difference appears to be the effect of estrogen on lipid metabolism. High levels of low-density-lipoprotein (LDL) cholesterol are associated with an increased risk of cardiovascular disease, whereas high levels of high-density-lipoprotein (HDL) cholesterol exert a protective effect. Estrogens increase HDL cholesterol and lower LDL cholesterol. The synthetic progestogens currently available in the USA have the opposite effect.

Postmenopausal women using unopposed estrogen replacement have a lower incidence of atherosclerotic lesions. They also have lower relative risks of death from myocardial infarctions and, possibly, of suffering a stroke. It is not clear if the effects of progestogens will negate some of these benefits.

EVALUATION

A thorough, directed history and physical examination are needed to evaluate and treat problems of the climacteric. In addition, laboratory studies and tests may be useful, if intelligently selected.

History

The pattern of the patient's menses should be clarified. While it is reasonable to reassure a woman that increasing irregularity in both the timing and the quantity of her menses is normal as she nears menopause, the clinician should remain alert for any history of intramenstrual or postmenopausal bleeding. Other causes for secondary amenorrhea should be considered, especially in women under age 40.

The clinician should then consider each of the systems that can be affected by estrogen deficiency. If symptoms are present, it is important to consider other causes as well.

The clinician should ask about the occurrence of hot flushes, which may be the patient's only symptom. Dyspareunia on initial penetration, vaginal or vulvar pruritus, and dysuria can all be attributed to urogenital atrophy. Bleeding may reflect friable, atrophic vaginal or cervical mucosa, but it is essential to eliminate the diagnosis of cancer. The clinician should inquire about stress urinary incontinence. Symptoms of and risk factors for cardiovascular disease should be sought.

Physical Examination

Gross inspection of the vaginal mucosa provides important clues to the hormonal status of the patient. Well-estrogenized mucosa is moist, rugated, and pink, whereas estrogen-deprived, atrophic mucosa is monotonously regular and may be pale or almost orange-red. It may also appear visibly dry. The atrophic cervix may be almost flush with the superior portion of the vagina, and its os may be stenotic.

A careful bimanual examination is essential. The rectovaginal examination is useful in assessing the smaller pelvic organs of the postmenopausal woman. A thorough breast examination should also be performed.

Laboratory & Other Studies

All women should have a Papanicolaou smear and a baseline mammogram. If there is any question about the menopausal status of the patient, FSH and LH levels should be assessed. An FSH:LH ratio of greater than 1 is virtually diagnostic of menopause.

Women placed on combination estrogen-progestogen therapy do not need an endometrial biopsy unless they have a history of intramenstrual or postmenopausal bleeding. However, if a woman on such therapy has bleeding at any time other than the withdrawal period of a cyclic regimen, an endometrial biopsy should be performed. If a postmenopausal woman has palpable adnexa or if her adnexa cannot be evaluated because of obesity, a pelvic ultrasonogram must be obtained to look for possible ovarian neoplasms.

Routine laboratory evaluation for osteoporosis is not generally indicated. For patients at high risk, dual-photon absorptiometry and quantitative computerized tomography (CT) are the most accurate modalities for assessing trabecular bone loss. Roentgenograms are not very useful because significant (20–50%) bone loss occurs before osteoporotic changes are visible.

THERAPY

Estrogen Replacement Therapies

A. Unopposed Estrogen Therapy: Originally, estrogens were prescribed without progestogens for hormone replacement therapy. However, such therapy clearly increases the patient's risk of endometrial carcinoma. For this reason, unopposed estrogens are prescribed only for women who have had a hysterectomy. The usual dosage is 0.625 mg of oral conjugated estrogens daily.

B. Cyclic Estrogen-Progestogen Therapy: The addition of a progestational agent, such as medroxyprogesterone acetate (MPA), negates the proliferative effect that estrogens have on the endometrium and reduces the incidence of endometrial cancer to at or below the level observed in controls.

A common replacement therapy regimen is 0.625 mg of oral conjugated estrogens daily for the first 25 days of the month with 10 mg of oral MPA added on days 16 through 25. The remaining days of the month the patient takes no hormones, during which time she usually experiences withdrawal bleeding. Some patients may have hot flushes during this withdrawal period, and for these women, 0.625 mg of oral conjugated estrogens daily, with 10 mg MPA on days 1 through 14, is useful. Some women may need more than 0.625 mg of conjugated estrogens to relieve symptoms.

C. Continuous Estrogen-Progestogen Therapy: The occurrence of withdrawal bleeding has been reduced by using a continuous daily regimen of 0.625 mg of conjugated estrogens and 2.5 mg of MPA. Irregular bleeding is common during the first 6 months, but all bleeding usually ceases after that.

D. Transdermal Estrogens: Conjugated estrogens are now available in a transdermal patch. Although this is a convenient method of administration, it has not been shown to have a beneficial effect on lipid metabolism. A progestogen should still be prescribed concomitantly unless the woman has had a hysterectomy.

E. Topical Vaginal Estrogens: Women whose main symptom is urogenital atrophy may benefit from the vaginal application of conjugated estrogens. One gram of conjugated estrogen cream is administered each night for 2 weeks, and 2–3 times a week thereafter. Vaginal estrogen therapy may be instituted along with systemic hormone replacement therapy for more rapid relief of urogenital symptoms and discontinued once systemic therapy has had an effect.

F. Initiation & Duration of Therapy: Because vasomotor symptoms and osteoporotic bone loss are greatest early in the climacteric, hormone replacement therapy is most effective when started as soon as symptoms occur (even if the woman is still menstruating). However, because there is evidence that even delayed hormone replacement may benefit lipid and mineral metabolism, it is a reasonable option even in the older postmenopausal woman. Moreover, preliminary data on cardiovascular effects support continuation of hormone replacement therapy throughout the patient's postmenopausal life.

Adjunctive Therapy

Alternative medications and therapies may increase the effectiveness of hormone replacements or may be substitutes if hormone replacements are refused by the patient or are contraindicated.

A. Calcium Supplements: Calcium supplements alone have little or no effect. Nonetheless, the addition of 1,000 mg of elemental calcium to a patient's diet will enhance the effect of hormone replacement on osteoporosis. Calcium supplements are contraindicated in the presence of nephrolithiasis.

B. Osteoclastic Inhibitors: Calcitonin has been approved for use in the USA by the FDA to treat osteoporosis but is currently available only in injectable form. Etidronate has not yet been approved, but recent studies suggest that it is safe and effective when administered orally in a cyclic manner.

C. Progestogens: Women who have contraindications to estrogen administration (see below) may benefit from MPA alone. Relatively high doses, 20 mg/d, of oral MPA or 150 mg of depot MPA every 3 months alleviate hot flushes and may also retard osteoporosis.

D. Clonidine: A centrally acting α-adrenergic agent, clonidine hydrochloride (0.1 mg orally, 3 times a day) is also effective therapy for hot flushes.

E. Modification of High-Risk Behaviors: Part of managing the effects of estrogen deprivation is the modification of high-risk behaviors. Increasing weight-bearing exercise and decreasing use of tobacco and alcohol may retard osteoporosis. The effects of behavior on cardiovascular disease are well known.

Contraindications, Complications, & Side Effects

A. Neoplasia: Currently, there is no convincing evidence that exogenous estrogens cause breast cancer. However, they can stimulate a preexisting, estrogen-sensitive, malignant condition. For this reason, a history of breast cancer is a *contraindication* to hormone replacement therapy. The evidence concerning adenocarcinoma of the endometrium is much clearer. Even though the carcinogenic effects of estrogen on the endometrium are reversed by addition of a progestogen, endometrial cancer and unexplained vaginal bleeding are contraindications to hormone replacement therapy.

B. Hypertension: Although some women taking high-dose oral contraceptives developed hypertension, no such association has been observed with hormone replacements. For this reason, hypertension is *not* a contraindication to hormone replacement therapy.

C. Thromboembolic Disease: Although women who used high-dose oral contraceptives experienced an increased risk of deep venous thromboses, no such increase has been observed in women who use hormone replacements. Although active thrombophlebitic or thromboembolic disease is a *contraindication* to hormone replacement therapy, a past history of these problems is not a contraindication unless such problems were associated with estrogen use.

D. Hepatobiliary: Estrogens affect hepatic metabolism in diverse ways. Estrogen-induced changes in hepatic excretory function appear to increase a woman's risk of developing cholelithiasis. Because estrogens are metabolized by the liver, exogenous estrogens are *contraindicated* in women with active liver disease. Prior history of liver disease is not a contraindication if normal liver function has returned.

E. Side Effects: The estrogens and progestogens used in hormone replacement therapy may also produce undesirable symptoms. Although the withdrawal bleeding that occurs when a woman is taking replacement hormones is usually accompanied by less dysmenorrhea and fewer premenstrual symptoms than a "natural" period, resumption of menses is unacceptable to some women. In most cases, this problem can be eliminated by switching to a continuous regimen. Estrogens may produce water retention and edema, and in severe cases, a thiazide diuretic may be needed. Breast tenderness may be caused by either estrogens or progestogens and is sometimes alleviated by reducing the estrogen dosage (to a minimum of 0.625 mg/d). Support bras may also help.

Although hormone replacements usually relieve climacteric headaches, some women report increased headaches when using hormone replacements. These symptoms usually respond to non-narcotic analgesics.

PROGNOSIS

The consequences of the menopause, while physiologically normal, can have wide-ranging detrimental effects on the physical well being of the postmenopausal woman. Almost all these effects can be reversed or reduced through hormone replacement therapy, at surprisingly little risk to most patients. Ultimately, each woman must decide whether she feels comfortable with the idea of hormone replacements, but it is the responsibility of the clinician to ensure that the risks and benefits are clearly discussed with all women for whom hormone replacement therapy is not contraindicated.

SUGGESTED READINGS

Dupont WD, Page DL: Menopausal estrogen replacement therapy and breast cancer. *Arch Intern Med* 1991;**151**:67.

Ettinger B: Overview of the efficacy of hormonal replacement therapy. *Am J Obstet Gynecol* 1987;**156**:1298.

Henderson BE et al: Decreased mortality in users of estrogen replacement therapy. *Arch Intern Med* 1991;**151:**75.

Stampfer MJ et al: Postmenopausal estrogen therapy and cardiovascular disease. Ten-year follow-up from the nurses' health study. *N Engl J Med* 1991;**325:**756.

Steinberg KK et al: A meta-analysis of the effect of estrogen replacement therapy on the risk of breast cancer. *JAMA* 1991;**265:**1985.

Disorders of Pelvic Support | 14

Victoria L. Tishman, MD

The pelvic organs are supported and maintained in their inter-abdominal position by the pelvic floor, which consists chiefly of muscle and ligamentous supports. Defects of pelvic support and the resultant clinical problems are seen commonly in general gynecologic practice. The pathogenesis, diagnosis, and management of these disorders are discussed in this chapter.

ANATOMIC CONSIDERATIONS

The levator ani is the chief muscular component of the pelvic floor. This muscle consists of a pair of broad flat muscle groups that extend from the pubis anteriorly to the coccyx posteriorly. Between these paired muscles is the urogenital hiatus, a slit through which the urethra, vagina, and rectum pass as they exit the abdominal cavity (Figure 14–1).

In addition to the muscular support of the pelvic diaphragm, the pelvic organs are also supported by a connective tissue layer, the endopelvic fascia. This layer of connective tissue gives rise to the ligamentous supports of the bladder, uterus, and rectum.

Disorders of pelvic support are the result of defects in the pelvic floor. For example, widening of the urogenital hiatus by childbirth can lead to herniation of the pelvic structures through this opening. Stretching or tearing of the ligamentous supports of the pelvic organs can lead to further herniation or descent of these organs.

DEFINITIONS

Disorders of pelvic support are described according to the organ primarily affected or displaced (Figures 14–2 through 14–4). For example, a **cystocele** is a protrusion of the bladder through

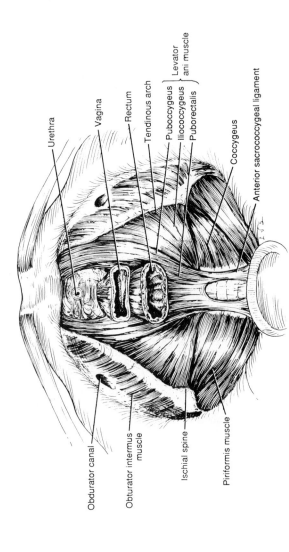

Figure 14-1. Pelvic diaphragm from above. *(Reproduced, with permission, from Pernoll ML [editor]:* Current Obstetric & Gynecologic Diagnosis & Treatment, 7th ed. Appleton & Lange, 1991.)

Urethra

Vagina

Rectum

Tendinous arch

Puboccygeus
lliococcygeus } Levator ani muscle
Puborectalis

Coccygeus

Anterior sacrococcygeal ligament

Obdurator canal

Obturator intermus muscle

Ischial spine

Piriformis muscle

152

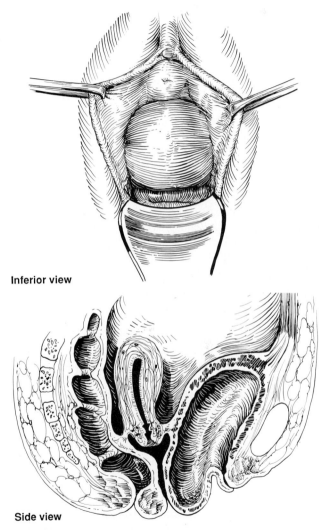

Inferior view

Side view

Figure 14–2. Cystocele. *(Reproduced, with permission, from Pernoll ML [editor]:* Current Obstetric & Gynecologic Diagnosis & Treatment, *7th ed. Appleton & Lange, 1991.)*

the pelvic floor and into the vaginal vault. (This defect is called a **cystourethrocele** if the urethra is also involved.) A **rectocele** is a protrusion of the rectum through the levator hiatus into the vaginal vault. An **enterocele** is a protrusion of the cul-de-sac and its contents into the vagina via the rectovaginal septum.

Uterine prolapse may occur as an isolated defect, but more commonly, it occurs in combination with one or all of the defects described above. Uterine prolapse is defined as descent of the cervix and corpus into the vaginal canal.

Vaginal vault prolapse is defined as descent of the vagina toward or through the introitus. This phrase is generally used to describe the vagina in the absence of a uterus, ie, after hysterectomy.

The severity of the defect is described with respect to the position of the displaced organ (Figure 14–5). A **first degree prolapse** is when the structure protrudes to the lower vagina, a **second degree prolapse** is when the structure protrudes to the introitus, whereas a **third degree prolapse** is when the structure protrudes through the introitus. **Procidentia** is defined as prolapse of the entire uterine corpus through the introitus.

ETIOLOGY

Obstetrical injury is often evoked as an explanation for disorders of pelvic support, since labor and childbirth may tear or stretch the muscular and fibrous supports of the pelvic organs. There is, however, a poor correlation between obstetrical history and the degree of relaxation observed. In fact, a small percentage of women with genital prolapse are nulliparous. To explain this discrepancy, anatomists have postulated a genetic predisposition for pelvic organ prolapse in some women.

In addition to childbirth, other conditions can increase a woman's risk of developing genital prolapse. For instance, the increased weight of the abdominal contents in obese women leads to stretching and weakening of the pelvic floor. Chronic coughing or straining at stool can contribute to this problem. Women who perform physical labor or weight-bearing exercise are also at increased risk. Finally, estrogen deprivation after menopause can lead to urogenital atrophy and loss of some of the connective tissue support.

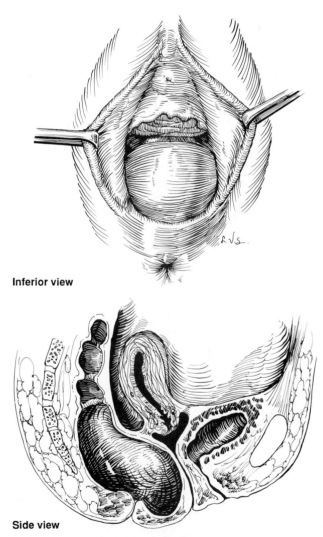

Inferior view

Side view

Figure 14-3. Rectocele. *(Reproduced, with permission, from Pernoll ML [editor]:* Current Obstetric & Gynecologic Diagnosis & Treatment, *7th ed. Appleton & Lange, 1991.)*

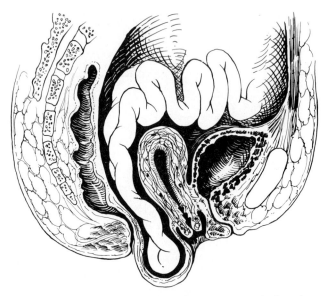

Figure 14–4. Enterocele. *(Reproduced, with permission, from Pernoll ML [editor]:* Current Obstetric & Gynecologic Diagnosis & Treatment, *7th ed. Appleton & Lange, 1991.)*

CLINICAL FINDINGS

Disorders of pelvic support are common, affecting almost one-third of parous women. The majority of these women will remain asymptomatic throughout their lives. Others may develop symptoms after childbirth, with increasing age, or after menopause. Among symptomatic women, their discomfort may not be proportional to the degree of prolapse, although a general correlation does exist.

A common complaint among women with pelvic organ prolapse is a vague feeling of pressure or fullness, especially with sitting or standing for long periods. Patients with more advanced prolapse may complain of a mass protruding up to the introitus. The protruding vaginal mucosa may become ulcerated secondary to chronic trauma, causing irritation and spotting. Some patients

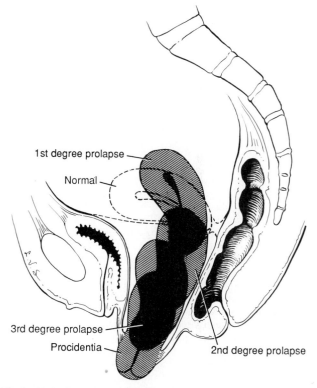

Figure 14–5. Prolapse of the uterus. *(Reproduced, with permission, from Pernoll ML [editor]:* Current Obstetric & Gynecologic Diagnosis & Treatment, *7th ed. Appleton & Lange, 1991.)*

may complain that their prolapse interferes with satisfactory coitus.

Patients may also complain of the secondary effects of pelvic relaxation. A woman with a large cystocele may have urinary dysfunction because of the anatomic displacement of her bladder. She may be unable to completely empty her bladder, thereby predisposing her to chronic urinary tract infection. Conversely, a cystourethrocele can also result in urinary incontinence, a condition discussed in Chapter 15.

A woman with a large rectocele may complain that she is unable to adequately empty her rectum on defecation. She may find that she can defecate more effectively by placing her fingers into her vagina to splint the posterior vaginal wall.

Some patients may be embarrassed by their symptoms and may be hesitant to complain to their physician. Therefore, when evidence of prolapse is noted on physical examination, the clinician should encourage the patient to discuss these types of complaints.

EVALUATION

The patient is best evaluated for disorders of pelvic support during a routine pelvic examination. When the patient is in the dorsalithotomy position, the examiner can look for evidence of prolapse by first inspecting the introitus for any visible prolapse. The patient should be asked to bear down, and the examiner should note any further degree of prolapse with straining.

An examination with the single blade of a vaginal speculum can further define the extent of a cystocele or rectocele. The examiner should detach the posterior blade from the speculum and use it to depress either the posterior or anterior vaginal wall. This technique allows inspection of the opposite vaginal wall.

When a rectocele is present and an enterocele is suspected, the examiner should insert the speculum blade posteriorly to displace the rectocele. The enterocele can then sometimes be seen superior to the rectocele, in the upper third of the posterior vagina. Frequently, the enterocele cannot be identified as a separate defect.

On bimanual examination, a bulging cystocele or rectocele can usually be palpated in the vault. In addition, a rectovaginal examination is an excellent way to detect a rectocele via palpation of a thinned and bulging rectovaginal septum.

Laboratory and radiologic studies are not useful in evaluating the patient with pelvic relaxation. The exception is the patient with urinary dysfunction, who should be evaluated further for problems of incontinence or retention, as described in Chapter 15. In addition, the patient with a chronic cough or chronic constipation may deserve evaluation for the primary problem.

TREATMENT

Medical Treatment

The choice of treatment depends on the patient's symptoms. In general, *no intervention* is indicated for asymptomatic pelvic relaxation.

The musculature of the pelvic floor may be strengthened by Kegel exercises, which are isometric contractions of the pelvic diaphragm. To instruct the patient in Kegel exercises, ask her to tighten the levator ani muscle voluntarily as if to stop the flow of urine. This contraction should be held for several seconds and then repeated several times. The patient should repeat this exercise several times a day. Some improvement should be evident after a few weeks.

In the postmenopausal woman, urogenital atrophy and loss of connective tissue support secondary to estrogen deprivation may improve with topical or systemic estrogen therapy.

Pessaries are useful in treating a woman with a symptomatic uterine prolapse or cystocele. A pessary is a device which, when inserted into the vagina, helps to support the pelvic structures. Many types of pessaries are available; most are made of plastic or of wire with a plastic coating (Figure 14-6). Pessaries currently available are of various shapes (eg, ring, arch, or ball). Most modern pessaries are inflatable or flexible. Each type comes in various sizes. Most pessaries are held in place within the vagina by the symphysis anteriorly and the perineal body posteriorly. As a result, a pessary may not be retained in a patient with little or no perineal support.

In fitting a pessary for a patient, choose a size that is held in place securely but does not place undue pressure on the vaginal walls. After the pessary is in place, the patient should stand and walk to be sure that the pessary does not become displaced. The patient should then return within one week to be reexamined for the fit and placement of her pessary. Thereafter, she should remove the pessary monthly (or return so that her clinician can remove it). The pessary should be washed in warm water and replaced with a lubricating jelly.

Surgical Treatment

When offered the choice between surgical correction and long-term pessary use, many healthy, active women will prefer the long-term benefits of surgical correction, Surgery should only be contemplated in a patient whose symptoms significantly impact on her daily life. Ideally, she should have completed her childbearing.

A high surgical failure rate is expected if a surgeon operates on women who are obese, chronically constipated, or who have a chronic cough. These factors should be addressed before surgery is contemplated.

Preoperatively, the patient should be evaluated for stress urinary incontinence, a condition that can be exacerbated by a surgical repair. If the patient is postmenopausal, estrogen therapy

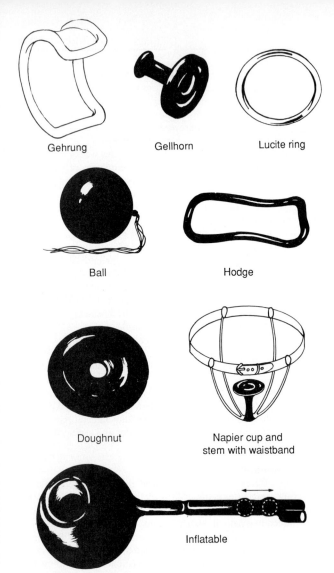

Gehrung

Gellhorn

Lucite ring

Ball

Hodge

Doughnut

Napier cup and
stem with waistband

Inflatable

Figure 14–6. Types of pessaries. *(Reproduced, with permission, from Pernoll ML [editor]:* Current Obstetric & Gynecologic Diagnosis & Treatment, *7th ed. Appleton & Lange, 1991.)*

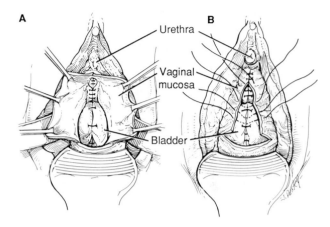

A

B

Urethra

Vaginal mucosa

Bladder

Figure 14-7. Repair of a cystocele. *A:* The vaginal mucosa has been separated from the bladder; the fascia is sutured in the midline for support. *B:* The trimmed vaginal mucosa is reapproximated and closed with suture. *(Reproduced, with permission, from Pernoll ML [editor]:* Current Obstetric & Gynecologic Diagnosis & Treatment, *7th ed. Appleton & Lange, 1991.)*

should be initiated in preparation for surgery. The purpose of this therapy is to reverse atrophic vaginitis, making the surgery technically easier.

A wide variety of surgical approaches are available for correcting defects of pelvic support. In choosing an operative approach, the surgeon must consider the nature of the patient's complaint, the severity of her condition, her age and overall health, and her wishes for future childbearing and coital function. Although a detailed discussion of operative technique is beyond the scope of this text, some of the more common approaches to repairing pelvic relaxation are reviewed below.

The procedure most frequently performed to correct disorders of pelvic support is an anterior and posterior repair, often combined with a vaginal hysterectomy. The anterior and posterior repair is designed to plicate the anterior and posterior vaginal walls. After completion of the vaginal hysterectomy, the anterior repair is begun. The vaginal mucosa is incised along the midline of the anterior wall. The mucosa is then undermined laterally, and the underlying paravesical fascia is drawn together in the midline (Figure 14-7). The vaginal mucosa is then trimmed and closed. A posterior repair is performed in a similar fashion. With a posterior repair, the levator ani muscles are plicated, thereby diminishing the size of the levator hiatus. During the posterior repair, an enterocele hernia sac is sometimes identified and removed.

In a patient whose medical condition would not permit this type of operation, a colpocleisis may be contemplated. This operation, also called a Le Fort procedure, partially closes the vagina and therefore is not appropriate for a patient who wishes to retain coital function.

Posthysterectomy vault prolapse is an uncommon complication of hysterectomy and presents serious problems for the patient. Pessaries are not usually effective because they are rarely retained. Several approaches have been proposed to deal with this problem. Two popular approaches include the sacrospinous suspension (a vaginal procedure in which the vagina is secured to the sacrospinous ligament) and the vaginal vault sacropexy (an abdominal procedure in which the vault is suspended from the sacrum). Vault prolapse after hystectomy is a complex surgical problem and should be managed by an experienced gynecologist.

SUGGESTED READINGS

Kegel A: Progressive resistance exercise in the functional restoration of the perineal muscles. *Am J Obstet Gynecol* 1948;**56**:238.

Mattingly RF, Thompson JD: *TeLinde's Operative Gynecology,* 6th ed. Lippincott, 1985.

Nichols DH, Randall CL: *Vaginal Surgery,* 3rd ed. Williams & Wilkins, 1989.

Gynecologic Urology | 15

Shari Thomas, MD

URINARY INCONTINENCE

Urinary incontinence is the uncontrolled loss of urine significant enough to cause social or hygienic consequences. The exact incidence of urinary incontinence is difficult to establish because many women believe that this problem is a normal consequence of childbirth or aging and are reluctant to seek medical attention. It is estimated that 12 million Americans experience incontinence and that up to one-third of all postmenopausal women suffer from this problem.

Urinary incontinence is clinically classified into 3 major types: (1) stress incontinence, (2) detrusor instability, and (3) overflow incontinence. **Stress incontinence** is the involuntary loss of urine during activities that increase intra-abdominal pressure. It denotes a symptom or clinical finding and occurs in 50–70% of patients. **Genuine stress urinary incontinence (GSUI)** refers to the urodynamic diagnosis of stress incontinence. It is the involuntary loss of urine occurring when, in the absence of a detrusor contraction, the intravesical pressure exceeds the maximum urethral pressure. **Detrusor instability** (urge incontinence, bladder instability) is the occurrence of spontaneous bladder contractions, usually during filling or other provocations, and is present in up to 30% of patients. Both forms of incontinence may occur together in up to 20% of patients. **Overflow incontinence** is loss of urine by overdistention of the bladder (hypotonic bladder condition) and occurs in 5–10% of patients. Other causes of urinary incontinence are infections, medications, vesicovaginal or vesicoureteral fistulas, and urethral diverticulum.

History & Physical Examination

In evaluating a patient with urinary incontinence, the most important information is derived from the history and physical examination, and this information must be correlated with specific diagnostic tests.

A. History: Information is gathered during a personal interview and supplemented by a detailed questionnaire completed by the patient before the office visit. The history includes a review of the precipitating factors that cause incontinence, for example, stress from coughing, laughing, sneezing, exercise, or sexual activity. If the symptom of **urge,** defined as a strong or sudden desire to void, is present, than the precipitating factors are noted and reproduced during urodynamic studies or cystometry. Common precipitating factors of urge incontinence are coughing, bouncing on heels in a standing position, changing from a supine to an upright position, or listening to the sound of running water. The duration of incontinence, volume of urine lost, and factors that relieve or worsen the process are also important to document.

Common symptoms associated with urinary incontinence are frequency, dysuria, nocturia, enuresis, postvoid fullness, dribbling, and hematuria. **Frequency** is defined as voiding more than 7 times a day and occurs with many types of incontinence. **Dysuria,** or pain on micturition, occurs in patients who have urinary tract infections and urethritis. **Hematuria,** the presence of gross or microscopic blood in the urine, occurs in patients with urinary tract infections, nephrolithiasis, and cancer. **Nocturia** is defined as waking up more than once to void during sleep, whereas nocturnal **enuresis** is defined as the loss of urine during sleep.

The patient should maintain a 24-hour urolog or voiding diary on a typical day (Table 15–1). The 24-hour urolog allows the clinician to assess the voiding pattern of the patient. During this interval, the patient records the time and volume of urine voided. The patient should be provided with a half-hat measurement device that fits in the toilet to easily record the amount voided. The patient also records episodes of urge, urge incontinence, and stress incontinence. Episodes of nocturia and frequency are readily discerned from this simple urolog. The urolog also indicates if the patient consumes large quantities of fluid or voids large volumes of urine, suggesting diabetes mellitus, diabetes insipidus, or psychogenic polydipsia.

The history of gynecologic surgery is important, especially previous bladder suspension surgery, hysterectomy, other pelvic surgery, or back surgery. Incontinent patients with previous bladder surgery are at high risk of subsequent surgical failure. These patients should be evaluated extensively by multichannel urodynamics before any treatment is initiated. Medical problems, includ-

Table 15-1. Example of a 24-hour urolog.

Time	Amount Voided (mL)	Activity	Leak Volume (approximate)	Urge Present	Amount of Intake (mL)

ing diabetes mellitus, multiple sclerosis, or Parkinson's disease, may also cause detrusor instability or a hypotonic bladder condition. Several medications affect the physiology of micturition and precipitate incontinence (Table 15-2).

B. Physical Examination: The physical examination includes a detailed pelvic examination, demonstration of urinary incontinence, and a Q-tip test (Figure 15-1). During the physical examination, urethral displacement is ideally quantitated using the Q-tip test, which is an objective description of the anatomic urethral defect. This test is performed by inserting a lubricated sterile cotton-tipped applicator into the urethra with the patient in the supine position. The applicator is pushed through the urethra past the urethrovesical junction, then pulled back until resistance is felt, at which point the cotton portion is resting directly adjacent to the urethrovesical junction. The angle of the applicator is measured against the horizontal plane parallel to the floor while the patient is at rest and during the Valsalva maneuver. A change of greater than 30° during straining indicates an anatomic defect. If the patient also has genuine stress urinary incontinence, the incontinence can be corrected surgically.

The pelvic examination also reveals any pelvic descent, specifically identifying a cystocele, rectocele, or enterocele and the degree of uterine prolapse (see Chapter 14). The patient is examined supine and either sitting or standing, if the supine position fails to demonstrate pelvic relaxation or incontinence. The patient is asked

Table 15-2. Medications that cause incontinence and their mechanisms of action.

Type of Medication	Symptoms	Urodynamic Findings
Anticholinergic β_2-adrenergic Antihistamine Tricyclic antidepressant	Urinary retention, overflow incontinence, hesitancy	Increased postvoid residual, increased bladder capacity
Cholinergic β-adrenergic blocking agent Prostaglandin $F_{2\alpha}$ Diuretic	Bladder spasm, urgency, urge, incontinence, nocturia, frequency, hesitancy, incomplete emptying	Increased bladder compliance, detrusor instability, decreased bladder capacity
α_1-Adrenergic blocking agent Lithium	Stress incontinence, nocturia, dribbling, frequency	Decreased urethral closure pressure
α_1-Adrenergic	Urinary retention, hesitancy, dysuria	Increased urethral closure pressure

to strain or cough in these positions in an attempt to demonstrate the leakage of urine.

Neurologic, cardiovascular, respiratory, and abdominal examinations are also performed. The neurologic examination includes an evaluation of the cranial nerves, cerebellar function, and motor and sensory tests, with emphasis on extremity weakness, sensation, and reflexes. The anal sphincter and perineal sensations may be selectively denervated from previous obstetric trauma and are specifically tested. On cardiovascular and pulmonary examination, pulmonary edema reveals the cause of nocturia and frequency if these are presenting complaints.

Diagnostic Tests

A. Urine Culture and Postvoid Residual: Before any invasive tests are performed, a urine culture is obtained on 2 separate occasions, and the postvoid residual is measured by catheterizing the bladder immediately after the patient micturates. Normally, the residual volume is less than 50 mL or 20% of the voided volume. Overflow incontinence, a hypotonic bladder condition, or incomplete emptying of the bladder, can be readily diagnosed by this simple method.

B. Cystometry: The cystometrogram measures the pressure-volume relationship during artificial filling of the bladder. Either carbon dioxide (CO_2) or water is used to fill the bladder, and the catheters used range from a simple Foley catheter, a double-lumen catheter, or a balloon pressure catheter to an electronic microtip catheter. Multichannel or complex cystometry consists of simultaneously measuring the intra-abdominal pressure, obtained from a pressure-sensitive catheter placed in the vagina or rectum, and the pressure in the bladder. The "true detrusor pressure" is then calculated by subtracting the intra-abdominal pressure from the intravesical pressure.

The 4 parameters evaluated during cystometry are **sensation, capacity, compliance,** and **contractility.** The first sensation of volume is perceived when the bladder is filled to 100–200 mL. A strong desire to void usually occurs at a volume of 300–400 mL, and maximum capacity occurs at 400–600 mL. The normal resting tone, or compliance, of the bladder, measured as pressure in cm H_2O, is approximately 2–14 cm H_2O. Any detrusor contraction that occurs during filling, spontaneously or with provocation, is diagnostic of detrusor instability.

The maximum bladder compliance is reached at volumes above the maximum capacity of 600 mL. Above this threshold, the bladder compliance diminishes, and the intravesical pressure may exceed 15 cm H_2O, initiating a bladder contraction, or the intravesical pressure may exceed the resting urethral pressure. This is the mechanism by which a hypotonic bladder induces overflow urinary incontinence. Once the bladder is relieved to a pressure below the maximum compliance, the leakage temporarily ceases.

It is essential to perform cystometry on all patients with urinary incontinence before surgical correction. Failure to identify detrusor instability results in an incorrect diagnosis and an incorrect treatment in 30% of patients.

C. Urethral Pressure Profile: Measurement of the intraluminal urethral pressure is the most widely accepted assessment of urethral function. This pressure can be recorded at rest, on coughing or straining, or during voiding. A transducer is pulled from the bladder neck down through the entire length of the urethra at a constant speed, and the pressure is measured continuously along the urethra. On a graph, these measurements form a bell-shaped curve, referred to as the urethral pressure profile (Figure 15–2).

The most important information derived from the urethral pressure profile is the maximum urethral closure pressure, which is the maximum urethral pressure minus the bladder pressure. The functional length of the urethra is measured by pulling the transducer at the same speed through the urethra as the chart speed is

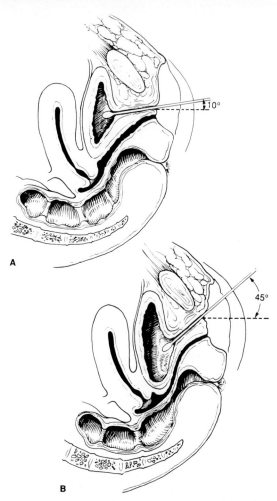

Figure 15–1. The Q-tip test for assessing urethral and bladder support. **A:** The resting angle of the cotton-tipped applicator is normal. **B:** With straining, the urethrovesical junction descends, causing the end of the stick to rotate upward. *(Reproduced, with permission, from Pernoll ML [editor]:* Current Obstetric & Gynecologic Diagnosis & Treatment, *7th ed. Appleton & Lange, 1991.)*

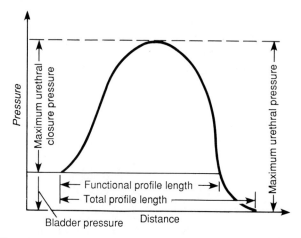

Figure 15–2. The urethral pressure profile (at rest) is recorded by measuring the intraluminal pressure along the length of the urethra. The pressure in the urethra is greater than the pressure in the bladder, resulting in urethral closure pressure. *(Reproduced, with permission, from Pernoll ML [editor]:* Current Obstetric & Gynecologic Diagnosis & Treatment, *7th ed. Appleton & Lange, 1991.)*

recording. The normal functional length ranges from 2.5 to 4.0 cm, but in patients with urinary incontinence, this length may be reduced. For a patient to maintain urinary continence, the urethral pressure must exceed the bladder pressure both at rest and during stress or during any increase in intra-abdominal pressure. The stress urethral pressure profile is obtained by continuously pulling the catheter through the urethra while asking the patient to cough intermittently. Equalization of pressure in the bladder and the urethra during stress in the absence of a detrusor contraction constitutes the urodynamic diagnosis of genuine stress urinary incontinence (Figure 15–3).

D. Radiographic Studies: Helpful radiographic techniques include plain films, intravenous pyelography, and cystourethrography. Plain films of the abdomen and pelvis can reveal congenital abnormalities, sacral agenesis, or spina bifida occulta, which result in neurologic incontinence problems. Intravenous pyelography,

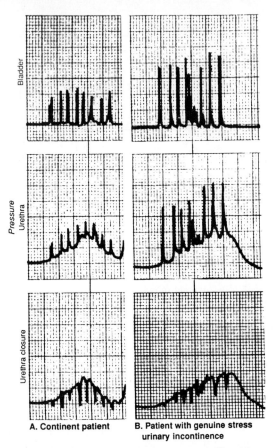

Figure 15-3. Stress urethral pressure profile. The patient coughs repeatedly as the pressure is recorded. **A:** Continent patient. Although the spikes recorded during coughing are higher in the bladder than in the urethra, a positive urethral closure pressure is maintained along the length of the urethra. No urinary loss was observed. **B:** Patient with genuine stress urinary incontinence. Pressure recorded during coughing is transmitted poorly to the urethra. By electronic subtraction, a zero or negative urethral closure pressure is demonstrated along the entire length of the urethra. Urinary loss was observed. *(Reproduced, with permission, from Pernoll ML [editor]: Current Obstetric & Gynecologic Diagnosis & Treatment, 7th ed. Appleton & Lange, 1991.)*

which outlines the urinary tract, is essential for patients who present with hematuria, gross or microscopic, or who have recurrent urinary tract infections. Cystourethrography involves first injecting radiopaque dye into the bladder and then x-raying the bladder and urethra with the patient in the lateral position, both voiding and straining. The cystogram obtained during voiding can identify the patient with urine refluxing retrograde into the ureters.

Bead-chain lateral cystourethrography is performed with the patient in the lateral position with a beaded chain in the urethra and bladder to observe the descent of the urethrovesical junction, both at rest and during straining; however, the Q-tip test is a simpler and less expensive way to achieve the same result.

Treatment

A. Nonsurgical Treatment:

1. Estrogen–Estrogen therapy benefits postmenopausal women with urinary incontinence caused by stress or detrusor instability. Vaginal estrogen therapy increases the blood flow, improves the tissue maturation index of the vaginal mucosa, and increases the maximum urethral closure pressure. Estrogen is instilled intravaginally, 1–2 g at bedtime, for 6 weeks and continued indefinitely on a maintenance dose of 2–3 times a week.

2. Kegel exercises–Kegel exercises often help patients with genuine stress incontinence because they strengthen the levator ani muscle and the pelvic floor diaphragm. The Kegel exercises are first performed by having the patient stop voiding in midstream by tightening the pelvic floor muscles. These exercises are then performed when not voiding and during stress.

3. Medications–Detrusor instability is best treated using anticholinergic agents or tricyclic antidepressants. Anticholinergic medications and tricyclic antidepressants increase bladder compliance and capacity and inhibit bladder contractility. The tricyclics also have α-adrenergic activity, which increases urethral closure pressure. Estrogen replacement therapy and Kegel exercises may also help patients with detrusor instability.

Patients with combined genuine stress incontinence and detrusor instability should be treated first with medications before surgery is attempted. Both genuine stress urinary incontinence and detrusor instability may be alleviated with surgery; however, surgery can also worsen detrusor instability.

4. Behavior modification–Biofeedback therapy, bladder retraining exercises, and coping strategies are advocated for patients with detrusor instability, genuine stress urinary incontinence, or both. Biofeedback therapy involves measuring the physiologic function of the pelvic floor muscles with electromyogram (EMG) electrodes, whose signals are amplified and simultaneously displayed to provide the patient immediate information on whether to tighten pelvic floor muscles or relax other muscles (eg, abdominal or gluteal muscles). During bladder retraining, the patient is placed on a voiding schedule, and the voiding interval is gradually increased to increase bladder capacity. Coping strategies include general relaxation and pelvic muscle exercises learned during biofeedback training.

The neurogenic bladder, commonly resulting from multiple sclerosis or diabetes, is best treated with bladder retraining exercises (having the patient void every 2–3 hours), biofeedback therapy, and cholinergic medication. Only on rare occasions should intermittent self-catheterization be required.

B. Surgical Treatment: Surgery for patients with genuine stress urinary incontinence includes 4 types of procedures: (1) abdominal procedures, using retropubic urethropexy (Burch or Marshall-Marchetti-Krantz procedure), (2) vaginal procedures, using a needle suspension technique (Pereyra, Raz, or Stamey procedure), (3) sling procedures or suburethral patches, and (4) artificial urethral sphincters. Anterior colporrhaphy, combined with Kelly plication, is not recommended for treating genuine stress urinary incontinence because more successful results are obtained using the first 3 procedures listed above. The principle of surgical repair in all these procedures is to elevate the urethrovesical junction to an intra-abdominal position. These techniques restore continence by allowing compression of the urethra by the pubovaginal portion of the levator ani muscle while the intra-abdominal pressure is increased. Vaginal needle suspension surgery may be preferred when a cystocele or rectocele also needs to be corrected.

Artificial urethral sphincters are used for patients who present with genuine stress urinary incontinence and no urethral descent. These patients usually have a low-pressure urethral sphincter.

URINARY TRACT INFECTIONS

Urinary tract infections are one of the most common types of infections in women. The incidence of bacteriuria in women is 5%, and up to 20% of all women will suffer from a urinary tract infection during their life span. Urinary tract infections are manifested as infections involving the bladder, referred to as **cystitis;** the kidney, **pyelonephritis;** or the urethra, **urethritis.** The most common organisms that infect the urinary tract are bacteria; infections with yeasts, viruses, or intracellular microorganisms, such as *Chlamydia, Mycoplasma,* or *Ureaplasma,* occur less often.

Cystitis is a superficial mucosal infection of the bladder wall. The clinical manifestations of cystitis are dysuria, frequency, urgency, nocturia, suprapubic discomfort, and low back pain. Less frequent symptoms are hematuria, a low-grade fever, or incontinence.

Pyelonephritis, an infection of the renal parenchyma, is sometimes characterized by high fever, chills, flank pain, nausea, and vomiting. Symptoms of cystitis may also be present during pyelonephritis and sometimes are the only symptoms in a patient with pyelonephritis. For this reason, recurrent cystitis should alert the clinician to a possible underlying (occult) pyelonephritis.

Pathogenesis

Urinary tract infections primarily ascend transurethrally from the periurethral area into the bladder or upper urinary tracts. Organisms can also be directly implanted during catheterization or instrumentation of the urinary tract.

Microbiology & Diagnosis

Escherichia coli is identified in 60–80% of symptomatic nonpregnant women with urinary tract infections. The organisms identified in the remaining patients are *Staphylococcus,* group D streptococci, *Klebsiella,* enterobacteriaceae, *Proteus,* and *Pseudomonas.*

Traditionally, the diagnosis of a urinary tract infection was based on finding "significant bacteriuria," which was defined as greater than or equal to 10^5 colony-forming units (CFU) per milliliter of urine. Unfortunately, only 50% of patients with symptoms of frequency and dysuria show significant bacteriuria. The remaining symptomatic patients have urine cultures that contain colony concentrations of 10^2–10^5 CFU/mL, nonpathogenic organisms, or organisms that require special culture media (eg, *Chlamydia, Mycoplasma,* or herpes (simplex), or no identifiable organism may be found.

The microscopic examination of a sediment of centrifuged urine should contain less than 5 epithelial cells per high-power field (HPF); otherwise, the specimen is considered to be a contaminated collection. The presence of bacteria, pyuria, or hematuria is noted. Bacteriuria is defined as the presence of any organisms per HPF on an *uncentrifuged* urine specimen, whereas pyuria is defined as the presence of more then 10 white blood cells per HPF. This value correlates with a bacterial count of greater than or equal to 10^5 CFU/mL. The presence of bacteriuria or pyuria on microscopic examination correlates with urine cultures containing more than 10^5 CFU/mL. Hematuria, the presence of red blood cells, is evident on microscopic examination in 40–60% of patients with acute cystitis. However, hematuria may also indicate other conditions (eg, cancer, collagen vascular disease, kidney stones, or trauma).

The biochemical tests developed to rapidly detect pyuria and bacteriuria are the Greiss test, which detects the presence of nitrites, and the leukocyte esterase test, which identifies by-products of white blood cells.

Interpreting culture results and urinalyses depends on the type of urine collection technique used. The 3 types of collection techniques are (1) clean-catch midstream (CCMS), (2) urethral catheterization, and (3) suprapubic bladder aspiration (Table 15–3). The CCMS method, although convenient, commonly yields erroneous results from contamination caused by bacteria in the periurethral area. For this reason, the patient needs precise instructions in obtaining a sample. Bacterial densities greater than 10^2 CFU/mL obtained by the CCMS method from a symptomatic patient are diagnostic of infection; however, in an asymptomatic patient, bacterial

Table 15-3. Culture diagnosis of urinary tract infection (UTI).

Collection Method	CFU/mL[1] Required to Diagnose UTI	
	Symptomatic Patient	**Asymptomatic Patient**
Clean-catch midstream	> 100	> 10,000
Straight catherization	> 100	> 100
Suprapubic bladder aspiration	Any organism	Any organism

[1] CFU/mL, colony-forming units per milliliter of urine.

Table 15-4. Antibiotic dosage regimens for treating urinary tract infections.

	Single-Dose Therapy	7- to 10-Day Therapy	Suppressive Therapy (3-6 months)
Trimethoprim and sulfamethoxazole	2 DS tablets[1]	1 DS tablet[1] every 12 hours	1 tablet[1] at bedtime
Trimethoprim	400 mg	100 mg every 12 hours	50 mg at bedtime
Nitrofurantoin	200 mg	100 mg every 6 hours	50 mg at bedtime
Amoxicillin	3 g	500 mg every 8 hours	No
Sulfisoxazole	2 g	500 mg every 6 hours	No
Cephalexin or cephradine	No	500 mg every 6 hours	No

[1]One DS (double strength) tablet contains 160 mg of trimethoprim and 800 mg of sulfamethoxazole; 1 tablet contains 80 mg of trimethoprim and 400 mg of sulfamethoxazole.

densities of greater than or equal to 10^4 CFU/mL are necessary to definitely diagnose an infection.

Treatment

Antibiotics used to treat symptomatic patients with urinary tract infections are listed in Table 15-4. Antibiotics are administered in 3 ways. The single-dose regimen is ideal for patients with superficial uroepithelial infection. The 7- to 10-day regimen is appropriate for high-risk patients, as defined in Table 15-5. Note

Table 15-5 Indication of high-risk patients.

Uncertain diagnosis
Recurrent urinary tract infection
Persistent symptoms (>7 days)
History of catheterization, instrumentation, or surgery
Pregnancy
History of medical diseases
History of gross hematuria
Age (<12 years or >65 years)
History of pyelonephritis

Table 15-6 Sources of persistent urinary tract infections.

Renal calculi
Fistula, vesicovaginal or vesicourethral
Ureteral duplication
Infected communicating cysts
Papillary necrosis
Foreign bodies
Ureteral reflux
Chronic pyelonephritis

that a culture analysis should be performed for high-risk patients before antibiotic therapy is begun. The 7- to 10-day regimen is also indicated when single-dose therapy fails to eradicate a superficial infection.

Long-term (4- to 6-week) therapy is indicated for patients with **persistent infection,** that is, when the same organism persists after the 7- to 10-day treatment is complete. In these cases, the patient often has subclinical pyelonephritis, which requires a detailed urologic evaluation, including cystography and intravenous pyelography. The most common source of bacterial persistence is infected renal calculi, in which bacteria persist within the interstices of the stone and are protected from the action of antimicrobial agents. Other sources of persistent infections are listed in Table 15-6.

Patients with **relapsing infection** and no demonstrable urologic abnormality may have low resistance to infections. Suppressive therapy for this problem is required (Table 15-4). **Reinfection** is defined as the occurrence of a different organism on culture analysis after the patient has undergone a 7- to 10-day course of therapy. This patient should be treated for 7–10 days with antibiotics sensitive to the causative organism.

Finally, a diagnosis of **chlamydial urethritis** or **urethral syndrome** should be considered in patients who present with symptoms of cystitis but no organism is identified by routine culture techniques.

SUGGESTED READINGS

Ostergard DR (editor): *Gynecologic Urology and Urodynamics: Theory and Practice,* 3rd ed. Williams & Wilkins, 1991.

Norton PA (editor): Urinary incontinence. *Clin Obstet Gynecol* 1990;
33:298.

Thiede HA (editor): Urogynecology. *Obstet Gynecol Clin North Am*
1989;**16**:709.

Wied GL (editor): Update on urogynecology: A symposium. *J Reprod Med*
1990;**35**:751.

16 | Benign Vulvar Lesions

Mitchell D. Creinin, MD

Vulvar itching and irritation are common gynecologic complaints, especially in postmenopausal women. Examinations of these patients often reveal white or red plaques. These lesions, when biopsied, are frequently found to be vulvar dystrophies. The term dystrophy was introduced by Jeffcoate in 1961 and is more appropriate than the nonspecific term **leukoplakia,** which simply means a white patch. Another lesion that is not a dystrophy but that produces similar symptoms is **Paget's disease.**

CATEGORIES

Vulvar dystrophies are classified into 3 categories (Table 16–1) according to the International Society for the Study of Vulvar Disease (ISSVD):

(1) **Squamous cell hyperplasia** (formerly **hyperplastic dystrophy**).
(2) **Lichen sclerosus.**
(3) Other dermatoses.

This classification is based on both gross and histopathologic changes. Lichen sclerosus with associated squamous cell hyperplasia was formerly known as a *mixed dystrophy;* currently, when these lesions are found simultaneously, both are reported. Lichen sclerosus is associated with coincident squamous cell hyperplasia in approximately 16% of cases.

When **vulvar intraepithelial neoplasia** (VIN, or cellular atypia) is also present, it is reported along with the corresponding vulvar dystrophy. The likelihood that a chronic vulvar dystrophy will develop a superimposed carcinoma is 1–5%. *The patient most likely to develop cancer is one with atypia at initial presentation.*

CLINICAL FINDINGS

Squamous Cell Hyperplasia

Squamous cell hyperplasias present as thick, pruritic, white or red plaques in a focal or multifocal pattern but are generally not

Table 16-1. Diagnosis and treatment of the most common vulvar dystrophies.

	Symptom	Histology	Treatment
Squamous cell hyperplasia (formerly hyperplastic dystrophy)	Pruritis Thick white plaques Focal or multifocal pattern	Hyperkeratosis Confluent rete ridges (acanthosis) Subcutaneous infiltration of chronic inflammatory cells	Fluorinated corticosteroid cream Crotamiton cream Burow's solution (6–8 weeks)
Lichen sclerosus	Pruritis Thin, atrophic skin (cigarette-paper) Diffuse Decreased labial size Scarring, fissures, contractures	Thin epithelium Presence or absence of hyperkeratosis Inflammation and collagenization of subcutaneous tissue	Testosterone cream Progesterone cream Continuous treatment
Vulvar intraepithelial neoplasia (VIN)	Pruritis, pain Slightly elevated white plaques or red nodules Multifocal	Background of squamous cell hyperplasia or, rarely, lichen sclerosus Abnormal maturation of epithelial cells Increased nuclear: cytoplasmic ratio	Laser ablation Wide local excision

diffuse. The areas of the vulva most commonly involved are the clitoris, labia minora, intralabial folds, and labia majora. These lesions reflect underlying histopathologic changes that are possibly caused by chronic irritation.

Lichen Sclerosus

Lichen sclerosus is a diffuse process causing a white color change with a parchment-like ("cigarette-paper") appearance. As with squamous cell hyperplasia, the presenting symptom is usually intense pruritis. The skin is thin and atrophic with decreased labial size, and scarring, fissures, or contractures are often present. The clitoral prepuce can be edematous with phimosis occurring late in the course of the disease. Similar lesions are found 18% of the time in extragenital areas, such as under the breast and on the lower abdomen. Lichen sclerosus can occur at any age from childhood to after menopause, but is usually asymptomatic until menopause.

Vulvar Intraepithelial Neoplasia

VIN has a variable clinical presentation. Lesions are usually multifocal, slightly elevated, white plaques, but they may also appear as red nodules or pigmented areas on the vulva. If red nodules are present, the lesion can easily be mistaken for Paget's disease or carcinoma in situ. Most lesions are posterior, predominantly in the perineal area. Itching is the primary symptom in 50% of patients; other common complaints are bumps, bleeding, and pain. These lesions are dysplastic when the vulvar epithelium shows abnormal maturation (nucleated cells at the epithelial surface) with increased mitotic activity and an increased nuclear:cytoplasmic ratio. The degree of dysplasia is defined in a manner similar to that for cervical dysplasia:

- VIN I: involvement of the lower third of the epithelium.
- VIN II: involvement including the middle third of the epithelium.
- VIN III: involvement including the upper third of the epithelium.

Because many features of these different lesions are similar, definitive diagnosis cannot be made based on clinical appearance alone; therefore, a biopsy of the lesions(s) is mandatory for histopathologic assessment.

DIAGNOSIS

The cornerstone of diagnosis of vulvar disease is **punch biopsy.** This biopsy is most easily accomplished using a Keyes punch to remove a core of specimen to the level of the dermis. Local anesthesia is essential and adequately produced with local infiltration of 1% lidocaine hydrochloride with epinephrine. If the vulvar lesions are not uniform in appearance, it is important to biopsy the different areas to ensure an accurate diagnosis.

Colposcopic examination of the vulva can be helpful in visualizing lesions that are otherwise unappreciable. However, colposcopy alone cannot discriminate between benign and dysplastic lesions; biopsy is necessary for diagnosis. Moreover, cytologic examination of the vulva with a Papanicolaou smear is not helpful because vulvar skin is thick and thus does not shed easily. However, if the lesion is ulcerated, cytologic examination may be helpful.

TREATMENT

Therapy can be instituted only after proper diagnosis of the lesion by biopsy. The patient is usually most concerned about relief of itching for which local care is as important as medical treatment to help relieve symptoms. Irritants should be avoided, including strong soaps and detergents, and the patient should use only cotton underwear. The physician needs to search for and treat other possible irritants, including **vulvovaginitis, urinary tract infections,** and **stress urinary incontinence** (see Chapter 15). For excoriated, weeping lesions, wet dressings with 5% aluminum acetate (Burow's) solution applied 3–4 times daily for 30 minutes can be used to relieve the pruritis.

Squamous Cell Hyperplasia

Squamous cell hyperplasia without atypia is treated with a fluorinated corticosteroid cream, eg, 0.05% fluocinonide, to relieve itching. The preparation should be applied as a cream rather than an ointment, because, although the cream is less potent, the ointment is moisture retentive and thus can worsen the symptoms. The cream is applied twice daily for 1–2 months until the itching is resolved and is often mixed with an anti-itching agent, such as crotamiton cream (Eurax). A combination of 7 parts corticosteroid cream and 3 parts Eurax is effective. Prolonged use of fluorinated corticosteroids can cause vulvar atrophy and contractures; thus, once symptoms have subsided, the cream is tapered off or changed to 0.1% hydrocortisone cream for maintenance therapy.

Lichen Sclerosus

Lichen sclerosus is treated with 2% topical testosterone propionate in petrolatum twice daily until the lesion is totally eradicated, which can take up to 4–6 months. Maintenance therapy with use of the ointment twice a week must be maintained indefinitely or the lichen sclerosus will return. The reported cure rate with this regimen is 93%. Side effects, mainly clitoromegaly and increased pubic hair growth, are due to the androgenic properties of testosterone. In the presence of severe pruritis, low-dose hydrocortisone cream or crotamiton cream can be added to help relieve symptoms. If cure is not accomplished or side effects become undesirable, 1–2% progesterone cream in petrolatum can be used.

When lichen sclerosus is present with foci of squamous cell hyperplasia (mixed dystrophy), therapy consists of a combination of fluorinated steroid cream and testosterone cream.

Vulvar Intraepithelial Neoplasia

When VIN is present, treatment is aimed at eradication of all lesions and possible coincident condylomata; this is usually accomplished by carbon dioxide laser ablation. This procedure requires general or regional anesthesia, and the lesions are ablated to a depth of 3–4 mm and heal in 2–3 weeks. However, lesions recur in about 30% of patients. An alternative treatment is wide local excision, which has the same cure rate as the more extensive skinning vulvectomy. Medical treatment using 5-fluorouracil cream can be considered. This option is 75% effective but can cause severe vulvar pain and edema and therefore may not be well tolerated.

PAGET'S DISEASE

Although not a vulvar dystrophy, Paget's disease is another potentially malignant lesion that causes vulvar irritation or itching; however, this lesion is usually erythematous and eczematoid, similar to diabetic vulvitis. This disease most commonly presents as a breast lesion that reflects underlying ductal malignancy. On the vulva, the lesion is usually intraepithelial but is highly associated with invasive cancer at other sites, most frequently involving the breast, cervix, or gastrointestinal tract.

Paget's disease of the vulva occurs most often in postmenopausal women, especially white women, with an average age of 65 years. Most patients complain primarily of itching, although some have only color change or discomfort. Lesions are erythematous with a white speckled appearance resulting from islands of hyperkeratosis. They are rarely well circumscribed and tend to spread, often in an occult manner. Grossly, the lesions are easily confused with cutaneous candidiasis or severe dermatitis.

Treatment involves both removal of the lesions as well as an extensive search for coincident cancers. Multiple biopsies are necessary to exclude invasive disease. Paget's disease is usually eradicated by wide local excision with a 2-cm margin. Clear margins are often difficult to obtain because this multifocal lesion usually extends beyond its clinically apparent borders. Even if the resection margins are free of disease, local recurrence remains a risk. Progression of benign Paget's disease to invasive adenocarcinoma of the vulva has been reported in less than 10% of patients. Patients that have been treated for Paget's disease need yearly follow-up with examinations for breast and gastrointestinal cancer and Papanicolaou smears of the cervix and vagina. When invasive cancer is present with Paget's disease, radical vulvectomy with lymphadenectomy is indicated.

SUGGESTED READINGS

American College of Obstetricians and Gynecologists. Vulvar dystrophies. *ACOG Technical Bulletin* No. 139, January 1990.

Friedrich EG: *Vulvar Disease.* 2nd ed. Saunders, 1983.

Kaufman RH, Friedrich EG, Gardner HL: *Benign Diseases of the Vagina and Vulva.* Year Book, 1989.

17 | Breast Disease

Deborah G. Grady, MD, MPH

Management of breast diseases is an integral part of the medical practice of gynecologists who are the primary health care providers for most women. Breast symptoms are among the most common complaints of women, and breast cancer is the most common cancer of women. The incidence of breast cancer is more than twice as high as the incidence of all pelvic cancers combined. The American Cancer Society estimates that in 1991 there will be 180,000 new cancers and 54,000 deaths from breast cancer among women in the USA. During their lifetime about one in every 10 women in the USA will develop breast cancer. Women fear breast cancer and dread the thought of mastectomy, radiation therapy, and chemotherapy. Gynecologists can address these fears by counseling their patients about breast health and by providing screening and diagnostic care.

Gynecologists should provide breast cancer screening programs for all patients, including physical examination, mammography, and instruction for performing breast self-examination. Gynecologists must be able to evaluate breast symptoms and abnormal physical findings, especially breast lumps, pain, inflammation, and nipple discharge. Finally, gynecologists should be able to treat most benign breast conditions.

SCREENING FOR BREAST CANCER

Screening for breast cancer includes an adequate history of factors that are associated with increased risk for breast cancer, a thorough physical examination of the breasts, instruction in breast self-examination, and in older women, mammography. The American Cancer Society recommends the following schedule of examinations:

(1) Breast self-examination monthly in women more than 20 years old.

(2) Breast examination by a health professional at least every 3 years between ages 20–40, then yearly thereafter.

(3) Baseline mammography at age 35–40, then every 1–2 years between ages 40 and 50, then yearly thereafter.

Risk Factors

Risk factors for breast cancer include increasing age, personal history of breast cancer, family history of breast cancer (especially in a mother or sister), nulliparity, first pregnancy after age 30, early age at menarche, late age at menopause, and history of breast biopsy for benign breast disease.

Physical Examination

Physical examination of the breasts includes inspection and palpation of the breasts and the axillary and supraclavicular lymph nodes (Figures 17–1 through 17–3). The breasts are inspected for symmetry or skin abnormalities with the patient sitting at rest, then with her hands behind her head and the chest thrust forward. Each breast is palpated while the woman is lying on her back with the ipsilateral hand behind her head. The second, third, and fourth fingers of the examining hand are used to gently and methodically examine each quadrant of the breast, the areolar area, and the axilla. The nipple is gently compressed in an attempt to elicit nipple discharge. Palpation is then repeated with the patient in the relaxed sitting position and then sitting and leaning slightly forward.

Self-Examination

All women should be taught how to perform breast self-examinations and counseled to examine their breasts monthly 2–3 days after menstrual bleeding stops (at this point in the menstrual cycle the breasts are least likely to be engorged or tender) or on the first day of the calendar month in postmenopausal women. Breast self-examination follows the procedures outlined for examinations by health care providers, except that women use a mirror to inspect their breasts and palpate each breast with the contralateral hand.

Mammography

Mammography is a radiologic evaluation of the breast that involves using a low, safe dose of radiation. Screening selected women with mammography has clearly been shown to reduce mortality from breast cancer and to identify cancers at an earlier stage.

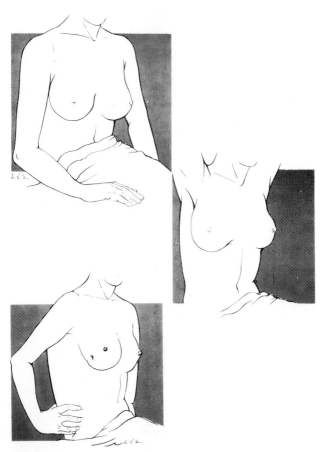

Figure 17-1. Inspection of breasts. Observe breasts with patient sitting, arms at sides and overhead, for presence of asymmetry and nipple or skin retraction. These signs may be accentuated by having the patient raise her arms overhead. Skin retraction or dimpling may be demonstrated by having the patient press her hand on her hip in order to contract the pectoralis muscles. *(Reproduced, with permission, from Wilson JL: Chapter 20 in* Current Surgical Diagnosis & Treatment, *4th ed. Dunphy JE, Way LW [editors]. Lange, 1979.)*

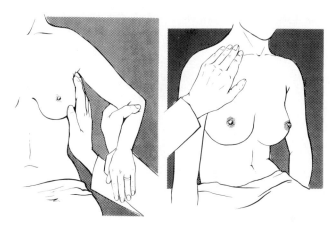

Figure 17-2. Palpation of axillary and supraclavicular regions for enlarged lymph nodes. *(Reproduced, with permission, from Giuliano AE: Chapter 20 in* Current Surgical Diagnosis & Treatment, *6th ed. Way LW [editor]. Lange, 1983.)*

EVALUATION & MANAGEMENT OF BREAST DISEASE

Breast cancer is clearly the most serious form of breast disease. The physician's primary task when evaluating a breast complaint is to differentiate breast cancer from benign disease. Unfortunately, benign breast diseases often mimic the symptoms of breast cancer. The most common breast complaints are lumps, pain, inflammation, and nipple discharge.

Breast Lumps

Lumps in the breast are of great concern because most patients with breast cancer present with a breast mass. Lumps in the breast are common: breast lumps are detected in as many as 50% of premenopausal women during physical examination. Most of these lumps are benign, but they are frightening to women who fear cancer. Evaluation of breast lumps often requires breast imaging and tissue sampling to establish the diagnosis.

A. Definitions: The following definitions are offered to avoid confusion. **Breast lumps** are masses in the breast noted on

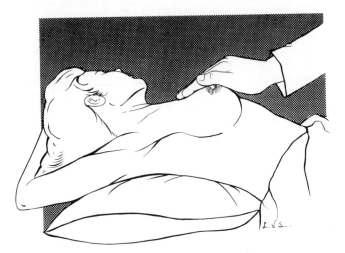

Figure 17-3. Palpation of breasts. Palpation is performed with the patient supine and arm abducted. *(Reproduced, with permission, from Giuliano AE: Chapter 18 in* Current Surgical Diagnosis & Treatment, *9th ed. Way LW [editor]. Appleton & Lange, 1991.)*

physical examination that may be either benign or malignant. **Benign breast disease** includes any breast abnomality that is not malignant. The results of the history, physical examination, and breast imaging may support the diagnosis of benign disease, but strictly speaking, benign breast disease is a pathologic definition applied only after the tissue of the mass has been analyzed. Benign breast disease encompasses a heterogeneous group of lesions, including **fibrocystic disease, fibroadenoma,** and other uncommon conditions, such as **mastitis, lipoma, traumatic fat necrosis,** and **galactocele.** Biopsies reveal that 90–95% of all benign breast diseases are fibrocystic disease or fibroadenomas. Fibrocystic disease is an ill-defined group of pathologic breast lesions, including cysts, fibrosis, adenosis, duct ectasia, hyperplasia, and papilloma. The incidence of fibrocystic disease increases with age, peaks at about the time of menopause, then declines. Clinically, women with fibrocystic disease often note multiple, tender nodules that are symmetrically distributed in both breasts. The nodules typically increase in size and become more painful just before the menses. Fibroadenoma is another pathologic type of benign breast tumor. It is common in women less than 30 years old and becomes less common with increasing age. Clinically, fibroadenoma usually occurs as a solitary, firm, rubbery, smooth, mobile mass. Findings from the history, physical examination, or mammogram may suggest fibrocystic disease or fibroadenoma, but strictly speaking, these terms should be used only to describe pathologic findings.

B. Medical History: The medical history includes a review of risk factors for breast cancer. If a breast lump has been noted by the patient, she should be asked how long it has been present, if it waxes and wanes with the menstrual cycle, and if there is associated cyclic tenderness. Nodules that have been present and unchanged for more than a year are usually benign, and cyclic symptoms suggest benign disease.

C. Clinical Findings: Physical findings are categorized as benign or suspicious for breast cancer. On inspection, skin dimpling or asymmetry of the breasts is suspicious. On palpation, benign breast lumps are usually multiple, bilateral, generally uniform, and symmetrically distributed nodules that may be slightly tender. The sensation on palpation is similar to the feeling of sliding the fingers over a mass of peas or grapes. The consistency of the nodules may vary from firm and rubbery to fluctuant. Clinicians often label these physical findings as "fibrocystic disease," but without histologic analysis, this condition should be called "lumpy breasts."

A breast lump is described as a dominant mass when the breasts are diffusely nodular, but one mass is clearly larger, firmer, or asymmetric in location. Dominant masses suggest breast cancer and require further evaluation. A lump is described as solitary if no other masses are present. In young women (< 25 years old), solitary masses that are smooth, rubbery, and mobile are most commonly found to be fibroadenomas on biopsy, but if a biopsy is not performed, such masses should simply be called solitary breast masses.

Thickening is another descriptive term used to refer to an area of the breast that feels more dense than the rest of the tissue. This thickening most commonly occurs in the upper outer quadrant of the breasts, an area where there is more glandular tissue than in the other quadrants. Benign thickening is roughly symmetric.

Dominant or solitary masses that are small and soft or cystic, smooth, and movable are more likely to be benign. Conversely, masses that are hard, irregular, or fixed and thickening that is asymmetric suggest breast cancer. Unfortunately, the clinical characteristics of these suspicious physical findings are not accurate enough to distinguish benign from malignant disease and further diagnostic tests are necessary.

D. Diagnostic Procedures: Routine laboratory tests are *not* helpful in evaluating breast nodules. Useful diagnostic procedures include mammography, fine needle aspiration, and excisional biopsy.

1. Diagnostic mammograms–Abnormalities detected on mammograms are classified as benign, malignant, or suspicious based on established radiologic characteristics. In the evaluation of a breast mass that is suspicious on physical examination, mammography has a sensitivity of about 80% and a specificity of approximately 90%. Overall, about 20% of women with palpable cancer will have a mammogram that shows no evidence of cancer, and this rate may be as high as 30% in younger women with dense breasts. *Note:* Mammography should be performed in the evaluation of a suspicious breast mass, but a negative mammogram alone should not delay or replace tissue sampling. The mammogram is useful to confirm the clinical suspicion of a malignant mass and especially to identify other nonpalpable suspicious areas in both breasts that might also require evaluation.

2. Fine needle aspiration (FNA)–FNA is a method for obtaining fluid and cellular material from a palpable mass. The results of cytologic examination of aspirated material are reported as malignant, benign, or suspicious. When the aspiration is performed and the findings are interpreted by an experienced cytologist, the false-negative rate (material from the FNA is described as benign when the lesion is malignant) is about 2%, a level that compares favorably with frozen section (0.7–4.9%) and excisional biopsy (1.4%). The false-positive rate (material from the FNA is described as malignant when the lesion is benign) approaches zero. When aspiration, fixing, or cytologic evaluations are performed by inexperienced personnel, the accuracy of the tests may fall to unacceptable levels. A clinician considering the use of FNA of breast lumps should check with the cytologist who evaluates the aspirates to ensure that the false-positive and false-negative rates are acceptable.

3. Excisional biopsy–In clinical settings in which expert FNA and cytologic evaluations are not available, the evaluation of a suspicious mass requires excisional biopsy. Biopsy is usually performed as an outpatient surgical procedure under local anesthesia with an attempt made to remove the entire mass. Subsequent risk status and treatment are based on pathologic diagnosis.

E. Evaluation Procedures & Treatment: If lumps discovered in the breast (Figure 17–1) are multiple, bilateral, diffuse, and symmetric, no further diagnostic testing is necessary. However, examination in women with lumpy breasts may be difficult, and it is important to emphasize the need for monthly breast self-examinations, regular physical examinations by a physician, and mammograms, as appropriate for age and risk factors. Women who present with a solitary or dominant mass or an area of asymmetric thickening should undergo mammography to evaluate the mass, to identify additional suspicious areas, and to provide a baseline for future examinations. Regardless of the results of the mammogram, material from the mass should be removed by FNA. If a solid mass is aspirated, cellular material should be sent for cytologic evaluation. If fluid is obtained at aspiration and the mass disappears, no further evaluation is necessary. However, if fluid is obtained by aspiration, but a palpable mass remains, the needle may have missed a solid mass next to a cyst or entered both a solid mass and a cyst, diluting the aspirated cells with benign cyst fluid. In this situation, the remaining solid mass should be immediately re-aspirated and material from the solid mass sent for cytologic analysis.

If the cytologic results indicate a malignant mass, the patient should be referred for surgical evaluation. If the cytologic results indicate a suspicious mass, an excisional biopsy should be performed. If the cytologic analysis indicates that the mass is benign and the mammogram does not show any features of cancer, the patient should undergo careful clinical evaluation at 6-month intervals. However, if the findings of the physical examination strongly suggest breast cancer or if the mammogram shows features suspicious for cancer, excisional biopsy should be performed even if results of the cytologic analysis indicate that the mass is benign.

Women with benign breast lumps generally need no treatment. Women with breast cancer should be referred to a breast surgeon for evaluation and removal of the cancer. Subsequent treatment is planned in conjunction with an oncologist.

Breast Pain

Breast pain and tenderness are probably the most common breast complaints. Benign breast disease is often associated with mild cyclic breast pain and breast swelling that intensifies in the premenstrual period, then improves during menses. This type of pain usually does not require treatment. Abstinence from methyl-xanthines (coffee, tea, chocolate, colas, theophylline) may decrease pain and lumpiness, but many women do not benefit from dietary change. Moderate salt restriction, mild diuretics, and nonsteroidal anti-inflammatory drugs are often effective. Patients who do not respond to these simple modalities may benefit from treatment with danazol, but this medication has substantial side effects that may not be reversible and should be administered only by a physician familiar with its use.

Most cancers are not painful unless the nodule is large, but a complaint of localized, constant breast pain should raise the suspicion of breast cancer regardless of the size of the mass. A painful solitary or dominant mass should be evaluated as outlined above.

Breast Inflammation

Mastitis is a general, somewhat vague, term used to describe any inflammation of the breast such as cellulitis or abscess. The differential diagnosis and treatment of cellulitis of the breast is the same as for other areas of the skin. Peripheral breast abscesses (located more than 1 cm from the areola) are usually caused by *Staphylococcus aureus* or streptococcal organisms; respond to incision, drainage, and antibiotic therapy; and generally do not recur or become chronic. Subareolar abscesses (within 1 cm of the areola) may be similar to a peripheral abscess, but half or more are a complication of mammary duct ectasia (thickening and inflammation of the large mammary ducts). In subareolar abscesses, the organisms isolated are more likely to be anaerobes than skin flora, and the abscess is likely to recur after simple incision and drainage, particularly if anaerobic organisms are not treated. Fistulas may form, and eventually, cure may require excision of the large duct system to remove duct ectasia.

Nipple Discharge

Nipple discharge is common. Many women can elicit nipple discharge by manipulation or squeezing of the nipple. Discharge that occurs only with manipulation is invariably benign. Discharge that is bilateral and from multiple mammary ducts is usually clear or milky. This type of discharge is generally physiologic, even when spontaneous, but occasionally is due to hyperprolactinemia (from a prolactin-secreting pituitary tumor or hypothyroidism). Women with spontaneous bilateral milky discharge (galactorrhea) should have serum prolactin and thyroid-stimulating hormone measured (see Chapter 21, Amenorrhea). Any discharge associated with a subareolar mass should be evaluated as described above for breast lumps. Nipple discharge that is spontaneous, unilateral, and from a single lactiferous duct may be due to breast cancer but is more often due to duct ectasia or papilloma. Patients with such discharge should be evaluated with mammography, and especially if the discharge is persistent and serous or bloody, surgical exploration of the large mammary ducts is indicated.

SUGGESTED READINGS

Hindle, WH: *Breast Disease for Gynecologists.* Appleton & Lange, 1990.

Health and Public Policy Committee, American College of Physicians: The use of diagnostic tests for screening and evaluating breast lesions. *Ann Intern Med* 1985;**103**:143.

Hermansen C et al: Diagnostic reliability of combined physical examination, mammography, and fine-needle puncture ("triple test") in breast tumors: A prospective study. *Cancer* 1987;**60**:1866.

Love SM et al: Benign breast disorders. In: *Breast Diseases.* Harris JR et al (editors). Lippincott, 1987.

18 | Women & Acquired Immunodeficiency Syndrome

Bonnie J. Dattel, MD

Thousands of women have been diagnosed as having acquired immunodeficiency syndrome (AIDS) since the disease was first recognized. However, women account for only 10% of the total reported AIDS cases. As discussed below, this small percentage may not accurately represent women who are infected with human immunodeficiency virus (HIV), the causative agent of AIDS, because AIDS symptoms are sometimes misdiagnosed as problems related to pregnancy or as strictly gynecologic problems. Health care providers are charged with specifically identifying both the risk factors for AIDS and the physical signs of the disease process in women, but they also face social and ethical dilemmas unique to women infected with HIV.

EPIDEMIOLOGY

AIDS primarily affects minority women of reproductive age: 75% of women infected with AIDS are between the ages of 13 and 39, and 50% are black while 20% are Hispanic. The major AIDS risk factors for women are intravenous drug use (52%) and heterosexual activity with infected men (31%). Acquisition of HIV from intravenous drug use is well established and continues to be the leading mode of transmission; however, it is anticipated that heterosexual transmission will account for more than 50% of AIDS cases in women in the 1990s. Fewer women (10%) are infected with HIV by transfusion because blood donor screening has been universally instituted; thus, this mode of transmission has been virtually eliminated. Transmission of HIV through sexual assault is clearly possible, but the prevalence of seroconversion after sexual assault is unknown.

PATHOLOGY

HIV is a retrovirus that infects cells with receptors for the T peptide. The virus enters such a cell (eg, T_4 lymphocyte or neural tissue) and is acted on by a reverse transcriptase that leads to production of DNA which is then incorporated into the infected cell's genome. More virus is produced, and the infection spreads. Infection with this retrovirus is cytopathic and not transforming, as is the case for herpes simplex virus or human papillomavirus.

TRANSMISSION

General Modes of Transmission
HIV is found in blood (specifically lymphocytes) and blood products, vaginal secretions, semen, and in lower concentrations in saliva, tears, breast milk, and urine. Viral transmission can occur through exposure to these infected substances, but the extent to which it occurs is largely unknown and depends on many cofactors not completely elucidated, such as the presence of other infections or concomitant drug use. Transmission during sexual activity in women is facilitated by the presence of genital ulcerative disease and by engaging in anal intercourse. Theoretically, trauma to either vaginal or rectal mucosa, such as a break in the mucosa that could occur during sexual assault, could also facilitate viral transmission. Although it appears that male-to-female transmission of HIV is more common, both female-to-male and female-to-female sexual transmission of HIV have been documented.

Perinatal Transmission of HIV
Despite the consequences to individual health for women infected with HIV, it is the potential for perinatal transmission of the disease that has received the most attention. Early in the history of AIDS, women were identified as being infected through retrospective analysis after their children were diagnosed with AIDS. Many of these women had subsequent pregnancies, and it is from these women that much of the initial information regarding perinatal AIDS was derived. Because about 80% of pediatric AIDS cases are the result of perinatal transmission, the consequences of a woman becoming infected with HIV are far-reaching.

Perinatal transmission of HIV from mother to fetus or neonate occurs in 17–65% of pregnancies, with most centers reporting a transmission rate of approximately 30%. HIV is thought to be transmitted to the fetus or neonate by two means: across the placenta (transplacental transmission) or by way of secretions during delivery (intrapartum transmission). Transplacental infection with HIV has been documented in abortuses (14 weeks and earlier) and in the placenta. Likewise, HIV has been recovered from vaginal and cervical secretions, thus establishing a potential mode for intrapartum transmission of infection. Epidemiologic evidence supports the hypothesis that both modes of perinatal transmission occur based on the fact that 2 groups of children are known to contract AIDS: (1) those clinically ill by 1 year of life, with a median age of 4.1 months, suggesting transplacental infection, and (2) those clinically ill at a median age of 6.1 years, suggesting that seroconversion and infection may have occurred at birth. In addition, neonates can be infected from maternally infected breast milk.

The risk of perinatal HIV acquisition is related to various cofactors that affect the mother, including continued intravenous drug use, concurrent infection with other viruses (eg, cytomegalovirus, herpes simplex virus, and hepatitis B virus), continued exposure to an HIV-infected partner, and maternal stage of the disease. These cofactors are similar to those reported for male cohorts for development of AIDS and are supported by the fact that 1:1 transmission does not occur nor does transmission always occur in subsequent pregnancies. *Note:* The mode of delivery does not appear to be related to transmission, because many infected children have been delivered by cesarean section.

As mentioned above, the stage of maternal disease, as indicated by CD4 counts, is reported to have a direct relation to perinatal transmission. These reports suggest that the lower the CD4 count—indicating a longer history or more advanced infection—the more likely it is that perinatal transmission will occur. However, this relationship has not held for many patients. Recent research indicates that antibodies to gp120 in maternal serum help prevent transmission of HIV from mother to fetus. Clearly, more research is needed to resolve this issue.

COURSE OF INFECTION

The natural history of infection with HIV is one of a relentlessly progressive immunologic disorder resulting in AIDS, a constellation of disorders reflecting immunocompromise. These disorders include opportunistic infections and cancers, such as *Pneumocystic carinii* pneumonia, candidiasis, and Kaposi's sarcoma. The temporal course of the disease involves a latency period after infection that averages 8–10 years, with approximately 50% of individuals developing AIDS at 10 years after seroconversion.

Much research has focused on predictors of disease advancement, including lymphocyte counts, particularly CD4 (T_4) counts. Several antigens, including the p24 antigen to HIV, gp120, and B_2-microglobulins can also be used as indicators to monitor the advancing disease state. At present, both clinical findings and a combination of laboratory values are best for following an individual patient.

The issue of maternal disease progression after pregnancy (term or interrupted) has been the center of much controversy because initial reports indicated a more rapid progression of AIDS in seropositive women followed after pregnancy. Interpretation of these data is hindered by lack of knowledge about both the seroconversion date and whether an infected child had been born previously, indicating that the women might have been in a more advanced stage of AIDS. More recent data, although still controversial, indicate that pregnancy has little effect on the course of disease progression.

DIAGNOSIS

To date there is no evidence that the course of AIDS is different in women and men, and the clinical manifestations of AIDS in women are similar to those reported for men. However, Kaposi's sarcoma occurs in only 1% of women with AIDS compared with 23% of men. *P carinii* pneumonia is the leading presenting opportunistic infection for both men and women with AIDS (60%).

Gynecologic manifestations of HIV disease or other systemic illnesses that occur with great frequency in women do not lead to the diagnosis of AIDS-related complex (ARC) or AIDS in women. However, frequent episodes of vaginitis, prolonged genital herpes outbreaks (> 3 months), rapid development of cervical cancer with human papillomavirus infection, and severe pelvic inflammatory disease all may be manifestations of immunocompromise in HIV-infected women. These disease processes, while compromising health and even leading to death, often do not result in an

AIDS diagnosis, thus compounding the potential bias for underreporting this disease in women.

However, one specific disease manifestation has been established as a presentation symptom of AIDS in women: chronic vaginal candidiasis. Among women with HIV infection, the presence of oral or chronic recalcitrant vaginal candidiasis has represented a more advanced stage of disease with severe immunocompromise. In fact, chronic vaginal candidiasis may precede the development of oral candidiasis in the natural history of HIV infection. Physicians should consider the diagnosis of AIDS in patients with chronic refractory vaginal candidiasis (1 year with ongoing antifungal therapy) so that proper therapy is not delayed.

MANAGEMENT

General Treatment

The clinical care of all HIV-infected individuals must be combined with psychologic and social support, risk factor reduction, and encouragement of "safe sex" practices. The universal infection control precautions listed in Table 18–1 should be used at all stages in the treatment of all patients, whether HIV-infected or not. Specific treatment modalities should be applied as clinically indicated for either pregnant or nonpregnant women. Such modalities include azidothymidine (AZT) therapy (100 mg orally 5 times a day) when CD4 counts are low (200–500 cells/μL), aerosolized pentamidine or trimethoprim and sulfamethoxazole (Bactrim, Septra) for *P carinii* pneumonia prophylaxis, and acyclovir for herpes simplex infection. The efficacy and side effects of compound Q, an experimental drug, are currently being studied in nonpregnant patients.

Treatment for Pregnant Women

The primary differences in treating parturient HIV-infected women are based on the additional changes brought on by pregnancy, the involvement of an additional patient (the fetus), and the intense clinical care provided during gestation.

The clinical management of HIV-infected women during pregnancy is similar to that of nonpregnant HIV-infected women except that the frequency and intensity of surveillance during gestation are increased. Pregnancy has been reported to involve altered cellular immunologic function and to increase susceptibility

Table 18-1. Universal infection control precautions.[1]

Universal precautions
1. Use of appropriate barrier precautions should be routine.
2. If contaminated, and also after gloves are removed, hands and other skin surfaces should be washed immediately.
3. Precautions should be taken to prevent injuries by needles, scalpels, and other sharp instruments or devices.
4. Although saliva has not been implicated in HIV transmission, mouth pieces, resuscitation bags, or other ventilation devices should be available in areas where need is predicted to minimize emergency mouth-to-mouth resuscitation.
5. Until their condition resolves, workers with exudative lesions or weeping dermatitis should refrain from all direct patient care and from handling patient care equipment.
6. Pregnant health care workers should be especially familiar with and strictly adhere to precautions to minimize the additional risk of perinatal infection.

Precautions for invasive procedures
1. Appropriate barrier precautions should be carried out, and gloves and surgical masks must be worn for all invasive procedures. All health care workers who perform or assist in vaginal or cesarean deliveries should wear gloves and gowns when handling the placenta or the infant until blood and amniotic fluid have been removed from the infant's skin and should wear gloves during post-delivery care of the umbilical cord.
2. Torn gloves should be removed and a new glove used as promptly as patient safety permits, and the injuring needle or instrument should be removed from the sterile field.

[1] Source: *ACOG Newsletter* (October 1987).

to and severity of infectious processes, although such reports have recently been questioned. A careful assessment during each prenatal visit should include direct evaluation of symptoms through a comprehensive review of systems and physical examination with particular emphasis on lymphadenopathy, oral and pharyngeal changes, and pulmonary auscultation. Laboratory assessment for these women must include parameters for monitoring disease progressions, such as CD4 counts in each trimester and the presence of sexually transmitted diseases (STDs) or other infections, such as toxoplasmosis and tuberculosis (Table 18-2).

The fetus needs to be evaluated with ultrasonography or non-stress testing and biophysical profile as clinically indicated (eg, when intrauterine growth retardation or maternal substance abuse is suspected). There has been no detectable adverse perinatal effect from HIV infection alone, including birth weight, gestational age,

Table 18-2. Laboratory assessment of the HIV-infected woman.

CBC with differential
Platelet count
Erythrocyte sedimentation rate (ESR)
CD4 count
Liver function tests
Serum immunoglobulin (IgC, IgA)
STD screening (gonoccocci, *Chlamydia*, VDRL)
Tuberculin test
Other (toxoplasmosis titers, cytomegalovirus [CMV])

head circumference, and malformation, when other maternal factors, such as intravenous drug use, have been considered. Therefore, the perinatal management for the HIV-infected woman during pregnancy should be directly based on individual clinical need. The intrapartum management for the mother and fetus in a pregnancy complicated by HIV infection differs only in that fetal scalp electrodes and fetal scalp sampling are best avoided if possible, as with other maternal infections, such as herpes simplex virus.

HIV-infected mothers should not breast feed their newborn infants because of the risk of transmitting HIV through breast milk, except when other neonatal food sources are unavailable.

The use of antiviral therapies, such as AZT, during pregnancy, intrapartum, or immediately postpartum is being investigated in terms of preventing perinatal transmission as well as improving the clinical course for both mother and baby. Compound Q has been shown to kill trophoblastic cells in vitro and therefore should not be used during pregnancy. No reports are yet available regarding the use of newer therapeutic options, such as the dideoxynucleosides didanosine and dideoxycytidine, during pregnancy.

PREVENTION & RELATED SOCIAL ISSUES

Because no vaccine is available, preventing HIV infection depends on continued screening of blood supplies, taking precautions in sexual practices, and implementing infection control procedures in health care settings.

Two particular dilemmas for HIV-infected women are sexuality and reproductive life. Condom use, widely recommended as a reasonable method to prevent HIV transmission, has evolved into a public education campaign directed at women. These recommendations do not take into account the female experience with condom use, nor do they recognize situations in which a woman's acquiescence to sex is expected and, when denied, may result in battering. Furthermore, much of the instruction regarding condom use concentrates on ways to make it more palatable to men—with the implication that the male sexual experience is primary.

Women also have the other complicating issue of reproductive options. Because of the perinatal transmission of HIV, the infected mother must examine her obligations regarding pregnancy and the future care of the child she is carrying and her other children should she become ill or die. Common issues concerning all HIV-infected individuals take on greater importance for the HIV-infected mother, particularly in the areas of housing, health care, child care, insurance, and employment. The issues surrounding perinatal transmission of HIV have led to a significant controversy regarding the reproductive rights of infected women. This controversy includes suggestions of mandatory testing, punishment (eg, imprisonment or termination of parental rights), and forced sterilization. However, it is not clear whether these recommendations would result in dramatic changes for women considering childbearing. For example, data from women choosing pregnancy termination or continuation indicate that HIV status had little effect on their decision.

HIV-infected women represent predominantly lower socioeconomic classes, many from cultural groups in which motherhood and childbearing are mainstays of self-esteem and in which the birth of a child may be their only legacy. The future goals for management of the AIDS epidemic must include attention to these specific issues generated by women in addition to medical therapeutic progress.

SUGGESTED READINGS

Bell BK: AIDS and women: Remaining ethical issues. *AIDS Educ Prev* 1989;**1**:22.

Cohen PT, Surde MA, Volberding PA: *The AIDS Knowledge Base.* Massachusetts Medical Society, 1990.

Minkoff HL: Care of pregnant women infected with human immunodeficiency virus. *JAMA* 1987;**258**:2714.

| # Domestic Violence, Rape, & Sexual Abuse

Susan Jan Hornstein

Domestic violence, rape, and sexual abuse are underrecognized problems with tremendous social and economic costs. While each issue requires individual treatment, there are numerous parallels in dealing with each type of abuse. The victims of these abuses are often reluctant to discuss their victimization, sometimes being secretive or even denying the problem. All these abuses are illegal. Effective records and documentation are often critical in proving civil or criminal cases.

DOMESTIC VIOLENCE

Domestic violence is the single most common cause of injury to women. It is estimated to occur in up to half of all familial relationships. Numerous social, emotional, and economic reasons compound the difficulties in accurately documenting the enormity of the problem. Domestic violence, wife battering, and spousal abuse are all terms used to name physical abuse occurring at the hands of an intimate partner, regardless of marital status. Battering occurs in same-sex relationships as well as heterosexual relationships. A batterer may continue to harass, pursue, and batter a victim even if both parties are not living together or even if the relationship has been terminated. The battering continuum includes verbal abuse, beatings, threats with weapons, use of weapons, and rape. Since the batterer has proved that he or she will maintain control through violence, subsequent threats of violence can be as traumatizing as the physical acts themselves.

General Characteristics

A 3-phase cycle of violence dictates the model for interaction between the battered wife and her abuser. The duration and intensity of each phase may vary from cycle to cycle, but the phases have been consistently documented and the cycle describes a predictable pattern.

Usually the longest, the first phase is a tension-building phase in which both partners become aware of the potential for "minor abusive incidents" to erupt into "full-scale violence." The victim employs many techniques to avoid this end. Ultimately, these techniques are unsuccessful, and the second phase, the battering phase, occurs. The battering phase usually lasts several hours and is characterized by its unpredictability. During the third phase, the abusive partner tries to atone for the violent behavior. The battered wife's assessment of her situation is at this time most distorted. She often invests in the belief that the battering will end and that the loving that her partner exhibits momentarily will continue into a relationship free of danger.

If no intervention occurs and if the relationship continues, the frequency and severity of the violence escalate. Repeated beatings manifest themselves either as specific injuries (that may not be recognized as being related to the battering) or as general health problems, such as anxiety, fear, stress, and depression. These problems are often present between the violent episodes, and suicide may be contemplated or attempted.

Response of the Victim

Many battered women repeatedly turn to health care providers for assistance. Some women may inform the practitioner of the cause of their injuries; many will not. Some victims may be so invested in denying their battering that they wait until their initial physical injuries begin to heal, then they seek help for an associated health problem, such as a sleep disorder or depression. The victim usually does not recognize that these conditions are symptoms of the battering, a result of the chronic anxiety of living with the ever-present threat of danger.

Typically, a battered woman experiences overwhelming feelings of guilt, fear, and shame. She is a product of learned helplessness, a feeling of powerlessness that becomes generalized to her entire life as a result of experiencing situations that are repeatedly out of her control. Denial is an important coping mechanism to avoid the hopelessness of the situation. Women who live with abuse or the threat of abuse may not define their batterer's behavior as abusive or violent.

Diagnosis & Treatment

The presence of even one of the symptoms outlined in Table 19-1 should arouse a physician's suspicions of battering. To con-

Table 19-1. Indications of domestic violence.

- The extent or type of injury (including burns) is inconsistent with the explanation.
- The patient frequently visits the emergency room or doctor.
- Multiple injuries are present in various stages of healing or there is evidence of previous injuries, such as scarring or fading bruises.
- Multiple injuries are present on the face, head, neck, or genitals.
- Injuries shift to the breast and abdomen during pregnancy.
- The patient defines herself as clumsy or accident prone.
- Psychosomatic or emotional complaints are reported, such as stress, hyperventilation, anxiety, depression, sleep disorders, or choking sensations.
- Alcohol abuse or drug dependency, especially of illicit medications (eg, tranquilizers, antidepressants, sedatives), is evident.
- The patient exhibits an exaggerated, startled response, is evasive, passive, or cries frequently.
- An over-protective partner accompanies the patient.
- Anger is directed inward, and the patient exhibits self-destructive behavior, especially suicidal tendencies.

firm a suspected diagnosis, it is important to first establish a rapport with the patient and then begin to ask nonjudgmental questions in a sympathetic and direct manner. The woman should be asked to describe her living arrangements, current and past relationships, how she gets along with her partner, if she and her partner argue, and whether the arguments involve loss of temper or physical confrontation. She should be asked to describe how she sustained the injuries. At this time it is appropriate to introduce a leading question such as, "It is not uncommon for a partner to hit his or her mate. Has this happened to you?" It is important for the clinician to acknowledge the problem and to affirm that it is unacceptable.

Most patients will be relieved at the opportunity to share their secret. Often, at this point, many women reveal histories of abuse. It is critical that the clinician help the patient review her options or refer her to appropriate social services. Community resources (temporary shelters, support groups, and other crisis centers), family, and friends should all be among the options considered. The physician may assist her in identifying her own strengths and potential resources and may help her to assess the level of danger that she and her children face.

However, the woman may not be emotionally or economically ready to leave her situation and may continue to deny the existence of battering. The decision of the patient must be respected, but resources should be provided nonetheless. Many women will return and be able to deal more directly with the problem. Patients may use referrals months or years later.

Careful documentation of the patient's visit is critical; injuries should be concisely and objectively described. In assessing these injuries, it is appropriate for the physician to use phrases such as "the patient states . . ." and ". . . is suggestive of . . . ." If the patient goes to court, the medical record may be the only evidence or documentation of the battering.

It is acknowledged that health care professionals who recognize domestic violence can and do assist in the prevention of further injuries, sexual assault, suicide, and homicide. Intervention can stop the generational cycle of violence.

RAPE

General Characteristics

Rape is a violent crime primarily directed against women. Rape is defined as a physical assault involving the genitalia of either the victim or the assailant. It is an expression of hostility, anger, and power. A rapist uses sexual acts to terrorize, humiliate, and hurt the victim. Numerous social myths surround rape. These misconceptions place responsibility for the crime on the victim. Women do not want to be raped nor do they enjoy it or encourage it. All rape victims are terrified; it is usually a life-threatening experience, which may be accompanied by physical injury.

Rape is a crime that affects all races, classes, and ethnic groups. Victims are often known by the assailant. They are vulnerable and isolated. They may lack knowledge about their rights and are likely to have feelings of shame, guilt, and embarrassment, resulting in a hesitancy to report the rape to the authorities. This reluctance can be compounded by unsympathetic or hostile authorities (eg, medical, legal, or law-enforcement personnel).

Response of the Victim

All victims suffer psychological trauma that is manifest in two phases: immediate and long term. The immediate, or acute, phase may last for a few days or several weeks. The patient's response varies based on the circumstances of the victim's attack, relationship to the assailant, the degree of force used, the length of time the victim was held against her will, and her life experience. The immediate phase may run the continuum of response from complete loss of emotional control (characterized by shaking and sobbing) to extreme emotional control, which may appear as withdrawal, detachment, or an overly calm manner. A common defense mechanism is also denial. The patient often experiences fear, disbelief, shock, anger, and guilt. Mood swings and rapid fluctuations in emotions are common. The victim may try to repress these feelings.

The long-term or chronic phase of the rape trauma syndrome may also be designated the reorganization phase. Significant changes in lifestyle and work patterns may occur (changes of job and residence). The patient may develop sexual dysfunction and problems with trust and relationships. Nightmares may continue, and phobias and sleep disorders may develop. This phase can be complicated if the rape resulted in a pregnancy or a sexually transmitted disease.

Medical Examination

The examination should be conducted as soon as possible with primary consideration for the emotional well-being of the patient while collecting substantiating evidence. Sensitive and supportive medical care can hasten a victim's recovery, support the emergence of healthy and healing coping skills, and assist the patient in a transition toward normal functioning. The patient's recovery can be severely affected by subtle insinuations that may further victimize the patient and capitalize on the myth that she is somehow responsible for the crime. Medical personnel should encourage patients to vent anxieties, express their feelings, and talk about their concerns and needs. Throughout the examination, the clinician should explain what is being done and why.

In addition to recording the history of the assault, the clinician needs to test for sexually transmitted diseases, document evidence of physical trauma, and obtain a detailed gynecologic history to determine the risk of pregnancy (Table 19–2). It is crucial that the medical examination be thorough and precise and that physicians follow set protocols and procedures for specimen collection because the examination provides critical information to law enforcement agencies and the judicial system. In this way the examination is an indirect but vital part of the rape prevention process.

A patient must consent to the medical examination for the collection of evidence. This consent means that the patient understands that evidence will be collected, preserved, and released to

Table 19-2. Management of the rape victim.[1,2]

Diagnosis and evaluation

A. Inform the police (with the patient's consent).

B. Obtain written informed consent for examination.

C. Obtain and record the history in the patient's own words. A tape recorder may be helpful. Obtain answers to other specific questions (if they have not already been answered). Record the general appearance and demeanor of the victim, and note whether clothing is torn or stained.

D. Collect and label relevant evidence, and protect the chain of evidence.
   1. Scrape under the fingernails, and also take trimmings from them.
   2. Comb pubic hair, and look for loose hairs from the assailant.
   3. Cut off a few pubic hairs and save them.
   4. Collect any other loose hairs or dried blood.
   5. Examine the perineum and other suspect areas with a Wood light (prostatic secretions are fluorescent even when dry).
   6. Examine a saline wet mount of vaginal secretions for spermatozoa; record their number and motility.
   7. Prepare 4 dried slides of vaginal contents (wash the vagina with saline if it is dry), and fix them with ether-alcohol.
   8. Collect vaginal aspirate or washings into a screw-topped specimen tube for acid phosphatase determination (a positive reaction indicates the presence of prostatic fluid ejaculate).
   9. Place a cotton swab of vaginal contents into a specimen tube (for typing of the blood group antigen in semen).
   10. Obtain material from the cervix for culture for gonococci and *Chlamydia*.
   11. Obtain urine for urinalysis (look for hematuria indicating genitourinary trauma).
   12. Photograph all external lesions, but only with the patient's written consent.
   13. If oral or rectal penetration has occurred, steps 5-9 should be repeated with specimens from those sites.

E. Perform a physical examination.
   1. Thoroughly examine the patient for signs of trauma, discharge, or bleeding; record the results of the examination; and photograph all lesions (the latter only with the patient's written consent).
   2. Perform a pelvic examination.
      a. Look carefully for signs of trauma to the external genitalia.
      b. Note and record whether the hymen is intact and whether any hymenal tags are fresh (indicating trauma) or healed.
      c. Using a warm, water-moistened speculum, carefully examine the vagina for lacerations. Rarely, peritoneal perforation may occur.

(continued)

Table 19-2. Management of the rape victim.[1,2] (*continued*)

Diagnosis and evaluation (*continued*)

   d. Evaluate the cervix for signs of preexisting pregnancy and trauma.

   e. Examine the rectal area. If penetration has occurred, proctoscopy may be advisable.

F. Obtain blood for blood chemistry studies (if indicated), a serologic test for syphilis, blood typing (to compare the alleged assailant's type with that of the victim), and pregnancy dating.

Treatment

A. Prevent sexually transmitted diseases. Treatment for gonorrhea, *Chlamydia,* and syphilis (Chapter 5) should be offered but not forced on the patient. Only about 3% of rapes result in gonorrhea, and only about 0.1% of cases result in syphilis. Follow-up cultures for *Neisseria gonorrhoeae* are essential. Perform a follow-up serologic test for syphilis 1 and 3 months after the rape.

B. Prevent pregnancy. Treatment for the prevention of pregnancy should be offered but not forced on the patient. Only about 1% of rapes result in pregnancy; the chances are much less if the victim is using an effective method of contraception. Give 2 Ovral tablets immediately and repeat in 12 hours. Advise the patient that nausea and vomiting may occur. Explain that abortion can be made available at a later time.

C. If the patient consents, report the incident to the proper authorities before the patient leaves the emergency department, since the police will want to question her. If the alleged victim is a child, the incident may be child abuse and should be reported to the appropriate child welfare authorities.

D. Start rape counseling immediately, preferably directed by experienced personnel who are part of an established rape counseling program.

E. Arrange follow-up; a definite appointment (time, place, and physician or clinic) should be made.

[1] This is a general outline; always refer to and follow the recommendations of regional authorities for evidence collection.
[2] Source: Mills J et al (editors): *Current Emergency Diagnosis & Treatment.* Appleton & Lange, 1990.

law-enforcement authorities. At any time during the examination, the patient has the right to refuse or terminate the examination.

Treatment

   Treatment must be performed in a nonjudgmental and respectful manner. The physician needs to treat injuries and infections and, if appropriate, sexually transmitted diseases; also, the possibility of pregnancy should be addressed. Medical follow-up may be necessary if pregnancy is suspected or if further tests or treatments for sexually transmitted diseases are warranted.

A trained support person can help guide a victim through the medical process. Help through crisis intervention and counseling should be made available along with referrals to rape crisis or trauma centers. The victim's partner, family members, and friends may also need assistance to cope with their own emotional responses and to be better equipped to understand and support the victim.

SEXUAL ABUSE

General Characteristics

Sexual abuse or sexual assault is defined as forced sexual activity or intimacy by one person on another. Sexual abuse includes the range of sexual contact from inappropriate kissing or fondling to masturbation, genital exposure, or intercourse. Sexual abuse of children is divided into two primary categories: abuse perpetrated by someone familiar to the victim (primarily incest) and abuse perpetrated by a stranger. The categories differ in several significant ways. Usually, abuse perpetrated by a stranger occurs in a single episode, the majority of the cases are reported to the authorities, and the victims are less likely to have the additional burden arising from the responsibilities and pressures of maintaining familial relationships (complicated by the abuser being a family member).

Incest, or sexual abuse involving a family member, constitutes the largest category of child sexual assault, approximately 80%. The majority of child sexual abuse involves a parent, step-parent, guardian, or relative. Father-daughter incest constitutes 75% of reported cases. Brother-sister incest is significantly less reported and probably accounts for the next largest category of incest. The remainder of sexual assault cases involve a family member, extended family, family friends, and acquaintances, such as neighbors or childcare personnel. Although boys and young men are also victims of sexual abuse, girls experience sexual abuse more often than boys.

Families in which incest occurs may appear outwardly normal. However, the families are often dysfunctional and beset by other problems, such as drug or alcohol abuse and battering. The mother or parent(s) may be cognizant of an incestuous situation but have agreed consciously or subconsciously to ignore the abusive behavior rather than jeopardize family relationships even more.

Response of the Victim

Most incest victims internalize responsibility for the abuse and become guilt-ridden. Children are often bribed and emotionally blackmailed to maintain silence about the abuse. They may be threatened with the responsibility of destroying the family if they reveal their secret.

Sexual abuse is humiliating and will destroy a child's self-image. An older child or adolescent experiencing sexual abuse may exhibit guilt, anger, inexplicable physical complaints, withdrawal, depression, and sleep disorders (Table 19–3). These children frequently have difficulty performing in school, and they may become sexually promiscuous or run away. Many of these dysfunctional behaviors continue into adulthood.

Diagnosis & Treatment

If any one of the indicators of sexual abuse listed in Table 19–3 is present, the clinician should begin detailed questioning. As with other forms of abuse, it is critical that the questions be specific, clear, and nonjudgmental. Affirmative answers need to be followed with more detailed questions to elicit the history of the abuse. At this point, the patient is usually relieved to tell her story. She may have never previously discussed her abuse. The clinician must be supportive and help the victim realize that the sexual abuse was not her fault, that she is not alone, and that her experience is shared by many others. The clinician interaction is a critical opportunity for the victim to understand that her abuse can be stopped

Table 19-3. Indications of sexual abuse in older children and adolescents.

- Withdrawal or depression.
- A sudden change in school performance: frequent absences, a drop in grades, arriving early or leaving late, refusing to dress for or participate in physical education classes.
- Spontaneous bouts of crying.
- Excessive bathing or poor hygiene.
- Sudden or new fears (eg, of family gatherings, or of males).
- Alcohol abuse or drug dependency.
- Self-destructive behavior, especially contemplating suicide.
- Extremely compliant or extremely aggressive behavior.
- Running away.
- An abnormal self-consciousness about one's body.
- Sudden acquisitions of gifts.
- An inability to relate to peers.

and its effect overcome. If the victim is still living in the abusive situation, the clinician can assist her to review options for safety, support, and legal intervention. Certain kinds of sexual abuse, such as abuse of children, require immediate reporting to local authorities.

Specific medical care includes treatment of any physical injuries and prevention of sexually transmitted diseases or pregnancy, if appropriate. Most communities offer legal and social services specifically designed to provide intervention and support for victims of sexual abuse and their families. The clinician can maximize intervention potential by becoming familiar with referral resources and using them.

SUGGESTED READINGS

Bass E, Davis L: *Courage to Heal. A Guide for Women Survivors of Child Sexual Abuse.* HarperCollins, 1988.

Burgess A, Wolbert E: *Rape and Sexual Assault: A Research Handbook.* Garland, 1985.

Martin D: *Battered Wives.* Volcano Press, 1986.

Walker LE: *Battered Wife.* Springer, 1984.

20 | Ethical Decision Making

Nancy Milliken, MD, & Elena A. Gates, MD

Over the last 20 years, the ethical aspects of medicine have increased in prominence both within the medical community and throughout society, partly because of medicine's increased ability to affect in dramatic ways the fundamental human processes of conception, birth, life, and death. Nowhere is this more evident than in the specialty of obstetrics and gynecology, whose practitioners assist in the creation of life through fertility techniques such as artificial insemination and in vitro fertilization. Obstetrician-gynecologists provide prenatal genetic diagnosis and counsel patients regarding their choices based on the information obtained. In addition, they address the issues of dying with their patients who have terminal pelvic cancers. Good decisions in all these areas require more than up-to-date medical knowledge; obstetrician-gynecologists must be sensitive to the ethical issues involved and understand the goals and values of all participants in the decision.

The 1983 President's Commission for the Study of Ethical Problems in Medicine clearly stated "the primary responsibility for ensuring that morally justified decisions are made lies with the physician." To make ethical medical decisions, practitioners in obstetrics and gynecology must acquire knowledge and skills in several areas. Each practitioner should develop an honest understanding of his or her own value system and how these values color his or her evaluation of the medical options in individual cases. He or she must have a knowledge of the fundamental principles of medical ethics and of the relevant cases in health law. Furthermore, the process by which each practitioner makes and implements ethical decisions should not be arbitrary but instead systematic and logically consistent. This chapter reviews several fundamental ethical principles and one approach to solving ethical dilemmas.

ETHICAL PRINCIPLES

Contemporary clinical decision making is based on several important ethical principles, which together constitute medicine's patient-centered professional ethic.

212

Beneficence

This principle requires health care professionals to enhance the well-being of patients to the best of their ability and to protect patients from iatrogenic harm. In the clinical setting, applying this principle often involves the difficult task of balancing medical benefits and risks. These medical benefits and risks should be defined objectively to avoid interpretations based on a physician's personal values, which may not be shared by the patient who will be affected. For example, a physician should not advise a woman over the age of 35 years that prenatal genetic diagnosis is unnecessary because the physician believes abortion is immoral.

Patient Autonomy

This principle requires a health care provider to honor a competent patient's informed decision about her medical care. This principle is based on the recognition that individual patients are free to choose how to live their lives based on their personal set of values. It is the patient who can best fit the medical goals advocated by her physician into the broader context of her life as defined by important personal relationships, religious beliefs, and individual aspirations. Physicians who disregard the values of their patients are called paternalistic. Physicians respect patient autonomy frequently in daily practice when they agree to management plans other than the ones they have recommended because of the preferences of their patients. Gynecologists often respect the decisions of ovarian cancer patients to forego the most aggressive and effective chemotherapy because of the desire to avoid severe side effects. An obstetrician who advises a woman with a history of life-threatening peripartum cardiomyopathy to avoid future pregnancy is prevented, out of respect for her autonomy, from doing anything that would interfere with her ability to conceive.

Justice

The principle of justice generally applies to relationships between individuals and between individuals and their society. Justice supports the right of individuals to claim what is due them. A just distribution of burdens and benefits is defined differently by different theories of justice. Some theories argue that this distribution should be based on characteristics such as merit, need, contribution, or effort; other theories declare that all benefits and burdens be distributed equally. In US society, for example, race, gender, or religion are not considered to be legitimate criteria for distribution of benefits such as education, housing, and employment. The principle of justice creates an obligation to treat equally those who are alike according to the agreed upon criteria. Selection of these criteria is an ethical exercise. Distribution of health care resources involves consideration of the principle of justice. Access to fertility assistance is currently decided largely on the ability to pay, which many consider an unjust criterion.

ETHICAL CONCEPTS

These ethical principles should guide the practice of medicine and are the basis of the following well-recognized concepts defining good patient care.

Informed Consent

Informed consent is the basis of much of the interaction between physician and patient today. The ideal of informed consent is to enable each patient to freely choose a medical or surgical treatment after adequate disclosure of the potential risks and benefits of the proposed treatment as well as those of alternative treatments or of no treatment at all. Put another way, the goal of informed consent is to protect patient autonomy. The right to informed consent or informed refusal is supported legally as well as ethically. In a now famous court case in 1914, Judge Cardozo stated "every human being of adult years and sound mind has a right to determine what shall be done with his own body."* Surgical consent forms usually include the elements of informed consent listed above. However, it must be emphasized that it is the comprehensive discussion of risks and benefits, not the piece of paper, that both legally and ethically ensures that a patient has the opportunity to give informed consent. Inherent in a patient's right to informed consent is her right to informed refusal of medical intervention. Thus, for religious reasons an informed patient can consent to laparotomy for a ruptured ectopic pregnancy while at the same time refuse the transfusion of all blood products, even if they are needed to save her life.

Capacity for Decision Making

A. Patient as Decision Maker: A patient must be capable of making decisions in order to exercise her right to informed con-

*Schloendorff v Society of New York Hospitals, 211NY 125,126: 105 NE92,93 (1914).

sent. Capacity for decision making requires the ability to understand information, evaluate it within the framework of a coherent set of personal values, and use it to make consistent decisions regarding medical treatment. A patient's capacity to make decisions can be determined by professionals at the bedside; a person's competence can be determined only by judges in a court of law. A person may be judged to be incompetent in one area of her life (eg, managing her finances) and still be deemed capable of making decisions regarding her health care.

B. Surrogate Decision Maker: If a patient is incapable of making her own medical decisions, a surrogate decision maker must be found. The physician does not automatically become the decision maker in this situation. Family members often make good surrogates; however, there can be circumstances in which their own self-interests would persuade them to make decisions counter to the best interests of the patient. The court may sometimes appoint a guardian. The surrogate decision maker should make decisions that respect the patient's wishes and protect and promote her best interests. In the ideal situation, the surrogate is guided by preferences the patient expressed before the development of her incapacity. Sometimes these preferences are formalized in a living will or durable power of attorney; often they are gleaned from a letter or remembered conversation. Physicians should be aware of the available legal processes in their states that allow patients to prepare directives in advance for medical care and should encourage their patients to use them. These mechanisms provide the best protection for an individual's autonomy in the health care system and can spare much unneeded agony for families of those patients who have lost their capacity to decide.

Confidentiality

Historically, physicians have made a commitment to keep information about their patients confidential, including both information provided by the patient and information uncovered by the physician during diagnostic procedures. This confidentiality and respect for patient privacy has been an essential element in the foundation of trust and respect that underlies the physician-patient relationship. Without this trust, the therapeutic effectiveness of the physician-patient relationship would be limited. There are situations in which protection of confidentiality could result in harm to a third party. For example, a patient infected with a sexually transmitted disease (STD) might refuse to inform her sexual partners, or a known carrier of a genetic disease might refuse to disclose this information to her partner with whom she plans to conceive. In general, the duty to maintain confidentiality takes precedence over other obligations. However, each state has laws covering the reporting of STDs for the protection of third parties. The laws covering human immunodeficiency virus infection vary from state to state and are often different from those for other STDs.

In caring for a pregnant woman, the obstetrician-gynecologist is confronted with the unique ethical challenge of balancing maternal health, maternal autonomy, and fetal health. Fortunately, these 3 elements are rarely in conflict, and the vast majority of pregnant women are prepared to assume significant risk to optimize the well-being of the fetus. However, on the rare occasion when the choice of a pregnant woman does confer some potential risk to her fetus, the obstetrician-gynecologist is obligated to inform the pregnant woman as to the consequences of her choices. The physician may be an advocate for fetal needs and enlist the aid of family members or other health care providers (eg, nurses, social workers, or psychiatrists) in persuading the pregnant woman to act on behalf of her fetus. At no time, however, should deceit or coercion be used to this end. The limitations and fallibility of medical knowledge should be acknowledged by the obstetrician-gynecologist, and any uncertainty about the diagnosis of fetal harm and prognosis of fetal benefit should be shared with the pregnant woman. Furthermore, it should be recognized that a statistically small degree of risk to the pregnant woman may be one that she legitimately may wish to avoid. As a competent adult, a pregnant woman has the right to make choices we allow any other competent adult, especially those that would preserve her bodily integrity.

Some people have advocated the use of court orders to force pregnant women to comply with medical recommendations. However, others believe that any use of force in the medical relationship will have destructive consequences, and patient autonomy and informed consent will lose their meaning. There is concern that, if force can be used, health care providers will be mistrusted by their patients, who may withhold important information for fear that it may be used against them or who may forego care altogether. For these reasons, in 1987 the American College of Obstetricians and Gynecologists stated in ACOG Committee Opinion 55: "Obstetricians should refrain from performing procedures that are unwanted by a pregnant woman" and "resort to the courts is almost never justified."

ETHICAL PROBLEM SOLVING

When physicians are confronted with ethical dilemmas in clinical medicine, the steps outlined in Table 20–1 can facilitate the decision-making process.

Table 20-1. Guidelines for resolving an ethical dilemma in clinical medicine.

Collect the clinical data
 Assess the clinical condition (diagnosis and prognosis) of the patient (and fetus if present).
 Evaluate the benefits and harms expected from alternative courses of action.
 Review the expected long-term outcomes of clinical alternatives in terms of the burden the patient will have to bear to benefit from each.
 Determine whether the clinical facts lead to consensus or uncertainty. Use consultants to clarify the medical facts and ensure that all options have been considered.
 Assess the personal and professional values that underlie the medical recommendations.

Understand Patient Choice
 Determine whether the patient has the capacity to make a health care decision.
 Ascertain whether the patient is informed of the medical facts.
 Ask the patient what her choices are and ensure that they are known to the medical team.

Identify ethical conflicts and prioritize the ethical principles
 Review the ethical principles that underlie each argument.
 Determine whether one of the principles is more important than the others and whether one course of action is more justified than another.
 Review other cases with similar ethical concerns for further information and insight. (The basic ethical question being considered is seldom a new one.) Ethics commentaries and the legal literature are sources for these cases. Hospital ethics committees are another valuable resource.

Choose the best option
 Choose an option that can be justified by recognized ethical principles.

Re-evaluate the decision after it is implemented
 Re-evaluate the major options in light of information gained during the implementation of the chosen course.
 Apply the lessons learned from the review in future decisions.
 Make your experience available to others (eg, an ethics committee is often ideal for disseminating such information).

SUGGESTED READINGS

Beauchamp TL, Childress JF: *Principles of Biomedical Ethics,* 3rd ed. Oxford University Press, 1989.

Elias S, Annas GJ: *Reproductive Genetics and the Law.* Year Book, 1987.

Ethics Committee of the American Fertility Society: Ethical considerations of the new reproductive technologies. *Fertil Steril* 1986;**46 (Suppl 1).**

The Hastings Center: *Guidelines of the Termination of Life-Sustaining Treatment and the Care of the Dying.* Indiana University Press, 1987.

The Hastings Center's Bibliography of Ethics: *Biomedicine and Professional Responsibility.* University Publications of America, 1984.

Jonsen AR, Siegler M, Winslade WJ: *Clinical Ethics: A Practical Approach to Ethical Decisions in Clinical Medicine,* 2nd ed. Macmillan, 1986.

Section III:
Endocrinology & Infertility

Amenorrhea | 21

Valerie L. Baker, MD, & Janice L. Andreyko, MD

DEFINITION

Primary amenorrhea is the absence of menses by age 16 in a woman who has normal growth and secondary sexual characteristics. Primary amenorrhea is also defined as the absence of menses by age 14 in a woman who does not have normal growth and secondary sexual characteristics. **Secondary amenorrhea** is the absence of menstrual periods for 3 cycles or for 6 months in a woman who has previously been menstruating.

To evaluate and treat amenorrhea, it is important to understand the physiology of menstruation. For menses to occur, the hypothalamic/pituitary gland/ovarian axis must function normally. Menstruation also requires an ovary that can produce the proper amount and sequence of estrogen and progesterone. The endometrium must be capable of responding to these hormones. Finally, the endocervix, vagina, and vaginal orifice must be open.

HISTORY

The history should include a review of menstruation (last menstrual period, bleeding pattern, cycle length and interval), recent pregnancy outcomes, and sexual activity. *Note:* The most common cause of amenorrhea is pregnancy, which must be excluded in any patient presenting with amenorrhea. It is important to know if the patient is taking medications, especially oral contraceptives and prolactin-increasing medications, such as phenothiazines, antihypertensives, and tricyclic antidepressants. Information regarding diet, physical activity, stress, and psychological functioning is needed. A review of systems should include inquiry about headaches, hot flushes, hirsutism (abnormal hair growth), galactorrhea, pattern of growth (for patients who have never had a period), and symptoms that indicate abnormal thyroid function, such as change in weight, sleeping patterns, appetite, or heat or cold intolerance.

PHYSICAL EXAMINATION

During the examination, the patient's secondary sexual characteristics are assessed, including breast development and pubic and axillary hair growth. These features indicate significant estrogen and androgen production. Changes in the patient's height and weight are also noted. If the growth spurt and secondary sexual characteristics are normal, it is likely that puberty is simply delayed, and the patient will usually go on to establish menses.

The staging of pubertal events in girls is outlined in Table 21-1. The first sign of puberty is an acceleration of growth followed by development of breast buds (thelarche) at a median age of 11.2 years. The most noticeable growth spurt (maximum rate of growth) occurs shortly after thelarche. Pubarche and axillary hair growth usually follow but may precede thelarche. Menarche is the last event in puberty, occurring at a median age of 13.5 years.

A pelvic examination is performed to confirm the presence of a patent vagina, normal uterus, and normal ovaries. Galactorrhea, thyromegaly, hirsutism, and signs of virilization (such as clitorimegaly) should be noted.

Table 21-1. Staging of pubertal events in girls.[1]

Event	Mean Age (yr)	Range
Breast budding	11.2	9–13.5
Pubic and axillary hair growth	11.7	9–14.5
Menarche	13.5	11–16
Adult-pattern pubic hair	14.4	
Adult breast development	15.3	

[1] Reproduced, with permission, from Seibel M: *Infertility: A Comprehensive Text.* Appleton & Lange, 1990.

LABORATORY STUDIES

As outlined in Figure 21–1, a pregnancy test is performed regardless of the patient's stated sexual activity. Other initial tests include measurement of prolactin, thyroid-stimulating hormone (TSH, thyrotropin), serum thyroxin (T_4), T_3 uptake, and possibly follicle-stimulating hormone (FSH) and luteinizing hormone (LH). If hirsutism or virilization is present, serum androgen levels are measured. If findings suggest Cushing's syndrome, corticotropin (adrenocorticotropic hormone, ACTH), dehydroepiandrosterone sulfate (DHEAS), and urinary free cortisol levels are obtained. Finally, if an anatomic abnormality is suspected, an ultrasonogram of the pelvis is obtained.

DIAGNOSIS & TREATMENT

High levels of serum prolactin may be associated with amenorrhea. The exact mechanism is still unknown, but possibilities include an inhibitory effect of prolactin on granulosa cell function or a direct inhibition of gonadotropin-releasing hormone (GnRH) release by hypothalamic dopamine.

Elevated Prolactin Levels

There are several causes of elevated prolactin levels. A nonsecreting pituitary tumor may elevate serum prolactin through a mass effect. Compression of the pituitary stalk may decrease dopamine availability to the anterior pituitary gland, resulting in increased prolactin secretion by the lactotrophs. Most often, an elevated serum prolactin is due to the presence of a prolactin-secreting tumor (**prolactinoma**). If prolactin is elevated, a computerized tomographic (CT) or magnetic resonance imaging (MRI) scan of the head should be obtained to exclude the presence of a pituitary tumor.

A prolactin-secreting adenoma is classified as a **microadenoma** if it is less than 10 mm in diameter or as a **macroadenoma** if it is greater than 10 mm in diameter. Although macroadenomas are rarely malignant, they can compress the optic chiasm, producing bitemporal hemianopia.

Bromocriptine, a dopamine agonist, is the usual treatment of choice for both macroadenomas and microadenomas. Bromocriptine binds to dopamine receptors and mimics dopamine's inhibition of prolactin secretion. It is usually more effective than trans-

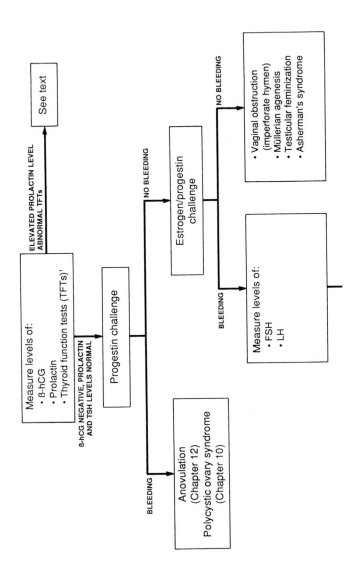

Measure levels of:
• β-hCG
• Prolactin
• Thyroid function tests (TFTs)[1]

ELEVATED PROLACTIN LEVEL
ABNORMAL TFTs

See text

β-hCG NEGATIVE, PROLACTIN AND TSH LEVELS NORMAL

Progestin challenge

BLEEDING

Anovulation
(Chapter 12)
Polycystic ovary syndrome
(Chapter 10)

NO BLEEDING

Estrogen/progestin challenge

NO BLEEDING

Vaginal obstruction
(imperforate hymen)
• Müllerian agenesis
• Testicular feminization
• Asherman's syndrome

BLEEDING

Measure levels of:
• FSH
• LH

222

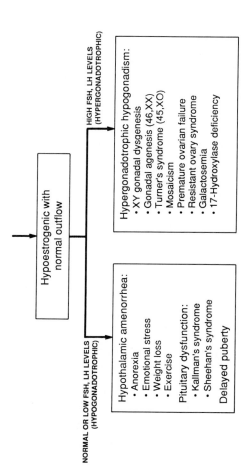

Figure 21-1. Diagnostic workup for amenorrhea. ¹Thyroid-stimulating hormone, T_4, T_3 uptake.

Hypoestrogenic with normal outflow

NORMAL OR LOW FSH, LH LEVELS (HYPOGONADOTROPHIC)

Hypothalamic amenorrhea:
  • Anorexia
  • Emotional stress
  • Weight loss
  • Exercise
Pituitary dysfunction:
  • Kallman's syndrome
  • Sheehan's syndrome
Delayed puberty

HIGH FSH, LH LEVELS (HYPERGONADOTROPHIC)

Hypergonadotrophic hypogonadism:
  • XY gonadal dysgenesis
  • Gonadal agenesis (46,XX)
  • Turner's syndrome (45,XO)
  • Mosaicism
  • Premature ovarian failure
  • Resistant ovary syndrome
  • Galactosemia
  • 17-Hydroxylase deficiency

sphenoidal surgery and eliminates surgical risks. The initial dose of bromocriptine is 1.25 mg at bedtime, but this amount is typically increased to 2.5 mg orally once or twice daily. Surgery is still the treatment of choice for nonsecreting tumors.

Pituitary tumors are usually slow growing but, in rare cases, become enlarged during pregnancy. A patient may receive bromocriptine during pregnancy if she develops headaches or visual changes.

Elevated Thyroid-Stimulating Hormone Levels

In primary hypothyroidism, serum thyroxine levels are too low to produce negative feedback on the pituitary and hypothalamus, resulting in elevated thyrotropin-releasing hormone (TRH) and TSH levels. TRH not only causes TSH secretion by the anterior pituitary but is also a prolactin-releasing hormone. In addition, TRH-induced prolactin release may result in amenorrhea. Hypothyroidism may be diagnosed by detecting elevated levels of TSH in serum. When hypothyroidism is treated with thyroxine, menses return. Hyperthyroidism may also produce amenorrhea but less often than hypothyroidism.

Progesterone Challenge

If the pregnancy test is negative and if the physical examination and all laboratory tests are normal, a progesterone challenge test is performed to assess the level of endogenous estrogen and the patency of the outflow tract (uterus and vagina). Medroxyprogesterone acetate (MPA), 10 mg orally daily for 5–7 days, or progesterone in oil, 200 mg intramuscularly once, is given.

A. Withdrawal Bleeding Occurs: As noted in Figure 21–1, if the patient bleeds within a week after completing the progesterone challenge, then it can be assumed that the outflow tract is patent and that there was proliferation of the endometrium by estrogen before the administration of progesterone. The diagnosis in this case is either anovulation (see Chapter 12) or polycystic ovary syndrome (PCO, see Chapter 10). Anovulation is a term usually reserved for patients who have no identifiable cause for absent or infrequent ovulation. The most likely cause is benign hypothalamic dysfunction that produces steady-state levels of gonadotropins and sex steroids (rather than the normal fluctuating levels).

An anovulatory patient may develop dysfunctional uterine bleeding, endometrial cancer, breast disease, infertility, or polycystic ovaries. Because of the risk of endometrial cancer, an endometrial biopsy is indicated if anovulation has been present for several years.

With an anovulatory patient, several treatment options are possible. A patient who desires contraception (which is needed because not all cycles will be anovulatory) may be given low-dose oral contraceptives. Alternatively, she may be given MPA, 10 mg orally daily for 10 days each month. If a patient desires pregnancy, ovulation may be induced. If at any time a patient with the diagnosis of anovulation who is taking oral contraceptives, progesterone, or hormone replacement does not experience withdrawal bleeding, a pregnancy test must be performed. If the patient is not pregnant, the diagnostic workup for amenorrhea must be pursued.

B. No Withdrawal Bleeding Occurs: If withdrawal bleeding does not occur, an estrogen/progesterone challenge test is performed.

Estrogen/Progesterone Challenge

Because endogenous estrogen levels may be low in patients who do not experience withdrawal bleeding after treatment with progesterone alone, the next step of the evaluation is to stimulate endometrial proliferation with conjugated estrogens (eg, Premarin), 2.5 mg orally daily for 21 days, with the addition of MPA, 10 mg orally daily on days 17 through 21. If withdrawal bleeding does not occur, the treatment is repeated using a higher dose of estrogen, beginning 1 week after the last dose of MPA.

A. No Withdrawal Bleeding Occurs: If withdrawal bleeding does not occur after the estrogen/progestin challenge is complete, an anatomic anomaly or an abnormal, scarred endometrium is present. Anomalies of müllerian duct development are common causes of primary amenorrhea. Asherman's syndrome, or a scarred endometrium, is a common cause of secondary amenorrhea.

1. Vaginal obstruction–An imperforate hymen or obliterated vaginal orifice may produce a hematocolpos or hematometra and cyclic pain. This diagnosis can usually be made by physical examination without an estrogen and progestin challenge.

2. Müllerian agenesis (Mayer-Rokitansky Kuster-Hauser syndrome)–In this condition, the vagina is absent, and the uterus may be normal or rudimentary. The ovaries are also normal, but urinary tract abnormalities may occur. If this condition is suspected, a karyotype is obtained, and the urinary tract is evaluated (eg, by intravenous pyelogram). An artificial vagina may be created by progressive dilatation or by surgery.

3. Testicular feminization (or androgen insensitivity syndrome)–Patients with testicular feminization have an XY genotype but a female phenotype. Because they lack normal receptors for androgen, they develop as females, despite normal male testosterone levels. They have a blind vagina and no uterus. Testes are present, often in the inguinal canal, and should be removed because of the risk of neoplasia. However, excision of the testes should be delayed until after puberty because the estrogen obtained by peripheral conversion of the androgens produced by the testes will feminize the patient at puberty.

4. Asherman's syndrome–Asherman's syndrome is the destruction and scarring of the endometrium, usually after curettage. Asherman's syndrome may also occur after uterine surgery (eg, cesarean section or myomectomy) or rarely as a result of severe pelvic infection.

If Asherman's syndrome is suspected, a hysterosalpingogram or hysteroscopy may help confirm the diagnosis. Asherman's syndrome is treated by dilatation and curettage (D&C) or, preferably, by lysis of adhesions at hysteroscopy. Then combinations of high-dose conjugated estrogens, 5.0 mg orally daily for days 1 through 21 of each month, and MPA, 10 mg orally daily for days 15 through 21, are given for 2 months.

B. Withdrawal Bleeding Occurs: If a patient does experience withdrawal bleeding after treatment with an estrogen and progestin and if the levels of the gonadotropins FSH and LH have not been measured, FSH and LH tests are performed approximately 2 weeks after the estrogen/progesterone challenge test is complete to allow gonadotropin levels to recover from steroid suppression. For a normal patient, the FSH level is 5–30 mIU/mL with an ovulatory midcycle peak about 2 times that of the baseline. The normal LH level is 5–20 mIU/mL with an ovulatory midcycle peak 3 times that of the baseline.

1. Low gonadotropin levels–Gonadotropin levels may be low or normal if a patient has **hypothalamic dysfunction,** a common cause of amenorrhea. The hypothalamus may not function normally in some patients with weight loss, anorexia nervosa, or with strenuous exercise (eg, marathon running). In general, decreasing the percentage of body fat below a critical level may lead to hypothalamic suppression.

Very low gonadotropin levels (which are rare) suggest a hypothalamic or, much less commonly, a pituitary defect in gonadotropin production. **Sheehan's postpartum necrosis** is an infarction and necrosis of the pituitary gland that occurs when its blood supply is interrupted at the time of an obstetrical hemorrhage. **Kallman's syndrome** is characterized by amenorrhea, anosmia, absent GnRH, and therefore low gonadotropin levels, and a normal female karyotype. Finally, low gonadotropin levels may occur in a teenage patient with benign delayed menarche.

2. Elevated gonadotropin levels–High gonadotropin levels (FSH > 40 mIU/mL, LH > 25 mIU/mL) are the result of ovarian failure and a lack of steroid feedback at the hypothalamus.

Several types of defects occur in the ovary. First, the gonads may fail to develop normally, a condition known as **gonadal dysgenesis.** In this condition, the gonad may be absent, may be only a streak of tissue, or may contain a Y chromosome. Gonadal dysgenesis is predominantly associated with abnormal genotypes (although it can occur in women with 46,XX). For example, patients with **Turner's syndrome,** having a 45,XO genotype, may have gonadal dysgenesis. These patients are typically short, with a webbed neck, shield chest, and possibly a coarctation of the aorta or renal anomalies.

If a patient with elevated gonadotropin levels is under 30 years of age, a karyotype is obtained. If she is a mosaic with a Y chromosome, the gonad is excised because there is a 25% chance that cancer will develop if a dysgenetic gonad is present. Gonadal tumors seldom appear after age 30, so older patients rarely need a genetic evaluation.

A second type of ovarian defect is **premature ovarian failure,** defined as loss of ovarian activity before age 35. It may be due to a rapid disappearance of follicles (premature menopause). Radiation, chemotherapy, infection, autoimmune disease, or chromosomal abnormalities may produce premature menopause. A second type of premature ovarian failure is the resistant ovary syndrome in which follicles are present but ovulation does not occur because the ovary lacks functioning gonadotropin receptors. If premature ovarian failure is suspected, a diagnostic workup for autoimmune disease is performed, including tests for antinuclear antibody, rheumatoid factor, complete blood count, erythrocyte sedimentation rate, thyroid function, thyroid antibodies, and 8 AM cortisol.

There are several rare causes of high gonadotropin levels. **Galactosemia** may lead to impaired gonadotropin activity or fewer oogonia. **17-Hydroxylase deficiency** leads to hypertension and lack of secondary sexual characteristics. Finally, cysts and benign and malignant tumors of the ovary can produce amenorrhea by interfering with normal ovarian tissue or by producing hormones that interfere with ovulation. These, however, do not cause elevation of gonadotropin levels.

SUGGESTED READINGS

Speroff L, Glass RH, Kase NG: *Clinical Gynecologic Endocrinology & Infertility,* 4th ed. Williams & Wilkins, 1988.
Yen SSC, Jaffe RD: *Reproductive Endocrinology: Physiology, Pathophysiology and Clinical Management,* 3rd ed. Saunders, 1991.

22 | Hirsutism

Rosemary Delgado, MD, & Janice L. Andreyko, MD

Hirsutism is the growth of excess coarse body hair in the female. It is often associated with excess androgen production and occurs in a male pattern hair distribution (face, chest, abdomen, or buttocks).

Hypertrichosis, on the other hand, is a generalized increase of soft, nonsexual hair. **Virilism** occurs when hirsutism is accompanied by clitoromegaly, voice deepening, frontal balding, or masculine changes in body habitus. This condition usually indicates a high degree of androgen production, eg, from an androgen-producing tumor.

ANDROGEN PRODUCTION

Testosterone is the major circulating androgen in females. It is produced by the ovaries (25%), adrenals (25%), and by peripheral conversion of another important androgen, androstenedione (50%). Androstenedione is produced by the ovaries (50%) and the adrenal glands (50%). Additional androgens include dehydroepiandrosterone (DHEA) and its sulfate (DHEAS), which are produced primarily by the adrenal glands (90–95%). These are weak androgens biologically but serve as markers for excess androgen production.

Most of the circulating testosterone is bound to a β-globulin sex hormone–binding globulin (SHBG), while 20% is loosely bound to albumin and the remaining 1–2% is free. It is the free and loosely bound hormone that is thought to be biologically active (ie, free to enter into and act on target tissues).

PATHOPHYSIOLOGY

Hirsutism is usually due to one of the following conditions:

(1) Increased androgen production by the ovaries or adrenal glands.

(2) Decreased production of SHBG by the liver, with resultant increase in bioavailable androgen.

(3) Increased sensitivity of the hair follicle to normal amounts of circulating androgen.

Causes of hirsutism are listed in Table 22–1.

EVALUATION

The initial evaluation should include a thorough history, especially the age at onset of hirsutism and rapidity of development, as well as length and regularity of menstrual cycles. This information is important because *rapid onset* of severe hirsutism suggests a neoplasm.

Physical examination should include documentation of hirsute areas and signs of virilism, as well as a pelvic examination to exclude the diagnosis of an ovarian mass.

During the initial laboratory evaluation, serum testosterone, androstenedione, and DHEAS levels should be obtained. If menstrual abnormalities or galactorrhea are present, serum prolactin, thyroid-stimulating hormone (TSH), luteinizing hormone (LH), and follicle-stimulating hormone (FSH) levels should also be measured.

Table 22–1. Causes of hirsutism.

Ovarian disorders
   Polycystic ovary syndrome
   Hyperthecosis
   Androgen-producing tumors
Adrenal disorders
   Congenital or adult-onset adrenal hyperplasia
   Cushing's disease or syndrome
   Androgen-producing tumor
Drugs
   Danazol
   Phenytoin
   Minoxidil
Other disorders
   Postmenopausal state
   Suppression of SHBG production by the liver (eg, obesity, acromegaly)
   Idiopathic hirsutism

Figure 22–1 outlines the evaluation of hirsute women with elevated testosterone or androstenedione levels. If the DHEAS level is normal but the testosterone or androstenedione levels are slightly elevated, **polycystic ovary syndrome** or a variant thereof is the likely diagnosis. In this case, ovarian suppression (eg, combination oral contraceptives) is usually beneficial. If testosterone or androstenedione levels are markedly elevated, an ovarian or adrenal tumor must be excluded by obtaining computerized tomographic (CT) or magnetic resonance imaging (MRI) scans of these organs.

Polycystic ovary syndrome is classically characterized by the triad of hirsutism, obesity, and oligomenorrhea or amenorrhea; however, patients are not necessarily very hirsute or obese. In this syndrome, the ovary produces increased amounts of androgens, which results in the peripheral manifestation of hirsutism. In the ovary, the androgens induce follicular atresia, which results in anovulation. The increased ovarian androgen production may be the result of increased stromal stimulation by elevated levels of LH (increased amplitude and frequency of LH pulses from the pituitary). The increased androgen produced by the ovaries is con-

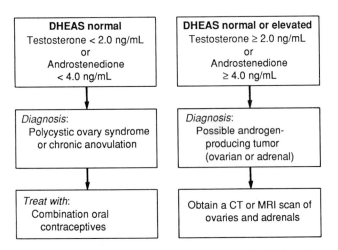

Figure 22–1. Evaluation of hirsute women with elevated testosterone and androstenedione levels.

verted to estrogen by the aromatase enzyme in peripheral adipose stroma. This increase in estrogen sensitizes the pituitary to gonado-tropin-releasing hormone (GnRH) and results in further increases in pituitary LH production, which stimulates the ovary to produce more androgen; thus, a "vicious cycle" is established that perpetu-ates itself. The cycle can sometimes be broken by weight loss (de-creased fat stroma) or temporarily by ovarian suppression (eg, oral contraceptive therapy), which decreases androgen production and reduces the symptoms of hirsutism. If the patient desires preg-nancy, the antiestrogen clomiphene citrate may be used (see Chap-ter 23).

Figure 22–2 outlines the evaluation of hirsute women with ele-vated DHEAS levels. When serum DHEAS is elevated, an adrenal androgen source is likely. An overnight dexamethasone suppres-sion test *excludes* Cushing's disease (a pituitary tumor that pro-duces corticotropin [adrenocorticotropic hormone, ACTH]) or syndrome (adrenal tumor) if serum cortisol levels are suppressed to less than 5 μg/dL.

When the serum cortisol level is suppressed to less than 5 μg/dL, the diagnosis is probably **late-onset adrenal hyperplasia.** The most common, but not exclusive, cause of this condition is a deficiency of the enzyme 21-hydroxylase in the adrenal gland. The pathway to cortisol formation has a relative block, and the precursor (17-hydroxyprogesterone) is present in an elevated concentration and is shunted into the androgen-forming path-way. Thus, the adrenal secretes increased amounts of androgens into circulation, which may result in hirsutism. Late-onset adre-nal hyperplasia resulting from a 21-hydroxylase deficiency is diagnosed when measured serum levels of 17-hydroxyprogester-one are elevated. Treatment consists of low doses of glucocorti-coid (eg, dexamethasone, 0.5 mg daily at bedtime) on a chronic basis.

When serum cortisol levels are not suppressed after an over-night dexamethasone suppression test, 24-hour urine free cortisol should be measured, and a high-dose dexamethasone suppression test should be performed. This test consists of administering 2.0 mg of dexamethasone orally 4 times a day for 7 days. If cortisol suppression does occur after the seventh day, it is unlikely that an adrenal tumor is present; rather, the diagnosis is probably a pituitary (ACTH) secreting adenoma. If cortisol suppression does not occur, an adrenal tumor must be ruled out.

If all androgen levels are normal, hirsutism is most likely due

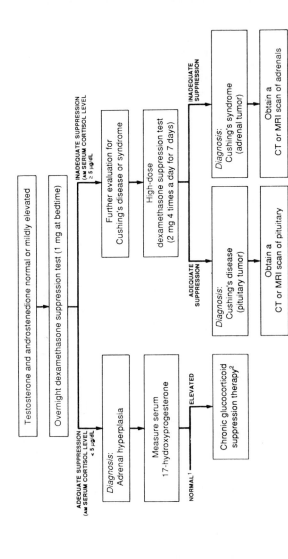

Figure 22–2. Evaluation of hirsute women with elevated dehydroepiandrosterone sulfate (DHEAS) levels. [1]Refer to reproductive endocrinologist for further evaluation. [2]Under the direction of a reproductive endocrinologist.

Testosterone and androstenedione normal or mildly elevated

Overnight dexamethasone suppression test (1 mg at bedtime)

ADEQUATE SUPPRESSION
(AM SERUM CORTISOL LEVEL < 5 μg/dL

INADEQUATE SUPPRESSION
(AM SERUM CORTISOL LEVEL ≥ 5 μg/dL

Diagnosis:
Adrenal hyperplasia

Further evaluation for
Cushing's disease or syndrome

Measure serum
17-hydroxyprogesterone

High-dose
dexamethasone suppression test
(2 mg 4 times a day for 7 days)

NORMAL[1]

ELEVATED

ADEQUATE
SUPPRESSION

INADEQUATE
SUPPRESSION

Chronic glucocorticoid
suppression therapy[2]

Diagnosis:
Cushing's disease
(pituitary tumor)

Diagnosis:
Cushing's syndrome
(adrenal tumor)

Obtain a
CT or MRI scan of pituitary

Obtain a
CT or MRI scan of adrenals

to increased end organ sensitivity to circulating androgen and may be treated with antiandrogens.

TREATMENT

Treatment is aimed at reducing ovarian or adrenal androgen overproduction or opposing the effect of androgens at the level of the hair follicle. Of course, any tumor that is discovered must be dealt with appropriately.

Since increased androgen production is most often from an ovarian source, oral contraceptives are usually used as initial treatment. They inhibit gonadotropin secretion, thus reducing gonadotropin-stimulated ovarian androgen production. Low-dose estrogen ($\leq$ 35 μg) pills are effective in suppressing androgens; therefore, higher dose pills are unnecessary. Generally, it is best to choose pills containing progestins that have minimal androgenic side effects (eg, norethindrone, ethynodiol diacetate). Usually, serum androgen levels are suppressed after 1 month of therapy, and clinical improvement in hair growth occurs after 5–6 months.

If, after 2 months, androgen levels are only minimally suppressed, an adrenal source of androgen production should be suspected and investigated, if this was not done initially. If there is a significant adrenal component to the source of androgen production and if a tumor has been excluded, treatment with glucocorticoids is indicated. In this case, prednisone, 5.0–7.5 mg/d, or dexamethasone, 0.5–0.75 mg/d, is given.

Alternative treatments to ovarian suppression by oral contraceptives are being investigated. These alternatives include the use of GnRH analogs, which inhibit pituitary gonadotropin secretion and thus inhibit gonadal steroid secretion.

Women who have normal circulating androgen levels and thus whose hirsutism is likely due to increased sensitivity of the hair follicle to androgen stimulation may be treated with antiandrogens. These medications prevent androgens from binding to their receptors. The most commonly used antiandrogen is spironolactone, in doses ranging from 100–200 mg/d. Side effects may include polyuria, irregular uterine bleeding, and, rarely, hyperkalemia. Antiandrogens may also be used in combination with oral contraceptives for more efficacious treatment in severe cases of hirsutism. Androgen production will be decreased and its effect at the end organ will be inhibited.

Cosmetic treatment is also an important adjunct to medical therapy. Electrolysis, shaving, or waxing removes coarse hair already present while the medical treatment will, in time, convert new hair growth from coarse to fine. Eventually, the need for cosmetic treatment will decrease.

SUGGESTED READINGS

Glass RH: Hirsutism. In: *Office Gynecology,* 3rd ed. Williams & Wilkins, 1988.

Speroff L, Glass RH, Kase NG: Anovulation. In: *Clinical Gynecologic Endocrinology & Infertility,* 4th ed. Williams & Wilkins, 1988.

Investigation of the Infertile Couple | 23

Janice L. Andreyko, MD

Infertility, defined as an involuntary reduction in the ability to conceive a pregnancy after 1 year of coitus, afflicts approximately 15% of couples in the USA. Normal monthly fecundity rate is 20–25%; 80% of fertile couples will achieve pregnancy in 1 year.

The following five major factors contribute to infertility:

(1) Male factor (35–40%).
(2) Tubal factor (20–25%).
(3) Ovulatory dysfunction (15–20%).
(4) Uterine and cervical factors (5–15%).
(5) Unexplained infertility (10–15%).

More than one factor may be involved in 10–15% of couples.

EVALUATION OF MALE FACTORS

History & Physical Examination

The history should include inquiries regarding past testicular injuries, undescended testes, mumps, orchitis, venereal disease, heat exposure, radiation, and chemical or toxin exposure. Drugs of particular concern include marijuana and anabolic steroids. Physical examination should include assessment for possible hypospadias, varicocele, or abnormal testicular size or consistency.

Laboratory Studies

A. Semen Analysis: Semen analysis should be performed after 2–3 days of abstinence. Normal parameters are listed in Table 23–1. A positive postcoital test result (forwardly progressing sperm in clear cervical mucus) is suggestive of a good sperm count and motility; however, the sperm count can only be accurately assessed by a formal semen analysis.

B. Sperm Antibodies: If there is clumping of sperm on semen

Table 23-1. Parameters of normal semen.[1]

Volume	2.5–6.0 mL
Count	≥ 20,000,000/mL
Motility	≥ 50% progressive motility
Morphology	≥ 60% normal forms
Liquefaction	≤ 30 min
Agglutination	Minimal
Infection	No white cells or bacteria

[1] Tested 2 hours after ejaculation.

analysis, sperm antibody tests may be performed. Sperm or serum may be evaluated; the presence of antibodies directly bound to the sperm has the most clinical significance.

C. Sperm Penetration Assay: The sperm penetration assay (SPA) is a test of the biological functioning of sperm. If human sperm are able to penetrate hamster eggs, they may be able to fertilize human eggs.

D. Endocrine Tests: Endocrine tests (serum levels of luteinizing hormone [LH], follicle-stimulating hormone [FSH], testosterone, and prolactin) as well as a testicular biopsy may be indicated if androgen status is clinically reduced.

EVALUATION OF FEMALE FACTORS

Tubal Factor

A. History and Physical Examination: Fallopian tubes are sometimes damaged as a result of venereal disease, pelvic inflammatory disease, or past use of an intrauterine contraceptive device. A history of a ruptured appendix may also suggest pelvic adhesive disease. Chronic pelvic inflammatory disease may also cause chronic pelvic pain. Physical examination is usually not very helpful, unless an inflammatory mass is present, which may be felt on palpation.

B. Hysterosalpingogram: In this procedure, radiopaque dye (water or oil based) is injected through the cervix into the uterus (Figure 23–1). The dye then flows through the fallopian tubes if they are patent or fills the tubes if a hydrosalpinx is present. The pelvis is imaged by x-ray. This procedure also provides information about the size and conformation of the uterus but does not evaluate the pelvis for the presence of adhesions. A hysterosalpingo-

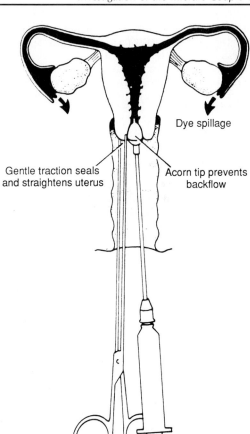

Figure 23-1. Hysterosalpingogram. *(Reproduced, with permission, from Seibel MM: Infertility: A Comprehensive Text. Appleton & Lange, 1990.)*

gram does not require anesthesia but does cause some pelvic discomfort. There is a small risk of aggravating pelvic inflammation, and antibiotic coverage is often used.

C. Laparoscopy: This outpatient surgical procedure requires a general anesthetic (Figure 23-2). A scope with a fiberoptic light source is introduced into the peritoneal cavity after insufflation of the abdomen with carbon dioxide. Insufflation is performed through a needle introduced into the abdomen under the umbilicus. The carbon dioxide minimizes the chance of trauma to an underlying viscus as the trochar is placed into the abdomen and also lifts the abdominal wall to allow visualization. Laparoscopy allows a thorough visualization of the pelvis to diagnose such problems as pelvic inflammatory disease and endometriosis. A considerable amount of surgery can be performed at the time of laparoscopy, especially with use of laser technology.

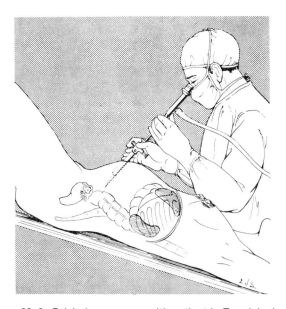

Figure 23-2. Pelvic laparoscopy with patient in Trendelenburg position. *(Reproduced, with permission, from Long AE: Chapter 5 in:* Current Obstetric & Gynecologic Diagnosis & Treatment, *4th ed. Benson RC [editor]. Lange, 1982.)*

D. Therapy: Depending on the degree of tubal damage and the age of the patient, she may benefit most from either tubal surgery or in vitro fertilization (IVF). When the fallopian tubes are patent and the damage is slight, lysis of adhesions may yield a pregnancy rate as high as 40% within 1 year. When the tubes are severely damaged, IVF results in a higher pregnancy rate than tubal surgery and reduces the chance of an ectopic pregnancy.

Ovulatory Dysfunction

A. History and Physical Examination: A history of irregular menstrual cycles strongly suggests oligo-ovulation or anovulation. A history of or physical finding of galactorrhea or hirsutism may suggest hyperprolactinemia or polycystic ovary syndrome.

B. Documentation of Ovulation: Documenting ovulation may include any or all of the following: basal body temperature monitoring, looking for a sustained rise of approximately 0.4° F after ovulation (Figure 23–3); measurement of serum progesterone (> 10 ng/mL) in the midluteal phase; and ultrasonographic documentation of the disappearance of the preovulatory follicle. Ovulation may be predicted based either on serum or urine measurement of the LH level to detect the LH surge or on sonographic identification of a dominant follicle.

Even if ovulation is occurring, the corpus luteum may not function adequately, resulting in a low luteal-phase progesterone level. Inadequate progesterone production may result in improper preparation of the endometrium for embryo implantation. This may be documented by endometrial biopsy, which will reveal a lining less advanced than it should be.

If anovulatory cycles are occurring or if there is evidence of an inadequate luteal phase, hormonal evaluation should include measurement of serum LH, FSH, prolactin, thyroid function, and, if there is evidence of hirsutism or virilism, serum androgen levels. Treatment may involve the use of such medications as clomiphene citrate.

Clomiphene citrate is a nonsteroidal agent taken orally that is used as an antiestrogen. It occupies nuclear estrogen receptors for long periods of time and reduces the concentration of estrogen receptors by inhibiting their replenishment. Therefore, the hypothalamic-pituitary axis cannot respond to the true endogenous estrogen level in the circulation. This effect results in increased FSH and LH release from the pituitary, which supports follicle maturation and the ovulatory process. The patients who respond best to clomiphene are anovulatory women with normal endogenous es-

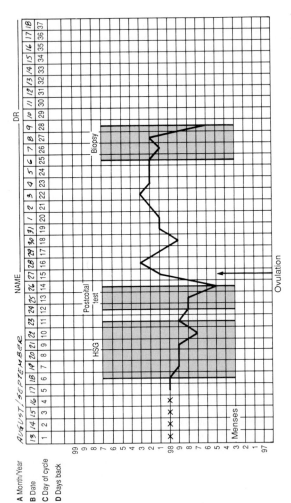

Figure 23-3. Basal body temperature chart demonstrates schedule for testing. (Modified and reproduced, with permission, from Seibel MM: Infertility: A Comprehensive Text. Appleton & Lange, 1990.)

trogen levels. Many of these patients are diagnosed with the polycystic ovary syndrome. In these patients, inappropriate gonadal-hypothalamic-pituitary feedback results in lack of consistent ovulation. Alteration of pulsatile gonadotropin secretion by the use of clomiphene results in ovulation in 80% of patients.

Clomiphene is usually begun on the fourth or fifth day of the menstrual cycle at a dose of 50 mg/d and is continued for 5 days. Ovulation should occur 1 week after the last pill is taken. If ovulation does not occur, the dose may be increased in subsequent cycles by 50 mg/d per cycle up to a maximum of 200 mg/d. The dose that results in ovulation may be repeated for 3–4 cycles before the patient is considered to have failed clomiphene treatment. Subsequent steps include addition of human chorionic gonadotropin (hCG) at midcycle to trigger ovulation or a change to human menopausal gonadotropin (Pergonal) treatment.

Ovulation after clomiphene treatment may be documented by monitoring basal body temperature, urine LH levels, or serum progesterone levels. The couple should be instructed to have sexual intercourse the day after the LH surge, as detected using an LH kit, or every second day for 1 week beginning 5 days after the last clomiphene dose. In well-selected patients, 80% ovulate, and half of these become pregnant in 3–4 cycles. The multiple pregnancy rate is 5%, most of which are twins. Side effects include hot flushes, headache, mood swings, visual symptoms, nausea, and bloating.

If hypothalamic amenorrhea is present or if clomiphene treatment is unsuccessful, the use of human menopausal gonadotropins (Pergonal) may be required. This treatment involves daily injections of Pergonal, each ampule of which contains LH and FSH. This method excludes any endogenous ovarian control of the cycle. Therefore, its use must be carefully monitored by serial ultrasonograms of the ovarian follicles and serial serum estradiol measurements. If too many follicles (usually more than 4) are developing or if serum estradiol is too high, ovulation should not be triggered (ie, hCG should not be given) to avoid the complications of multifetal pregnancy and hyperstimulation. Even with close monitoring, the multiple pregnancy rate with Pergonal treatment is 20–25%.

Ovarian hyperstimulation syndrome includes ovarian enlargement with abdominal bloating, discomfort, and weight gain. As a result of this syndrome, the ovaries leak fluid into the peritoneal cavity, and severe cases may involve ascites, pleural effusions, and intravascular hypovolemia with oliguria and thrombosis. The most severe cases can be life threatening. Laboratory evaluation reveals hemoconcentration, rising blood urea nitrogen, hyperkalemia, and acidemia. Treatment involves bed rest, analgesia, and monitoring of electrolytes, weight gain, and urine output. Intravenous crystalloid and colloid therapy is usually used. *Pelvic examinations must be avoided* to prevent rupture of the enlarged, fragile ovaries. The syndrome resolves in approximately 7 days if the patient is not pregnant and 2–3 weeks if she is.

The recent availability of the gonadotropin-releasing hormone (GnRH) pump allows administration of GnRH in a pulsatile fashion to mimic its release from the hypothalamus and stimulate pulsatile release of LH and FSH from the pituitary. Thus, the GnRH pump is a useful alternative for treating hypothalamic amenorrhea.

Uterine & Cervical Factors

A. History: Inquiry should be made regarding previous uterine surgery (eg, dilatation and curettage), which could result in endometrial scarring (Asherman's syndrome), and cone biopsy of the cervix, which could compromise mucus production.

B. Hysteroscopy: A hysteroscopy is an examination of the uterine cavity with a fiberoptic scope using a distention medium, such as carbon dioxide or high-molecular-weight dextran (Figure 23–4). If a uterine septum, adhesions, polyps, or small fibroids are present, they can be surgically removed through the hysteroscope.

C. Postcoital Test: This test allows not only some assessment of sperm quality but also evaluation of the quantity and quality of the cervical mucus. The mucus is aspirated from the endocervix at midcycle, just before anticipated ovulation, approximately 10–12 hours after coitus. The mucus is placed on a slide and examined for clarity, the distance it can be stretched (spinnbarkeit), and the presence of progressively motile sperm. As the mucus dries, it should form a fern pattern, indicating the influence of preovulatory levels of estrogen. Table 23–2 lists the criteria for cervical mucus evaluation. When the mucus quality is poor, it may sometimes be improved by oral administration of estrogen or it may be bypassed by intrauterine insemination of washed sperm.

UNEXPLAINED INFERTILITY

This term is used when no cause for infertility can be demonstrated, as is the case with about 15% of infertile couples. With

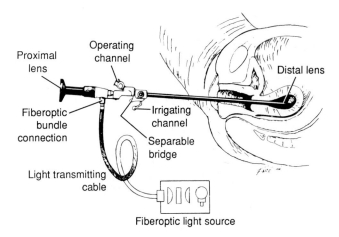

Figure 23-4. Diagram of hysteroscope in use. *(Reproduced, with permission, from Valle RF, Sciarra JJ: Minn Med 1974; 57:892.)*

advancing technology, explanations will likely be forthcoming. Currently, treatment for unexplained fertility is empiric. Some women respond to ovulation induction (eg, clomiphene or hMG) combined with intrauterine insemination of washed sperm at the time of ovulation. However, some couples require assisted technologies, such as gamete intrafallopian transfer (GIFT) or in vitro fertilization to assist conception. Still other couples may conceive with no intervention at all, but require a longer time than most couples to do so.

Table 23-2. Rating system for evaluating cervical mucus.

	Assigned Value[1]			
	0	**1**	**2**	**3**
Amount (mL)	None	0.1	0.2	0.3
Spinnbarkeit (cm)	None	1-4	5-8	9
Ferning	None	Atypical	2+	3+
Cellularity	11	6-10	1-5	Occasional
Viscosity	4+	3+	2+	1+

[1]After the scores are added together, the mucus is rated as follows: optimal = 15; 10 = favorable; 5 = hostile.

Table 23-3. Typical evaluation of an infertile couple.

Primary procedures
    History and physical examination
    Documentation of ovulation
    Semen analysis
    Postcoital test
    Demonstration of tubal patency, usually by hysterosalpingogram
Secondary procedures (guided by results of primary procedures)
    Ultrasonographic monitoring of cycle
    Hormonal evaluation
    Endometrial biopsy
    Sperm antibody test
    Sperm penetration assay
    Laparoscopy
    Hysteroscopy

A typical evaluation of an infertile couple follows the steps outlined in Table 23-3. The evaluation must also include an assessment of how much investigation and treatment the couple wishes to pursue. All investigations and treatment alternatives must be discussed thoroughly, and the treatment must be individualized. Once diagnoses are established, probabilities of success of different treatments must be presented to the couple so that informed choices can be made and so that the couple will embark on treatment with realistic expectations.

SUGGESTED READING

Seibel MM: Workup of the infertile couple. In: *Infertility: A Comprehensive Text.* Appleton & Lange, 1990.

Recent Advances in Infertility | 24

Janice L. Andreyko, MD

GONADOTROPIN-RELEASING HORMONE ANALOGUES

Gonadotropin-releasing hormone (GnRH) is a 10-amino acid protein synthesized by the hypothalamus of the brain. It is responsible for the release of luteinizing hormone (LH) and follicle-stimulating hormone (FSH), both of which are important in the regulation of gonadal function. Therefore, GnRH is the brain peptide that governs steroid hormone production by the gonad and ovulation itself in females. It is secreted in a pulsatile fashion, which is necessary to ensure proper pituitary and gonadal function.

Since GnRH was first synthesized in 1971, more than 2000 analogues of GnRH have been synthesized, some agonistic and some antagonistic. The original incentive for developing the agonists was to treat anovulation. Because the half-life of native GnRH is only 4–8 minutes, it was hoped that long-acting agonists would be more practical. However, the potent agonists that were developed had a paradoxical effect of initially stimulating the release of LH and FSH, but then inhibiting release of these gonadotropins when used on a chronic basis. The receptors for GnRH on the pituitary gland become desensitized, and the secretion of LH and FSH decreases. This property of the agonistic analogues has led to their subsequent testing and use for many conditions in men, women, and children (Table 24–1). However, there are two areas in which GnRH analogues have been specifically used to treat infertile women: for treatment of endometriosis (which may be associated with infertility) and for ovulation induction. Both topics are discussed below.

Because these compounds are proteins, they are broken down by gastric secretions and therefore have little activity if given orally. The most common methods of administration are by daily subcutaneous injections, by long-acting monthly depot injections, or by nasal spray.

Table 24-1. Clinical uses of GnRH analogues.

Women	Men	Children
Treatment of endometriosis, uterine fibroids, hirsutism, and premenstrual syndrome. Augmentation or induction of ovulation.	Treatment of Metastatic carcinoma of the prostate.	Treatment of precocious puberty.

Endometriosis

GnRH agonists are highly successful in treating endometriosis. In all studies pelvic pain and pain with periods were reduced. Objectively, the extent of endometriosis was assessed before and after treatment by laparoscopy. This method of directly viewing the pelvis showed significant reduction in the amount of disease after use of GnRH agonists.

In one double-blind study, women were divided into 3 groups and received daily doses of either 400 or 800 μg of the GnRH analogue nafarelin or 800 mg of danazol. The extent of disease was reduced equally in all 3 groups with an average 43% reduction. Eighty percent of patients were asymptomatic or only minimally symptomatic after the first month of treatment. Of the women enrolled in the trial who desired pregnancy, 52% of those receiving 800 μg/d of nafarelin were successful, as were 30% of those taking the 400-μg dosage and 36% of those taking danazol. These differences were not statistically significant.

Side effects of the GnRH analogue are those primarily due to hypoestrogenemia: 90% report hot flashes, whereas others complain of vaginal dryness, headaches, and mood swings. Bone densitometry by quantitative computerized tomography and dual-photon absorptiometry have shown decreases in bone mass, but these changes were reversed after treatment was discontinued.

Ovulation Induction or Augmentation

In addition to their usefulness in in vitro fertilization (IVF), GnRH analogues are useful to induce ovulation in patients who do not undergo IVF. Because use of agonistic analogues results first in a release of gonadotropins from the pituitary gland before suppression is achieved, protocols of ovulation induction were developed that capitalize on this phenomenon. This "flare" phase has been used in conjunction with exogenous gonadotropins in patients who were resistant to or required large doses of exogenous gonadotropins in order to ovulate.

In addition, patients with disordered endogenous gonadotropin secretion (eg, patients with polycystic ovary syndrome) may benefit from suppression of endogenous gonadotropins before initiation of exogenous gonadotropin therapy.

IN VITRO FERTILIZATION

The first child resulting from IVF was born in 1978 in England. Since then, thousands of children have been born throughout the world as a result of IVF. The initial indication for IVF was tubal disease, and this condition remains the principal reason for which IVF is sought as a treatment. However, other indications now include endometriosis, male factor infertility, and unexplained infertility.

The essential steps in a successful IVF cycle include ovulation induction with monitoring of follicle size and serum estradiol levels, oocyte retrieval, oocyte fertilization and division, embryo transfer to the uterus, and successful implantation.

Ovulation Stimulation

Most protocols have involved use of human menopausal gonadotropins with FSH and LH (Pergonal) or clomiphene plus Pergonal given concomitantly. More recently, the use of GnRH agonists plus Pergonal has eliminated premature LH surges and resulted in increased numbers of mature oocytes at retrieval. The GnRH agonist may be given as a subcutaneous injection or as a nasal spray. Pergonal is administered by daily intramuscular injections.

Monitoring of the Cycle

The cycle is usually monitored by sequential ultrasounds to assess ovarian follicle size and number. In the last few years, endovaginal transducers have become available that allow precise ultrasonographic ovarian assessment because the transducer is placed almost adjacent to the ovaries. Serum estradiol levels are also monitored by a rapid radioimmunoassay, which provides same-day results. The goal of stimulation is to achieve a lead follicle that is 17 mm in diameter with at least 3–4 other follicles with a diameter of

14–15 mm or greater. Serum estradiol levels should be approximately 300 pg/mL per follicle greater than 14 mm in diameter.

Once the above criteria are achieved, a single dose of 5,000 or 10,000 units of human chorionic gonadotropin (hCG) is administered to induce final follicular maturation.

Oocyte Retrieval

Oocytes are retrieved approximately 35 hours after hCG injection, about 1 hour before the anticipated time of ovulation. Initially, oocytes were retrieved laparoscopically, but with the advent of the endovaginal ultrasound transducer, follicles are now usually aspirated using endovaginal ultrasonography to guide the needle (Figure 24–1). A sterile needle is placed alongside the transducer, and the needle is passed through the vaginal wall into each ovary. Once the needle is in the ovary, follicles are aspirated in succession. This technique does not require anesthesia; analgesia and sedation with short-acting narcotics and sedatives are sufficient. The majority of patients feel minimal discomfort.

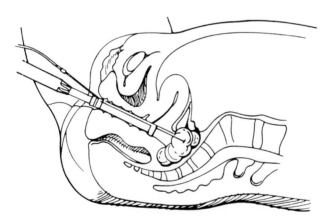

Figure 24–1. Oocyte retrieval. In the transvaginal approach, under vaginal ultrasound guidance, a needle is passed through the posterior vaginal wall, traversing a small amount of tissue, into the ovarian follicle, where it is used for aspiration. *(Reproduced, with permission, from Stangel JJ [editor]: Infertility Surgery: A Multimethod Approach to Female Reproductive Surgery. Appleton & Lange, 1990.)*

Oocyte Culture

The skill of an embryologist is required to identify the oocyte under magnification. After eggs are identified, they are inseminated approximately 4–12 hours later, depending on the maturity of the oocyte. Sperm are first washed with culture medium, then approximately 50,000–100,000 are added to each Petri dish containing an oocyte.

The day after insemination, the eggs are examined for evidence of fertilization (presence of two pronuclei). They are examined again the following day for signs of cleavage and are then transferred to the uterus.

Embryo Transfer

Embryos are most commonly transferred between the 4- and 8-cell stage, approximately 48 hours after retrieval. The chance of success increases with the number of embryos transferred, and usually up to 6 embryos are replaced. Multiple pregnancy rates are approximately 30% with 4–6 embryos. Couples are given this information when making a decision as to how many embryos to transfer at one time. They are made aware of complications of multifetal pregnancies as well as the availability of a technique called fetal reduction in which, for example, a triplet pregnancy may be reduced to a twin pregnancy. In experienced hands, the fetal reduction procedure has a 5–10% chance of resulting in loss of the total pregnancy. If this procedure is acceptable to a couple, they will usually choose to have a higher number of embryos (eg, 6 instead of 4) transferred.

The luteal phase of the cycle is supported with sequential hCG injection or intramuscular progesterone injections.

If extra embryos are present, they may be cryopreserved for transfer to the uterus in a future cycle. Success rates for this procedure are approximately 5–10%.

Overall, success rates for clinical pregnancies and delivery of healthy newborns vary tremendously between programs. Currently, the most successful programs have rates of approximately 30% clinical pregnancy per embryo transfer. The live birth rate in the USA (ie, the national average in 1988) is 12% per cycle in which embryos are transferred.

GAMETE INTRA-FALLOPIAN TRANSFER (GIFT)

GIFT is a technique offered to couples when the female partner has at least one patent, normal fallopian tube. In addition, it is usually offered to patients with unexplained infertility. In this procedure, ovulation is induced in the same manner as that for IVF, but the oocytes are retrieved by means of laparoscopy or minilaparotomy. The oocytes are then placed with the partner's sperm into a transfer catheter. The catheter is gently introduced into the distal 3 cm of the fallopian tube, and the gametes are discharged into the tube (usually 2 eggs/tube). The eggs and sperm are then allowed the opportunity to fertilize in the natural environment of the tube, and the embryos progress to the uterus. Success rates with this technique have been slightly higher than with IVF. Ectopic pregnancies occur 3–8% of the time. If many oocytes are retrieved, some may still be fertilized in vitro and later transferred to the uterus, or they may be frozen for replacement in a subsequent cycle.

SUGGESTED READINGS

Andreyko JL et al: Therapeutic uses of gonadotropin-releasing hormone analogs. *Obstet Gynecol Surv* 1987;**42**:1.

Henzl MR et al: Administration of nasal nafarelin as compared with oral danazol for endometriosis. *N Engl J M* 1988;**318**:485.

Speroff L, Glass RH, Kase NG: In vitro fertilization. In: *Clinical gynecologic Endocrinology & Infertility,* 4th ed. Williams & Wilkins, 1988.

Section IV:
Gynecologic Oncology

Vulvar & Vaginal Cancer | 25

Kris Strohbehn, MD, & Lisa G. Sandles, MD

INTRAEPITHELIAL NEOPLASIA

Etiology & Classification

Current research links carcinogenic changes in the squamous epithelium of the female genital tract to certain stimuli. The term "field response" comprises the simultaneous changes in the cervical, vulvar, and vaginal epithelium that can occur in response to these stimuli. Recent evidence links sexually transmitted viruses, especially specific types of human papillomavirus (HPV), to changes in the epithelium of these organs.

Classification

Depending on severity, these changes are classified as mild, moderate, or severe dysplasia. These types of dysplasia are also termed type I, II, or III intraepithelial neoplasia, respectively. In the cervix, these changes have been characterized as premalignant states, some of which develop into frankly invasive carcinoma (see Chapter 4). Although studies linking vulvar intraepithelial neoplasia (VIN, Chapter 16) and vaginal intraepithelial neoplasia (VAIN) to invasive carcinoma are inconclusive, most researchers believe that the behavior is similar. If left untreated, some of the cases of VIN and VAIN will progress to frankly invasive cancer.

Symptoms & Signs

VAIN is often asymptomatic and consists of multifocal lesions that usually occur on the upper third of the vagina. The Papanicolaou smears of patients with VAIN are frequently abnormal. In one-half of patients with VAIN, another genitourinary site is involved with dysplasia or carcinoma.

Diagnosis

Diagnosis of the lesions is confirmed by colposcopically directed biopsy, which is performed with Kevorkian-Younge or Tischler punch biopsy forceps. Postmenopausal women should be treated with topically applied estrogen cream for 2 weeks before colposcopic examination to better define the abnormal areas.

Treatment

The most effective treatments are as follows: (1) local excision of the lesion (if unifocal); (2) laser ablation; (3) topical 5-fluorouracil application; or (4) total vaginectomy with split-thickness skin graft for more extensive lesions. Acetic acid (3%) or Schiller's solution (iodine) is painted in the vagina to highlight the areas that should be biopsied.

VULVAR CANCER

Incidence

Vulvar cancer is rare. It is the fourth most common malignant neoplasm involving the female reproductive tract, following endometrial, cervical, and ovarian cancers. Vulvar cancer most frequently occurs in elderly women, and the average age at detection is 65 years. Nonetheless, 15% of vulvar cancers occur in patients younger than 40 years of age.

Histology

The most common histologic type of vulvar cancer is **squamous cell carcinoma,** which represents 90% of all cases. **Melanoma** of the vulva accounts for 4–5% of vulvar cancers, but 15% of all cases of melanoma in women occur primarily in the vulva. Approximately 8% of carcinomas located on the vulva are metastases.

Etiology

The cause of vulvar cancers is unknown. Recent evidence links certain types of human papillomavirus to vulvar carcinoma.

Symptoms & Signs

The most common symptoms of vulvar cancer are as follows: pruritis, an asymptomatic mass, an ulcer, vulvar discharge, or dysuria; vulvar pain and bleeding can occur in the advanced stages. Physical signs on examination may include a polypoid mass, a plaque, or an ulcer. The lesions may be white, red, or even hyperpigmented. There may be an associated inguinal adenopathy. It is important to perform a complete gynecologic examination to exclude the possibility that the tumor is metastatic from the vagina, cervix, or urethra.

Diagnosis

Any questionable lesion on the vulva should be biopsied. The dermatologic rule "when in doubt, biopsy" is especially pertinent regarding the vulva. The biopsy is best performed using a Keye's punch biopsy (4 or 6 mm). The area to be biopsied should be infiltrated with 1–2% lidocaine after cleaning with povidone-iodine. The most suspicious areas should be biopsied. When heterogeneous lesions are present, several areas should be sampled. Colposcopy is useful for locating the most suspicious areas to biopsy if a gross lesion is not visible.

Staging

The staging of vulvar carcinoma is shown in Table 25–1.

Workup

After vulvar cancer has been diagnosed, further evaluation and preoperative workup should include the following: (1) a full history and complete physical examination, including close inspection of the skin, rectovaginal examination, and careful palpation of the inguinal regions to check for lymph node metastases; (2) complete blood count, serum chemistry panel, and urinalysis; (3) electrocardiogram; (4) chest radiograph; (5) barium enema, proctosigmoidoscopy, and cystoscopy, as indicated; and (6) abdominal-pelvic computerized tomographic (CT) scan if inguinal nodes are suspicious for metastases.

Treatment

Treatment of vulvar cancer traditionally has involved en bloc radical vulvectomy with dissection of the pelvic nodes for stages I and II. Because of the many complications of a radical vulvectomy, many physicians currently advocate a less radical procedure for stage I carcinoma of the vulva. Patients with this stage of cancer are unlikely to have pelvic node involvement and can be treated with inguinal node dissection and local radical excision of the tu-

Table 25-1. International Federation of Gynecology and Obstetrics (FIGO) staging of carcinoma of the vulva.[1]

Stage 0 Tis	Carcinoma in situ, intraepithelial carcinoma.
Stage I TI N0 M0	Tumor confined to the vulva or perineum—2 cm or less in greatest dimension. No nodal metastasis.
Stage II T2 N0 M0	Tumor confined to the vulva or perineum—more than 2 cm in greatest dimension. No nodal metastasis.
Stage III T3 N0 M0 T3 N1 M0 T1 N1 M0 T2 N1 M0	Tumor of any size with: (1) adjacent spread to the lower urethra or the vagina, or the anus, or (2) unilateral regional lymph node metastasis.
Stage IVA T1 N2 M0 T2 N2 M0 T3 N2 M0 T4 Any N M0	Tumor invades any of the following: Upper urethra, bladder mucosa, rectal mucosa, pelvic bone or bilateral regional node metastasis.
Stage IVB Any T, Any N, MI	Any distant metastasis, including pelvic lymph nodes.

[1] 1988 revision.

mor. Many physicians believe that inguinal node dissection need only be ipsilateral if the primary lesion is unilateral. If 2 or more nodes are found to be positive after unilateral inguinal dissection, then bilateral inguinal lymph node dissection and pelvic irradiation are recommended.

For stage II and III disease, radical vulvectomy is recommended. Radiation therapy is used adjuvantly for extensive inguinal node involvement or with pelvic node involvement. For stage IV vulvar carcinoma, radiation therapy is used pre- or postoperatively and may be combined with chemotherapy. Preoperative chemotherapy and radiation therapy may reduce the extent of surgery that is subsequently required. Total pelvic exenteration is an option in rare instances.

Complications

Complications of treatment are directly correlated to how extensive the surgery, radiation, or combination therapy is. Complications include (1) psychosexual dysfunction and disturbances of body image; (2) wound breakdown (in approximately one-half of all radical operations); (3) lymphedema, especially when pelvic nodes are dissected; and (4) stress urinary incontinence.

Prognosis

The 5-year survival rates for stages I and II are approximately 90% and 80%, respectively. These survival rates decrease significantly for stages III and IV.

The prognosis of vulvar cancer is strongly associated with lymph node metastases, the likelihood of which correlate with the depth of tumor invasion, the size of the tumor, presence of vascular space invasion, and the histologic grade. Five-year survival rates are about 90% for patients with stage I or II tumors with negative inguinal nodes but decrease to about 50% if inguinal nodes are positive. The spread of vulvar cancer is fairly systematic and follows the lymphatic drainage of the vulva.

Lymphatic drainage is usually to the ipsilateral nodes, although it can also involve the contralateral side, especially if the tumor is midline. The lymph drains via the mons pubis and then follows the superficial inguinal nodes to the deep femoral nodes (including an important anatomic landmark, **Cloquet's node**—the most cephalad deep femoral node, just below the inguinal [Poupart's] ligament) and finally to the deep pelvic nodes. The pelvic lymph nodes are involved about 20% of the time when the excised inguinal nodes are positive for cancer. As noted above, pelvic nodal involvement is related to the size of the tumor, depth of invasion, and inguinal nodal metastases. The 5-year survival rate falls to about 20–25% if pelvic node metastases are present.

Other Vulvar Cancers

Malignant melanoma is the second most common type of vulvar cancer. It usually arises from a junctional or compound nevus. It is frequently located on the labia minora or clitoris. Prognosis is related to size of the lesion and the depth of invasion. The prognosis is extremely poor unless it is diagnosed very early. The staging is based on Clark's or Breslow's classification of malignant melanoma, which can be found in most medical oncology or dermatology texts. Treatment usually involves radical vulvectomy and pelvic lymph node dissection, although more conservative approaches are advocated for the lower stage lesions.

Other rare vulvar cancers include **basal cell carcinoma, adeno-**

carcinoma (including Bartholin's gland), **verrucous carcinoma** and **sarcoma of the vulva;** further information on these rare tumors is beyond the scope of this review and can be found in the references listed as suggested readings.

VAGINAL CANCER

Incidence

Primary vaginal cancer is extremely rare. Vaginal cancer is most often secondary to extension or metastasis from a tumor from another source. These metastatic tumors may arise from the cervix, endometrium, ovary, urethra, vulva, bladder, rectum, and gestational trophoblastic neoplasia. A tumor in the vagina is considered to be a primary vaginal cancer only if these other sites are excluded as the primary source of the cancer.

Histology

Squamous cell carcinoma is the most common type of vaginal cancer; sarcoma, melanoma, and adenocarcinoma (including clear cell) occur rarely.

Etiology

The cause of squamous cell vaginal cancer is unknown but may be linked to human papillomavirus. Predisposing factors include a prior history of invasive or preinvasive carcinoma of the cervix, prior pelvic radiation, and smoking.

Clear cell adenocarcinoma of the vagina has been linked to maternal ingestion of diethylstilbestrol (DES) and subsequent in utero exposure to the fetus. The estimated risk of developing clear cell carcinoma in an exposed individual is approximately 0.1%. The usual age at diagnosis ranges from 14 to 30 years old. Medical follow-up for daughters exposed to DES is discussed in Chapter 4. Adenocarcinoma may also arise from foci of endometriosis.

Symptoms & Signs

Symptoms include a persistent bloody vaginal discharge, which is usually painless. Vaginal cancer can also present as a vaginal mass or ulceration. The lesions are most frequently located on the upper half of the vagina.

Diagnosis

Diagnosis is confirmed by biopsy.

Staging

    The staging of vaginal cancer is outlined in Table 25–2.

Treatment

    Surgical treatment of vaginal cancer plays a limited role. Radical hysterectomy, vaginectomy, and pelvic node dissection can be performed for the very early stages involving the upper vagina. A vulvectomy is performed if the lower third of the vagina is involved. Most physicians recommend radiation therapy for the early stages. Radiation is the only indicated therapy for stages III and IV, although total pelvic exenteration is occasionally performed for certain cases of stage IVA disease.

    The treatment of clear cell carcinoma is similar to that for other vaginal cancers but with emphasis on preservation of vaginal and ovarian function when possible, given the young age of these patients. The 5-year survival approaches that of cancers of the cervix and upper vagina.

Prognosis

    The 5-year survival rate is about 40–50% for all types of vaginal cancer. Recently, this 5-year survival rate has improved signifi-

Table 25-2. Staging of carcinoma of the vagina[1]

Preinvasive carcinoma	
Stage 0	Carcinoma in situ, intraepithelial carcinoma.
Invasive carcinoma	
Stage I	The carcinoma is limited to the vaginal wall.
Stage II	The carcinoma has involved the subvaginal tissue but has not extended to the pelvic wall.
Stage III	The carcinoma has extended to the pelvic wall.
Stage IV	The carcinoma has extended beyond the true pelvis or has involved the mucosa of the bladder or rectum. A bullous edema as such does not permit allotment of a case to stage IV.
Stage IVA	Spread of the growth to adjacent organs.
Stage IVB	Spread to distant organs.

[1]American Joint Committee for Cancer Staging and End-Results Reporting: Task Force on Gynecologic Sites: Staging System for Cancer at Gynecologic Sites, 1979.

cantly, with some centers reporting a 90% 5-year survival for stage I disease.

The spread of vaginal cancer usually follows the lymphatic drainage according to the following general rules: the upper third drains in the same pathways as the cervix; the middle third may drain to any pelvic nodes, and may follow lymphatic drainage of the rectum or bladder; the lower third usually drains in the same route as the vulva (ie, to the inguinal nodes).

Other Vaginal Cancers

Melanoma, verrucous carcinoma and sarcomas of the vagina are extremely rare. Two rare vaginal tumors, sarcoma botryoides and endodermal sinus tumor, occur in the first few years of life. These tumors are discussed in the suggested reading references.

SUGGESTED READINGS

Berek JS, Hacker NF: *Practical Gynecologic Oncology.* Williams & Wilkins, 1989.

DiSaia PJ, Creasman WT: *Clinical Gynecologic Oncology,* 3rd ed. Mosby, 1989.

Kurman RJ: *Blaustein's Pathology of the Female Genital Tract,* 3rd ed. Springer-Verlag, 1987.

Karen K. Smith McCune, MD, PhD, & Lisa G. Sandles, MD

EPIDEMIOLOGY

Incidence

Cervical cancer is the eighth most common cause of cancer-related death in women of all ages in the USA, with 15,000 new cases of cervical cancer diagnosed each year. In the world, cervical cancer is the most common cancer in women. The incidence is decreased by screening populations using cervical cytologic studies (Papanicolaou smear, see Chapter 4); the incidence is 4.5 per 100,000 in screened populations and 29 per 100,000 in unscreened populations. In addition, the disease tends to be detected at an earlier stage in screened populations.

Risk Factors

The following factors are associated with an increased risk for **squamous cell carcinoma** of the cervix: early age at first coitus; more than 4 sexual partners; a history of genital warts (human papillomavirus [HPV] infection); smoking; race (eg, blacks are at greater risk than whites); and an immunocompromised host. The sexual history of the partner is also important, including the number of his sexual partners, whether a previous partner has had cervical cancer, and whether he has a history of penile cancer. The incidence is higher in minorities and women from low socioeconomic status; the incidence is very low in Amish, Jewish, Mormon, and Muslim women.

Risk factors for **adenocarcinoma** of the cervix are different than those for squamous tumors and include nulliparity, diabetes, older age, and in up to 20% of cases, HPV. **Clear cell carcinoma,** one of the histological variants of adenocarcinoma, is often associated with in utero exposure to diethylstilbestrol (DES).

Etiology

Squamous cell carcinoma appears to be caused by cervical infection with HPV. HPV is a double-stranded DNA virus with a genome of approximately 8000 base pairs. More than 60 subtypes of the virus have been identified, and they are distinguished by their propensity to grow in restricted distribution, such as on the hands, soles of the feet, larynx, or genital tract. The most common HPV subtypes found in the genital tract are 6 and 11, which cause genital warts, and 16, 18, 31, 33, 35, 45, 51, 52, and 56, which are associated with cervical intraepithelial neoplasia (dysplasia) and cervical squamous cell cancer.

Multiple lines of evidence support the causal association of HPV with cervical cancer. Epidemiologically, the risk factors for cervical cancer correlate with those for a sexually transmitted disease. In biochemical assays, more than 90% of cervical squamous cell carcinomas contain viral DNA. Viral DNA is also found in some adenocarcinomas of the cervix, although not as often as in squamous cell carcinomas. The prevalence of HPV in young, sexually active populations may be as high as 20-25%; therefore, it is obvious that, in the vast majority of cases, the infection is controlled through immunological means, and other events must be required for development of cervical cancer.

Screening

Because approximately 20% of Papanicolaou smears are falsely negative in patients with cervical cancer, the cervix must be carefully inspected during annual pelvic examinations. If abnormalities are found on the cervix, they are biopsied or the patient should be examined by an experienced colposcopist (see Chapter 4).

CLINICAL FEATURES

Symptoms

The most common symptom is abnormal bleeding, including hypermenorrhea, intermenstrual bleeding, postcoital bleeding, and postmenopausal bleeding. Any abnormal bleeding in both reproductive-aged and postmenopausal women must be investigated by performing a Papanicolaou smear and by carefully examining the cervix. (In postmenopausal women, an endometrial biopsy should also be performed). Abnormal vaginal discharge is a less common complaint. Pain indicates more advanced disease, as does weight loss, anorexia, urinary frequency, or loss of urine or stool through the vagina. Cervical cancer is asymptomatic in 8-10% of patients and is often first detected during a pelvic examination or as a result of abnormal findings on a Papanicolaou smear.

Findings

Cervical cancers may appear as exophytic, smooth, or ulcerative. There may be no visible tumor on the ectocervix, but the cervix may be distended by a large endocervical lesion, creating a barrel-shaped cervix. The tumor may extend onto the vagina or be palpable lateral to the cervix on rectovaginal examination (parametrial extension). Finding a fixed mass during a bimanual examination suggests that the tumor extends to the pelvic side wall. The presence of urine or feces in the vagina indicates the extension of the tumor into the bladder or rectum associated with a fistula. Ascites is rare in cervical cancer. It is also unusual for cervical cancer to spread to the ovaries, so the presence of an adnexal mass suggests a separate process. In extremely advanced disease, the supraclavicular nodes may be involved, more often on the left than on the right.

Diagnosis

Diagnosis must be based on biopsy specimens. If an obvious lesion is visible during the physical examination, it must be biopsied directly, and cone biopsy is contraindicated because of the risk of severe hemorrhage. If no lesion is seen grossly but the Papanicolaou smear is abnormal, colposcopy must be performed to detect abnormal areas for biopsy. If the results of the colposcopic examination are negative, a cone biopsy must be performed. It is important to obtain a histologic diagnosis, even in the presence of a gross tumor, because of the different clinical behaviors of the various cell types and to confirm that the cervix is the site of origin.

Natural History

Cervical cancer tends to infiltrate locally into the parametria and vagina and to spread into the pelvic lymph node chains (hypogastric, external iliac, and obturator). Spread initially occurs laterally as a result of fascial planes anterior and posterior to the cervix. However, in advanced disease, the bladder or rectum is invaded. Next, the growth spreads to the common iliac or aortic lymph nodes, and finally tumors may spread to distant organs, such as the lung and liver, by hematogenous routes. In advanced disease, death may result from uremia due to ureteral obstruction, anemia secondary to hemorrhage, bowel obstruction, respiratory failure as a result of pulmonary metastases, or pulmonary emboli.

HISTOLOGY

The most common cell type is squamous cell carcinoma, which accounts for approximately 75% of all cervical cancers. These tumors are assessed histologically by the degree of differentiation, with grade 1 being well differentiated and grade 3 poorly differentiated.

Adenocarcinoma accounts for approximately 25% of cervical cancers. Histologic subtypes include **endocervical** and **endometriod** patterns, clear cell, and **adenoma malignum** (very well differentiated endocervical adenocarcinoma). Mixed patterns of adenosquamous carcinoma can occur. Rare cell types are the **neuroendocrine** and **carcinoid (small cell) carcinomas. Verrucous carcinoma** is an indolent, locally invasive, warty growth that rarely metastasizes but shows stromal invasion. **Metastatic tumors** from the endometrium and ovaries can also occur in the cervix.

STAGING

Staging is based on the natural course of the disease: stage I is confined to the cervix, stage II extends onto the vagina or into the parametria, stage III extends to the pelvic side wall, and stage IV involves the bladder or rectum (IVA) or distant disease (IVB) (Table 26–1 and Figure 26–1). Note that staging is based on clinical assessment. The evaluation for patients with cervical cancer is outlined in Table 26–2. Careful bimanual and rectovaginal examinations need to be performed to assess the degree of lateral spread of the tumor.

Although staging is determined clinically, additional studies, such as computerized tomographic (CT) scans or magnetic resonance imaging (MRI) scans, are often used to determine the true extent of disease on which treatment is based. If CT or MRI scans reveal enlarged pelvic or periaortic lymph nodes, samples should be biopsied using CT-guided needle aspiration. When the results of fine needle aspiration biopsies of suspicious lymph nodes detected on radiographic images are either negative or inconclusive, surgical exploration of para-aortic lymph nodes may be indicated. If surgical staging is performed before radiation therapy is administered, the extraperitoneal, rather than the transperitoneal, approach is advocated to reduce complications, such as bowel obstruction.

Table 26–1. International Federation of Gynecology and Obstetrics (FIGO) staging of cervical cancer.

Stage I	Lesion is confined to the cervix (extension to the uterus should be ignored).
IA	Microscopic disease or visible lesion with minimal invasion.
IA1	Minimal microscopically detected invasion.
IA2	Invasion less than 5 mm deep and 7 mm wide.
IB	Lesions with dimensions greater than stage IA2 lesions.
Stage II	Carcinoma extends beyond cervix but not onto the pelvic side wall. Involves parametria or upper two-thirds of the vagina.
IIA	Involves upper two-thirds of the vagina.
IIB	Involves parametria.
Stage III	Carcinoma extends onto pelvic wall or involves the lower one-third of the vagina. Includes all cases with hydronephrosis or nonfunctioning kidney.
IIIA	Involves lower one-third of the vagina but no extension onto the pelvic side wall.
IIIB	Extension onto the pelvic side wall or hydronephrosis.
Stage IV	Carcinoma extends beyond pelvis or invades bowel or bladder mucosa.
IVA	Spread of growth to adjacent organs.
IVB	Spread of growth to distant organs.

The diagnosis of microinvasive cancer (stage IA) must be based on the results of a cone biopsy with negative margins. Simple cervical biopsy specimens are not sufficient because more advanced disease may be missed. Although the international system classifies a lesion as microinvasive if its depth of invasion is 5 mm or less (measured from the basement membrane), the Society of Gynecologic Oncologists (SGO) in 1974 adopted 3 mm as the depth for defining microinvasive disease, with more than 3 mm of invasion being treated as invasive cancer. This classification is supported by the fact that, if the depth of invasion is 3 mm or less, the risk of lymph node metastases is less than 1%; between 3 and 5 mm of invasion, the risk of node metastases is about 7–8%. In addition, for a lesion to qualify as microinvasive according to SGO criteria, there must be no vascular or lymphatic space involvement, and the entire lesion must be encompassed on a cone biopsy (ie, cone margins are negative). Most gynecologic oncologists also re-

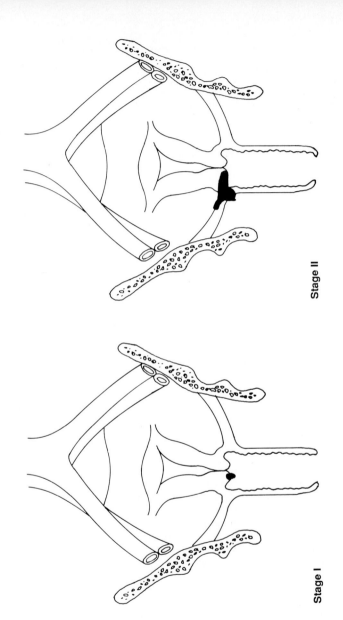

Stage II

Stage I

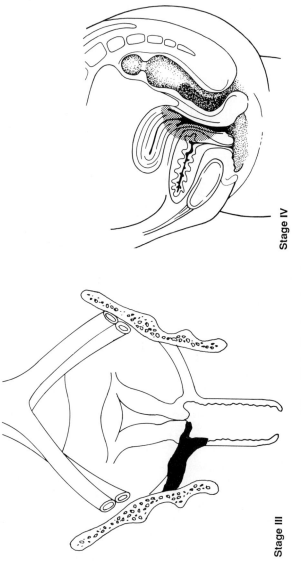

Stage IV

Stage III

Figure 26-1. Staging of cervical cancer (Table 26-1).

Table 26-2. Pretreatment evaluations of patients with cervical cancer.

All Patients	Patients With Advanced Disease
Pelvic, bimanual, rectovaginal examinations	Cystoscopy
Biopsies, colposcopy	Proctosigmoidoscopy
Stool guaiac	CT scan of upper abdomen[1]
Chest x-ray	
Liver function tests	
Serum calcium	
Intravenous pyelogram, or CT with contrast,[1] or MRI[1]	

[1] CT and MRI scans are only diagnostic tools; the information they provide is not used in the staging. Enlarged lymph nodes should be aspirated by fine needle or biopsied at the time of surgery.

quire that the tumor be nonconfluent, meaning that no focus of invasion larger than 1 mm^2 is present.

Note that the above SGO definition is applicable *only* to squamous cell lesions. There is currently no universally accepted definition for microinvasive adenocarcinoma of the cervix.

TREATMENT

Stage IA (Microinvasive) Lesions (Squamous Lesions Only)

Simple hysterectomy is adequate therapy for a stage IA squamous lesion if the following criteria are met: the lesion is less than 3 mm deep with no vascular or lymphatic space involvement, the pattern of invasion is nonconfluent, and all of the lesion is encompassed by cone biopsy.

Stage IB & IIA Tumors

Two options are available for treating stage IB and small stage IIA tumors: (1) radical hysterectomy with lymph node dissection or (2) pelvic irradiation. The cure rates are the same, and the complication rates are equivalent. Thus, the selection of the treatment modality depends on patient variables (Table 26-3).

A. Radical Hysterectomy: The basic principle of radical hysterectomy (Meigs-Wertheim operation) is wide dissection and excision of the cardinal and uterosacral ligaments adjacent to the cervix to remove a wide area surrounding the tumor, which potentially

Table 26-3. Comparison of surgical and radiation treatment for stage IB and IIA cervical cancer.

Surgery: radical hysterectomy and lymph node dissection
  Advantages
    Preserves ovarian function in young women.
    Preserves the vagina.
    Radiation therapy remains an option in case of recurrence.
  Disadvantages
    Leads to bladder or bowel dysfunction (usually temporary).
    May cause ureteral damage and pulmonary embolus.
    Contraindicated in obese patients and patients with multiple
      medical problems.
Radiation therapy
  Advantages
    Eliminates the need for surgery.
    Can be safely used in obese patients and those who are poor
      surgical risks for medical reasons.
  Disadvantages
    Multiple visits are required.
    Contraindicated for acutely psychotic or uncooperative patients.
    May cause vaginal dryness or dyspareunia.
    May cause radiation enteritis.
    Contraindicated in the presence of a pelvic kidney, diverticulitis,
      tubo-ovarian abscess, or adnexal mass.

---

contains early metastases. A 2- to 3-cm-wide margin of vagina is removed. The pelvic lymph nodes (hypogastric, external iliac, and obturator) and lower common iliac nodes are completely dissected. If nodal involvement is found or if surgical margins are positive, pelvic irradiation is delivered postoperatively, although it is not clear that such therapy affects survival. Complications of this operation include ureteral stricture or fistula, bladder or bowel dysfunction (usually transient), venous thrombosis and pulmonary embolus, lymphocysts, lymphedema, and vaginal shortening.

B. Radiation Therapy: Radiation treatment currently consists of delivery of high-energy photons that are absorbed by tissue and converted into electrons and radicals, causing chemical damage inside cells. The most damaging and lethal changes occur in DNA, resulting in impaired mitosis. The presence of oxygen in tissues enhances the damage of radiation by causing increased production of radicals and irreversible damage to the DNA. Cells are most sensitive to radiation damage during mitosis, hence mitotically active tissues are more sensitive.

Radiation can be delivered by external beam (**teletherapy**) or by local application to tissues (**brachytherapy**). Two types of brachytherapy are available for the cervix: intracavitary radiation therapy involves inserting a tandem into the cervix and adjacent vaginal ovoids (Fletcher-Suit applicator) into which radiation sources are loaded; interstitial application (Syed perineal template) consists of inserting needles into the cervix and parametria through which radiation sources are loaded. A Syed template is used for bulky or asymmetrical lesions that cannot be adequately treated using a standard Fletcher-Suit system.

Radiation doses are limited by the tolerance of the surrounding tissues. The cervix is very radioresistant and can tolerate doses in excess of 10,000 rads. Doses delivered to the pelvis are limited because the bowel and bladder can withstand radiation levels of only 6,000–7,000 rads. The goal in treating cervical cancer is to deliver as much radiation as possible internally as brachytherapy. If the tumor is large or asymmetric, teletherapy is applied first to shrink the tumor so that brachytherapy can then be applied.

Radiosensitizers are chemicals that enhance the damaging effect of radiation. Hydroxyurea administered in conjunction with radiation therapy has been demonstrated to improve outcome compared with radiation treatment alone. Cisplatin, a chemotherapeutic agent, is also being studied as a radiosensitizer.

Complications of radiation therapy are related to effects on the surrounding irradiated tissues and consist of enteritis with diarrhea, proctitis, cystitis, bowel fibrosis and obstruction, bowel or bladder fistulae, vaginal stenosis and dyspareunia, and hematologic suppression.

Stage IIB Through Stage IV Tumors

Currently, treatment of stage IIB, III, and IV tumors consists primarily of radiation therapy. Staging laparotomy can be helpful to assess the highest level of lymph node involvement. In cases of distant spread of disease, palliative therapy is indicated and consists of radiation to painful areas and liberal use of analgesia. Until recently, chemotherapy was thought to have limited usefulness in treating cervical cancer and thus was usually reserved for patients who did not respond to radiation treatment and who were not candidates for exenteration. In these cases, the best results have been obtained with regimens containing cisplatin. Lately, however, chemotherapy has also been used initially to treat locally advanced (stage IIB–IVA) lesions before subsequent radiation therapy or surgery.

Recurring Cancer

Recurrences of cancer in the central pelvis in patients who have undergone radiation therapy can be treated with pelvic exenteration, with a 30–50% 5-year survival rate. This is a radical operation that involves removal of the bladder, which requires ureteral diversion into an ileal or transverse colon loop (anterior exenteration); removal of the rectum and anus with construction of a colostomy (posterior exenteration); and removal of part or all of the vagina with myocutaneous flaps to create a neovagina if preservation of sexual function is desired. Total pelvic exenteration combines the anterior and posterior operations.

Contraindications to exenteration include extrapelvic metastases, extension of the tumor to the pelvic side wall, poor surgical risk, sciatic nerve involvement, and psychological reluctance to deal with the subsequent altered body image.

Follow-Up

After treatment for cervical cancer, surveillance should consist of a visit every 3 months for a careful physical examination, Papanicolaou smear and pelvic examination, and a yearly chest x-ray. After 2 years without recurrence, the patient is seen every 6 months for the same assessment. A periodic CT scan is used by some physicians.

PROGNOSIS

Squamous Cell Carcinoma

Overall, the 5-year survival rate for all stages of squamous cell carcinoma is 50%. The best guide for predicting the outcome is the stage of the disease at diagnosis (Table 26–4). Survival rates decrease 30–50% when metastases to lymph nodes occur. The extent of vascular space involvement, the depth of invasion, and the size of

Table 26–4. Survival of patients with squamous cell carcinoma of the cervix according to the stage of disease at diagnosis.

Stage	Survival Rate 5 yr After Treatment (%)
I	60–90
II	60–75
III	30–35
IV	10
Overall	50

the tumor also correlate well with the predicted outcome. The grade of the tumor does not correlate as well with the outcome.

Adenocarcinoma

Generally, adenocarcinoma is detected somewhat later than squamous cell carcinoma because abnormal endocervical cells are not as easily detected on Papanicolaou smears. In addition, the lesions are often not seen during examinations because they are located in the endocervical canal. For these reasons, the 5-year survival rate is lower than that for squamous cell carcinomas, with the overall survival rate being about 50%. Stage, nodal involvement, vascular space involvement, depth of invasion, and size and grade of tumor correlate with outcome.

CERVICAL CANCER DURING PREGNANCY

The incidence of cervical cancer during pregnancy is approximately 1 per 2000 pregnancies; conversely, approximately 1 in every 34 cases of cervical cancer are diagnosed during pregnancy or within 1 year postpartum. Symptoms are similar to those in nonpregnant women.

If the fetal age is 20 weeks or less, treatment is usually indicated. Early lesions (stage IB) can be treated either with radiation therapy or radical hysterectomy and bilateral pelvic lymph node dissection. More advanced lesions are treated with radiation therapy. Spontaneous abortion usually occurs shortly after initiation of radiation therapy. If the fetal age is more than 20 weeks, treatment may be delayed until the fetus is viable. Treatment may then consist of cesarean section with immediate radical hysterectomy and bilateral pelvic lymphadenectomy or cesarean section followed by radiation therapy.

SUGGESTED READINGS

Droegemueller W et al: Chapter 27 in: *Comprehensive Gynecology,* Mosby, 1987.

Hacker NF et al: Carcinoma of the cervix associated with pregnancy. *Obstet Gynecol* 1982;**59:**735.

Henson D, Tarone R: An epidemiologic study of cancer of the cervix, vagina, and vulva based on the Third National Cancer Survey in the United States. *Am J Obstet Gynecol* 1977;**129:**525.

Mattingly RF, Thompson JD: Chapter 32 in: *TeLinde's Operative Gynecology,* 6th ed. Lippincott, 1985.

Endometrial Cancer | 27

Michael L. Pearl, MD

EPIDEMIOLOGY

Adenocarcinoma represents more than 90% of endometrial cancers and is the most common gynecologic cancer in the USA. Occurring more frequently than ovarian and cervical cancer combined, it ranks fourth (33,000 estimated new cases in 1991) among all cancers in women, behind breast (142,000 cases), colorectal (78,000 cases), and lung (54,000 cases) cancers. Predominately a postmenopausal disease, the average age at diagnosis is 58 years. Only 2–5% of cases are diagnosed in women under 40 years of age; however, 20–25% of patients are premenopausal.

The etiology of endometrial cancer is unknown, but a large body of clinical evidence implicates unopposed estrogen as a major factor. There is a well-documented association between the use of exogenous estrogen and the development of endometrial hyperplasia and subsequent adenocarcinoma. In addition, disorders characterized by chronic endogenous estrogen production in the absence of progesterone have a high incidence of associated adenocarcinoma.

Several factors have been observed to be correlated with an increased risk of development of endometrial cancer (Table 27–1).

ENDOMETRIAL HYPERPLASIA

Endometrial hyperplasia results from prolonged estrogen stimulation of a susceptible endometrium in the absence of progestational effects. This disorder tends to progress through a continuum from simple to complex to atypical hyperplasia. **Cytologic atypia** is the single most important factor when assessing the risk of progression to carcinoma.

Abnormal uterine bleeding or vaginal discharge are the most common symptoms. The diagnosis is made through histopatho-

Table 27–1. Associated risk factors for endometrial cancer.

Hormones
Exogenous
Endogenous
Obesity
Nulliparity
Diabetes
Anovulation
Late menopause
Pelvic irradiation

logic evaluation of endometrial tissue obtained by biopsy or by dilatation and curettage. The appropriate treatment depends on many factors, including the type of hyperplasia and the patient's reproductive status (Figure 27–1). For peri- and postmenopausal women who are good surgical candidates, total abdominal hysterectomy and bilateral salpingo-oophorectomy is recommended for atypical hyperplasias and for hyperplasia without atypia if it is recurrent. In patients for whom surgery is contraindicated, treatment with progestins is indicated. Progestins are continued indefinitely, and periodic evaluation by endometrial biopsy is recommended because of the possibility of recurrent or persistent disease.

ENDOMETRIAL CARCINOMA

Clinical Features

A. Symptoms: Postmenopausal bleeding is the presenting complaint in more than 90% of cases of endometrial cancer. Occasionally, a purulent, blood-tinged discharge is the initial symptom. Pain is a late complaint, often correlating with metastatic disease.

The best guideline to follow in assessing postmenopausal bleeding is to assume that the bleeding is caused by endometrial cancer until proved otherwise. About 20% of patients with postmenopausal bleeding will have endometrial cancer. Additional causes of postmenopausal bleeding include atrophic changes in the vagina or endometrium, cervical or endometrial polyps, and other gynecologic cancers. In younger women, endometrial cancer almost invariably presents as abnormal uterine bleeding. In these women, persistent or recurrent abnormal bleeding should prompt an evaluation for endometrial cancer.

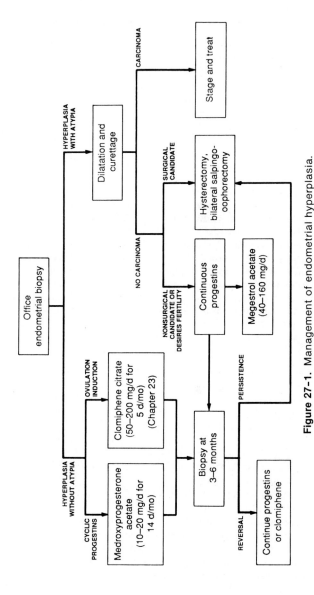

Figure 27-1. Management of endometrial hyperplasia.

273

B. Physical Examination: The general examination is often unremarkable, although obesity, hypertension, and the stigmas of diabetes may be associated findings. During the pelvic examination, the vaginal vault and cervix rarely demonstrate anything other than bleeding from the os. During the bimanual and recto-vaginal examinations, the physician should evaluate the cervix for consistency; the uterus for size, shape, and mobility; the adnexa for masses; and the parametria for nodularity or induration. Careful palpation of the vagina is indicated to exclude vaginal metastases, which may be mucosal or submucosal.

C. Diagnosis: Histologic examination of endometrial tissue is necessary to diagnose endometrial cancer. For most patients, the initial evaluation can be performed on an outpatient basis. A Papanicolaou smear should be obtained, followed by endocervical curettage and endometrial biopsy. These steps are necessary to identify occult cervical carcinoma, or extension of endometrial cancer into the cervix. Formal dilatation and curettage (D&C) is mandated for any abnormality short of frank malignancy, inadequate evaluation due to cervical stenosis or insufficient tissue, or poor patient tolerance. The persistence of symptoms despite normal findings during the office examination also necessitates a D&C.

Pathophysiology

Adenocarcinoma of the uterus arises from endometrial glands. It may develop from preexisting hyperplasia or arise *de novo*. As adenocarcinoma grows, it invades the myometrium and may involve the cervix. Lymphatic spread to parametrial, pelvic, para-aortic, or inguinal nodes may occur. The risk of nodal metastasis depends on the tumor stage and grade, the depth of myometrial invasion, and whether the cervix is involved. Hematogenous spread to the lungs occurs infrequently and rarely to the liver or bone. Peritoneal implants may develop from transtubal or transmural spread. Once in the peritoneal cavity, endometrial carcinoma behaves similarly to ovarian cancer.

Classification & Staging

The majority of endometrial carcinomas are adenocarcinomas. Primary squamous cell carcinomas are extremely rare and highly malignant. The histologic type significantly affects the prognosis.

The stage is assigned on the basis of surgical-pathologic findings (Table 27–2). The majority of endometrial cancers (75%) are

Table 27-2. International Federation of Gynecology and Obstetrics (FIGO) surgical-pathologic staging of endometrial cancer.

International classification (staging)	
Stage 0	Atypical hyperplasia or carcinoma in situ.
Stage I	Confined to the uterine corpus.
IA	Limited to endometrium.
IB	Invasion of less than half of the myometrium.
IC	Invasion of more than half of the myometrium.
Stage II	Tumor extends to the cervix.
IIA	Endocervical gland involvement.
IIB	Cervical stromal invasion.
Stage III	Tumor extends outside the uterus but is confined to the true pelvis.
IIIA	Serosal or adnexal invasion or positive cytologic washings.
IIIB	Vaginal metastases.
IIIC	Metastases to pelvic or para-aortic lymph nodes.
Stage IV	Tumor extends outside the pelvis or invades the bladder or rectum.
IVA	Tumor invasion of bladder or bowel.
IVB	Distant metastases, including intra-abdominal or inguinal lymph nodes.
Histologic classification (all stages)	
Grade 1 (G1)	5% or less of nonsquamous or nonmorular solid growth pattern.
Grade 2 (G2)	6–50% of nonsquamous or nonmorular solid growth pattern.
Grade 3 (G3)	More than 50% of nonsquamous or nonmorular solid growth pattern.

stage I at the time of diagnosis. Once assigned, the stage cannot be altered. For optimal management, it is important that the initial staging be thorough, especially for apparently early disease.

Treatment

The optimal therapy for patients with endometrial cancer, especially stage I, remains controversial. Historically, stage I endometrial cancer in the USA has been treated with intracavitary radiation followed by immediate hysterectomy and bilateral salpingo-oophorectomy. Although this protocol remains a mainstay of therapy, there has recently been a shift toward initial surgical-pathologic staging. With this type of staging, patients at high risk for recurrence can be identified and therapy can be individualized.

A. Stage I (Confined to the Uterine Corpus): After the abdomen is opened with a vertical, midline incision, peritoneal washings are obtained for cytologic analysis, and the abdomen is carefully explored for evidence of metastases. Extrafascial total abdominal hysterectomy with bilateral salpingo-oophorectomy is the cornerstone of therapy. When patients have grade 1 (G1) or grade 2 (G2) tumors and less than one-third of the myometrium is involved, any palpable suspicious pelvic or para-aortic nodes are removed. For more advanced cases, hysterectomy is followed by selective pelvic and para-aortic lymphadenectomy.

When patients have G1 or G2 tumors and less than one-third of the myometrium is involved but the cytologic analyses of nodes and peritoneal tissue are negative, no further therapy is required. All other patients with more advanced disease frequently receive postoperative radiation therapy. According to this protocol, only 25–50% of patients will require postoperative therapy.

Radiation therapy is also indicated when pelvic or para-aortic node metastases are present. The risks and benefits of giving radiation therapy in patients who have deep myometrial invasion without nodal metastases are currently being evaluated. In this study, patients are selected randomly to receive either no further treatment or radiation therapy.

At the time of surgical staging, tumors should be evaluated for the presence or absence of estrogen and progesterone receptors. Such evaluation is important for two reasons: (1) prognostically, because patients who test positive for estrogen and positive for progesterone receptors have a better prognosis, and (2) therapeutically, because tumors that have estrogen and progesterone receptors are much more likely to respond to hormonal (progestin) therapy.

B. Stage II (Tumor Extends to the Cervix): There is a greater propensity for lymphatic spread when the tumor extends into the cervix, and therapy must encompass likely sites of metastasis. Stage IIA disease is managed similarly to stage I, grade 3 tumors. Clinically overt cervical involvement may be managed by radical hysterectomy or with preoperative pelvic radiation therapy, followed by simple hysterectomy, bilateral salpingo-oophorectomy, and para-aortic lymphadenectomy.

C. Stage III (Tumor Outside the Uterus but Confined to True Pelvis): Gross extrauterine disease is treated by tumor-reductive surgery. Patients with vaginal or parametrial involvement are treated with pelvic radiation followed by tumor-reductive surgery. Residual disease in both circumstances is treated with extended field radiation therapy or systemic therapy with hormones or cyto-toxic drugs.

D. Stage IV (Tumor Outside Pelvis or Invades Bladder or Rectum): Patients who are able to tolerate surgery should undergo tumor reduction, followed by systemic therapy with hormones or cytotoxic drugs. Patients with distant metastases or those who are too ill to undergo surgery are treated with systemic hormones or chemotherapy and palliative radiation therapy.

E. Hormonal Therapy: Numerous studies have documented the efficacy of progestins in treating advanced or recurrent endo-metrial carcinoma. Patients with extensive or recurrent disease and measurable levels of hormone receptors may be treated with high-dose progestins, either megestrol acetate, 80 mg orally 3 or 4 times a day, or medroxyprogesterone acetate, 50–100 mg orally 3 times a day. The maximum clinical response may not be seen for several months, and treatment should continue as long as the disease is stable. The measured hormone receptor content of the tumor is an important indicator of the response rate to hormonal therapy.

F. Chemotherapy: Patients with advanced or recurrent dis-ease who are not candidates for surgical or radiation therapy may be offered combination chemotherapy. Currently, the most active agents are cisplatin and doxorubicin.

G. Peritoneal Cytology: In approximately 10–15% of clinical patients with stage I disease, peritoneal cytologic test results are positive. The incidence increases with increasing grade, depth of invasion, and stage. The appropriate management of endometrial carcinoma with positive peritoneal cytologic findings remains un-settled because of insufficient data regarding recurrence risk and treatment. Currently, intraperitoneal ^{32}P (a radioactive isotope), whole abdominal radiation therapy, or progestins are often used.

H. Recurrent Disease: Approximately 70% of recurrences occur within 3 years after initial treatment. Local recurrences (pel-vic wall, vagina, parametrium) are most common in nonirradiated patients. In contrast, distant metastases (lung, abdomen, liver, or bone) are more frequent in patients who received radiation therapy with their primary therapy.

Local failures are treated with surgery, radiation, or a combi-nation of the two. Distant disease is treated with hormonal or cyto-toxic agents. Selective irradiation may be beneficial for palliation of brain or bone metastases.

Prognosis

Survival rates vary with the stage and grade of carcinoma (Table 27–3). Other significant prognostic factors include depth of

Table 27-3. Endometrial carcinoma distribution and survival by stage and grade.

Stage	Distribution (%)	5-year Survival Rate (%)
I	74.3	74.2
G1	39	81
G2	38	74
G3	23	50
II	14.7	57.4
III	7.2	29.2
IV	2.7	9.6

invasion, histologic type, vascular space involvement, positive peritoneal cytologic results, and nodal and adnexal metastases. In addition, many patients have serious concomitant medical disorders that contribute to the mortality rate.

SARCOMAS

Sarcomas are heterogeneous, highly malignant tumors that constitute 3–5% of all uterine cancers. The etiology is unknown, but 5–10% of women with mixed mesodermal sarcomas (tumors with both carcinoma and sarcoma components) have a history of prior pelvic irradiation. Sarcomas occur most frequently in the postmenopausal period but may affect any age group, including infants.

Functionally, the uterine sarcomas may be divided into 3 groups: (1) leiomyosarcomas, (2) stromal sarcomas, and (3) mixed mesodermal tumors. They are staged similarly to endometrial carcinomas (Table 27–2).

Postmenopausal bleeding is the most frequent symptom, but abdominal pain or distention and awareness of a pelvic mass are common. Often, the diagnosis is made following routine surgery for leiomyomas.

Therapy consists of total abdominal hysterectomy, bilateral salpingo-oophorectomy, and bilateral pelvic lymphadenectomy. Patients with advanced or recurrent disease are treated with radiation or chemotherapy.

Overall, the prognosis for patients with uterine sarcoma is dismal. More than 50% of stage I cases recur, and long-term survival with advanced disease is exceedingly unusual.

SUGGESTED READINGS

DiSaia PJ, Creasman WT: *Clinical Gynecologic Oncology,* 3rd ed. Mosby, 1989.

Kurman RJ (editor): *Blaustein's Pathology of the Female Genital Tract,* 3rd ed. Springer-Verlag, 1987.

Morrow CP, Townsend DE: *Synopis of Gynecologic Oncology,* 3rd ed. Churchill Livingstone, 1987.

28 | Ovarian Cancer

Michael L. Pearl, MD

EPIDEMIOLOGY

Ovarian cancer is the second most common cancer of the female genital tract. However, it is the most lethal, accounting for more than 50% of all deaths from gynecologic cancer. The American Cancer Society estimated that, in 1991, 20,700 new cases of ovarian cancer would be diagnosed and that 12,500 women would die of this disease. The mortality from ovarian cancer is greater than that from cervical and endometrial cancers combined. Only 35% of women diagnosed with ovarian cancer survive 5 years.

CLINICAL FEATURES

Symptoms

Early ovarian cancer is usually asymptomatic, or symptoms are so vague that they are not recognized by either the patient or her physician. Symptoms occur with progressive enlargement of the tumor and invasion of the surrounding structures. The presenting complaints are often of short duration and most commonly consist of abdominal distention and pain. Less frequently, abnormal vaginal bleeding may occur. Vague abdominal symptoms, including dyspepsia, mild anorexia or nausea, and indigestion may precede other symptoms by many months. *Note*: Any woman more than 40 years old with otherwise unexplained gastrointestinal symptoms should be evaluated for ovarian cancer. Encroachment of the tumor may also lead to urinary frequency, constipation, or dyspareunia.

Physical Examination

The results of the physical examination may be completely normal with early disease. The classic finding of abnormal distention associated with an abdominopelvic mass is a late occurrence.

During the pelvic examination, the lower genital tract usually has a normal appearance, although the vagina may be displaced by an extrinsic mass. An adnexal mass may be palpated during the bimanual examination. Characteristics that suggest malignancy include **bilaterality, fixation, an irregular contour,** and **a solid component.** It is important to feel for nodularity in the cul-de-sac or parametria that may represent tumor studding. *A palpable ovary in a postmenopausal woman is abnormal and needs immediate evaluation.*

With advanced disease, the patient may appear cachectic and chronically ill. The supraclavicular, axillary, and inguinal nodes should be palpated for metastases. Marked ascites is often present, although it may be difficult to distinguish from a large cystic mass. An "omental cake," or mestastic disease in the omentum, may be palpated anteriorly. Pleural effusions and lower extremity edema frequently occur. The thyroid gland, breasts, and rectum must be carefully examined for primary tumors metastatic to the ovary.

Diagnosis

The definitive diagnosis of ovarian cancer is based on findings on surgical exploration. The complete preoperative evaluation is outlined in Table 28–1. For those patients with suspected advanced disease, the preoperative preparation should include a mechanical and antibiotic bowel preparation, as well as prophylaxis against thromboembolic disease (eg, minidose heparin, sequential inflatable stockings).

Table 28-1. Preoperative evaluation for ovarian cancer.

Careful history
Complete physical examination
Mammogram
Pelvic examination with Papanicolaou smear
Complete blood count, urinalysis, and chemistry panel
Tumor markers
   For epithelial tumors: CA125, carcinoembryonic antigen (CEA)
   For germ cell tumors: human chorionic gonadotropic (hCG), alpha-
      fetoprotein (AFP), and lactic acid dehydrogenase (LDH)
Chest x-ray
Pelvic sonogram
Intravenous pyelogram (IVP)
Barium enema and gastrointestinal (GI) series (if indicated)
Computerized tomographic (CT) or magnetic resonance imaging (MRI)
   scan (if indicated) (CT may replace IVP and pelvic sonogram)

PATHOPHYSIOLOGY

The ovary gives rise to a wider variety of tumors than any other organ (Table 28–2). The primary ovarian cancers are divided into epithelial tumors, germ cell tumors, and sex cord–stromal tumors. The overwhelming majority (about 80%) of ovarian cancers in the USA are epithelial in origin.

Nearly every type of cancer has been reported to metastasize to the ovary. The most common types originate in the gastrointestinal system, breast, or pelvic organs. Other, less frequent, sources of metastases include carcinoid, lymphoma, and melanoma.

Once the cancer has reached the surface of the ovary, it can directly invade the adjacent structures. More commonly, viable tumor cells are shed directly into the peritoneal cavity and implant at multiple sites on the peritoneal serosal surfaces. Transdiaphragmatic spread may occur by lymphatic drainage to produce pleural or mediastinal disease. Lymphatic metastasis occurs primarily to the para-aortic nodes, as well as to the external iliac and hypogas-

Table 28-2 Classification of ovarian cancers.

Epithelial tumors
   Serous
   Mucinous
   Endometriod
   Clear cell
   Brenner
Germ cell tumors
   Dysgerminoma
   Endodermal sinus tumor
   Teratoma
   Embryonal carcinoma
   Choriocarcinoma
   Polyembryoma
   Mixed germ cell tumors
   Gonadoblastoma
Sex cord-stromal tumors
   Granulosa stromal cell
     Granulosa cell
     Thecoma or fibroma
   Sertoli-Leydig stromal cell
     Sertoli cell
     Leydig cell
   Gynandroblastoma
Metastatic tumors

tric nodes. Hematogenous dissemination occurs primarily in advanced disease. Lung and liver are the most common sites, followed by kidney, bone, adrenal glands, and spleen.

EPITHELIAL TUMORS

Epidemiology

The incidence of epithelial ovarian cancer is highest in industrialized countries. Over the past 50 years, the incidence of ovarian cancer has steadily increased in the Western world. The lifetime risk that women born in the USA will develop ovarian cancer is 1 in 70 (1.4%). The risk steadily increases with age, with a mean age at diagnosis of 60 years. Factors associated with an altered risk of ovarian cancer are listed in Table 28–3.

The cause of epithelial ovarian cancer is unknown. According to one current model, epithelial inclusion cysts form following microtrauma from incessant ovulation or through incorporation of foreign bodies. Stimulation of these cysts by elevated levels of gonadotropins or estrogens leads to differentiation, proliferation, and malignant transformation. The actual stimulus for malignant transformation remains unidentified.

Clinical Descriptions

A. Serous Carcinoma: Papillary serous carcinoma is the most common malignant epithelial tumor, representing 50% of all ovarian epithelial cancers. Grossly, they are primarily cystic and multilocular, with some solid components. The cyst fluid is usually

Table 28-3. Associated risk factors for ovarian cancer.

Increased risk
Family history of ovarian cancer
History of breast cancer
Nulliparity
Delayed pregnancy
Talc use
Obesity
Coffee consumption (> 4 cups/day)
Blood type A
Unopposed postmenopausal estrogen replacement
Reduced risk
Oral contraceptive use

turbid or bloody. Microscopically, the neoplastic epithelium resembles that of the fallopian tube. Psammoma bodies are common. These tumors grow rapidly, with early peritoneal spread. Bilateral involvement occurs in 33% of stage I tumors and is more frequent in advanced stages. Elevated CA125 levels are present in up to 80% of women with advanced serous cancers and are useful for monitoring disease progression.

B. Mucinous Carcinoma: Mucinous carcinoma accounts for 15% of the malignant ovarian epithelial tumors. Grossly, mucinous tumors are cystic and multilocular, with some solid components. They are often larger than the serous tumors, with reported cases as large as 50 cm in diameter. The cyst fluid varies from watery to gelatinous in consistency. Microscopically, the neoplastic epithelium resembles that of the large bowel or, rarely, the endocervix. Bilateral involvement occurs in less than 25%. Elevated carcinoembryonic antigen (CEA) levels are present in approximately 65% of patients with mucinous tumors and are useful for monitoring disease progression.

C. Endometrioid Carcinoma: Endometrioid carcinoma represents 10–15% of all malignant ovarian epithelial tumors. Grossly, they are cystic but frequently have solid components partially filling the lumen. Microscopically, the neoplastic epithelium is identical to that of typical endometrial adenocarcinoma. Squamous components, either benign or malignant, are common. Frequently, these tumors arise in foci of ovarian endometriosis, and they may coexist with endometrial adenocarcinoma. In such cases, because it may be impossible to determine the primary site, the tumors are considered dual primaries rather than metastatic. They are usually unilateral and locally invasive with late peritoneal spread.

D. Clear Cell Carcinoma: Clear cell carcinoma constitutes 5% of all malignant ovarian epithelial tumors. Grossly, they consist of a mixture of cystic and solid components. Microscopically, the neoplastic epithelium resembles cells of mesonephric origin. Frequently, they are admixed with elements of other epithelial tumors, primarily endometrioid and serous carcinomas. Bilateral involvement occurs in 40% of malignant clear cell tumors. They are locally invasive, with late peritoneal spread.

E. Brenner Tumors: Malignant Brenner tumors are very rare, representing less than 0.1% of all malignant ovarian epithelial tumors. Grossly, they are large and partially cystic, with the cystic components usually containing polypoid masses. Microscopically, the neoplastic epithelium consists of nests of cells similar to Walthard's inclusions found on the surface of the fallopian tube, mesosalpinx and mesoovarium, or in the ovarian hilus. They are usually unilateral.

F. Borderline Tumors: Borderline tumors are histologically intermediate between clearly benign and truly invasive tumors. Nearly 75% of borderline tumors are stage I at diagnosis. They are characterized by an absence of stromal invasion but with some features of malignancy. They follow an indolent course with infrequent, late recurrences, and the prognosis for long-term survival for patients is good, despite residual or recurrent disease.

Staging

Ovarian cancers are classified on the basis of surgical-pathologic findings (Table 28–4). Once assigned, the stage cannot be changed.

Treatment

A. Surgery: Surgery is the primary form of treatment in almost all therapeutic programs. A complete staging laparotomy is crucial to correctly determine the stage and to assess the need for adjuvant therapy (Table 28–5). The goal of surgery is debulking, that is, removal of the primary tumor and all tumor nodules greater than 2 cm in diameter without unduly jeopardizing the patient's life. Survival and response to chemotherapy is correlated with the volume of disease remaining after initial surgery.

"Second-look" procedures may be performed after a planned course of chemotherapy to assess whether a patient with a complete clinical response is pathologically free of disease.

Conservative surgery to preserve reproductive function in young women is indicated only for those rare patients with a surgically staged IA, low-grade tumor who strongly desire children. These patients should be followed closely and encouraged to complete their childbearing early. Subsequently, they should have their internal gynecologic organs removed.

B. Chemotherapy: Various systemic agents are active against ovarian cancer. For patients with advanced disease, combination chemotherapy using drugs with differing methods of action and toxicities is more efficacious than single-agent therapy. Cisplatin-based protocols offer the highest response rates.

Intraperitoneal administration is an alternative route that exposes the peritoneal cavity to high concentrations of drug. In addition, agents such as cisplatin are readily absorbed into the circulation, providing systemic exposure.

Table 28-4. International Federation of Gynecology and Obstetrics (FIGO) staging of ovarian cancer (1989).

Stage I	Growth limited to the ovaries.
IA	Growth limited to one ovary; no ascites containing malignant cells. No tumor on the external surface; capsule intact.
IB	Growth limited to both ovaries; no ascites containing malignant cells. No tumor on the external surface; capsule intact.
IC	Growth limited to one or both ovaries and with one of the following: tumor on the surface of one or both ovaries; ruptured capsule; ascites that contain malignant cells; or positive peritoneal cytology.
Stage II	Growth involving one or both ovaries with pelvic extension.
IIA	Extension or metastases to the uterus or fallopian tubes.
IIB	Extension to other pelvic tissues.
IIC	Tumor at either stage IIA or IIB and with one of the following: tumor on the surface of one or both ovaries; ruptured capsule(s); ascites that contain malignant cells; or positive cytology.
Stage III	Tumor involving one or both ovaries with peritoneal implants outside the pelvis or positive retroperitoneal or inguinal nodes.
IIIA	Histologically confirmed microscopic seeding of abdominal peritoneal surfaces. Nodes negative.
IIIB	Histologically confirmed implants of abdominal peritoneal surfaces, none exceeding 2 cm in diameter. Nodes negative.
IIIC	Abdominal implants larger than 2 cm in diameter or positive retroperitoneal or inguinal nodes.
Stage IV	Growth involving one or both ovaries, with distant metastases. Parenchymal liver metastases equal stage IV.

Patients who fail first-line chemotherapy generally respond poorly to second-line chemotherapy. Clinical responses are uncommon and short.

Prognosis

The prognosis for patients with ovarian cancer depends on the clinical stage, the histological type and the grade, age, and volume of residual tumor after surgery. Of these variables, the volume of residual tumor is the most important. Despite considerable progress over the past 20 years, the prognosis for patients with advanced disease has not improved significantly. Ovarian cancer remains the leading gynecologic cause of death in Western countries.

Table 28-5. Components of surgical staging.

Evaluation procedure
  Staging laparotomy
Surgical procedures
  Vertical incision
  Peritoneal washings for cytologic evaluation
  Meticulous exploration
  Excisional biopsy of suspicous lesions
  Peritoneal biopsies (including right and left colic gutters, anterior
    and posterior cul-de-sac, and diaphragm)
  Appendectomy
  Removal of primary tumor along with total abdominal hysterectomy
    and bilateral salpingo-oophorectomy
  Infracolic omentectomy
  Selective pelvic and para-aortic lymphadenectomy
  Debulking (as indicated)

Germ Cell Tumors

Germ cell tumors account for 15–20% of all primary ovarian tumors and are predominately a disease of young women, with a median age at diagnosis of 19 years. Frequently, these tumors occur as a rapidly enlarging abdominal mass causing significant pain. Except for dysgerminomas, the majority are unilateral.

Clinical Descriptions

A. Dysgerminoma: Dysgerminomas are the most common malignant germ cell tumors, representing 40% of all germ cell cancers. Almost 75% occur during the early reproductive years, and they are rarely found after 35 years of age. They are the most frequent tumors encountered in association with gonadoblastomas and intersex states. They are characterized by bilaterality (15–30%), occasional recurrence after many years, and a predilection for lymphatic spread. Similar to their male homologues, testicular seminomas, dysgerminomas are exquisitely radiosensitive, accounting for the excellent survival rates for patients with these tumors. Even with stage III disease, the 5-year survival rate approaches 80% with appropriate therapy. Recently, chemotherapy has largely replaced radiation therapy as the primary treatment modality because chemotherapy allows for the preservation of ovarian function in many patients.

B. Endodermal Sinus Tumor: Endodermal sinus tumors are highly malignant tumors that occur almost exclusively in young women. They are the second most common germ cell tumor, accounting for 22% of germ cell cancers. The median age at diagnosis is 20 years. They grow rapidly, with a propensity for spontaneous rupture leading to a hemoperitoneum. They often occur as a component of mixed germ cell tumors. Combination chemotherapy has dramatically improved the prognosis of patients with endodermal sinus tumors, with a 50% 2-year survival rate for stage III disease.

C. Teratoma: Teratomas arise from a single germ cell. All 3 cell layers—endoderm, mesoderm, and ectoderm—are represented. These tumors consist of either mature or immature elements. Their malignant potential is related to the presence of immature elements.

Immature teratomas represent 20% of malignant germ cell tumors. They are the third most common malignant germ cell tumor. Neural tissue is the most frequent malignant component, but mesenchyme, cartilage, and other nonneural epithelia are also found. The prognosis depends on the stage and grade of the tumor and the presence of other germ cell tumor components.

Malignant elements, predominately squamous in origin, are found in 1–2% of otherwise benign dermoids. The majority of patients (85%) who have teratomas with malignant elements are more than 40 years of age.

D. Embryonal Carcinoma: Embryonal carcinoma is a highly malignant ovarian germ cell tumor that is similar to embryonal carcinoma of the testis. These tumors almost always occur as components of mixed germ cell tumors. The median age at diagnosis is 15 years. Patients with embryonal carcinoma often present with isosexual precocious puberty or other abnormal hormonal manifestations.

E. Choriocarcinoma: Teratomatous choriocarcinomas are exceedingly rare cancers that usually occur as a component of mixed germ cell tumors. Pure tumors can be diagnosed with certainty only in the prepubertal period. They are often associated with isosexual precocious puberty. Unlike gestational choriocarcinomas, teratomatous choriocarcinomas respond poorly to chemotherapy.

F. Polyembryoma: Polyembryomas are extremely rare and usually occur as components of mixed germ cell tumors. These tumors are not sensitive to radiation, and their response to chemotherapy is uncertain.

G. Mixed Germ Cell Tumors: These tumors account for 10–15% of all germ cell cancers. The majority consist of dysgerminomas or immature teratomas mixed with endodermal sinus tumors. The prognosis for patients with mixed germ cell tumors depends on the stage and the most malignant element found in the tumor.

F. Gonadoblastoma: Gonadoblastomas occur almost exclusively in patients with dysgenetic ovaries. Approximately 25% occur in phenotypic males. Because they have a propensity to produce malignant germ cell tumors (often dysgerminomas), they should be removed as soon as they are diagnosed.

Treatment

The majority of germ cell tumors are stage I at diagnosis. In these cases, appropriate therapy consists of peritoneal cytologic evaluation, unilateral salpingo-oophorectomy, subtotal omentectomy, and selective node examination. Pre- and postoperatively, it is important to monitor the available tumor markers (Table 28–6). The majority of patients require postoperative combination chemotherapy.

The exception to this protocol is the dysgerminoma because of its propensity for lymphatic spread. After a peritoneal cytologic evaluation is obtained, unilateral salpingo-oophorectomy and, if indicated, wedge biopsy of the contralateral ovary are performed. A subtotal omentectomy is done, as is selective pelvic and para-aortic lymphadenectomy. Nodal disease is treated with radiation or, more recently, with chemotherapy. Intraperitoneal disease is managed with combination chemotherapy.

Patients with advanced disease are treated with cytoreductive surgery, followed by combination chemotherapy.

Table 28-6. Markers for ovarian germ cell tumors.

Tumor	Lactic Acid Dehydrogenase (LDH)	Human Chorionic Gonadotropin (hCG)	Alpha-Fetoprotein (AFP)
Dysgerminoma	Positive	Positive or negative	Negative
Endodermal sinus tumor	Positive or negative	Negative	Positive
Immature teratoma	Positive or negative	Negative	Positive or negative
Embryonal carcinoma	Positive or negative	Positive	Positive

SEX CORD–STROMAL TUMORS

Sex cord–stromal tumors are uncommon, accounting for 5% of all primary ovarian tumors. They are often hormonally active, producing estrogen, progesterone, testosterone, or corticosteroids. Consequently, they often are evident as a result of a hormonal imbalance, the effects of which depend on the age of the patient. The majority of sex cord–stromal tumors are benign, although the granulosa-theca cell and Sertoli-Leydig cell tumors act as borderline malignancies. They are predominantly unilateral and solid.

Granulosa-Theca Cell Tumors

These tumors consist of a mixture of granulosa and theca cells. More than 50% occur in postmenopausal women. They have a propensity to rupture with development of intraperitoneal bleeding and acute onset of pain. They are frequently estrogen-producing, leading to isosexual precocious puberty in young girls and abnormal bleeding in older women. As a consequence, associated endometrial abnormalities, ranging from hyperplasia to adenocarcinoma, are common. Approximately 85% are stage I at presentation. Recurrences tend to be late, averaging 10 years after treatment. The 5-year survival rates range from more than 95% for stage I to 25% for stage IV.

Sertoli-Leydig Cell Tumors

Sertoli-Leydig cell tumors account for less than 1% of all primary ovarian tumors. They consist of a mixture of Sertoli and Leydig cells. The average age at diagnosis is 25 years. The majority of Sertoli-Leydig cell tumors are androgenic, although they may also produce estrogens or be hormonally inactive. Patients classically present with evidence of hirsutism or virilization, that is, acne, deepening of the voice, clitorimegaly, and increased libido. The majority of these tumors are stage I at diagnosis. The five-year survival rate for stage I tumors approaches 90%.

Treatment

For women past reproductive age, total abdominal hysterectomy and bilateral salpingo-oophorectomy is the preferred treatment. In young women with early disease who wish to preserve their fertility, unilateral salpingo-oophorectomy is appropriate. Postoperative chemotherapy should be considered when the results of peritoneal cytologic evaluations are positive and for tumors more than 10 cm in diameter, granulosa-theca cell tumors with rupture, poorly differentiated Sertoli-Leydig cell tumors, or any tumors more advanced than stage I.

SUGGESTED READINGS

DiSaia PJ, Creasman WT: *Clinical Gynecologic Oncology,* 3rd ed. Mosby, 1989.

Kurman RJ (editor): *Blaustein's Pathology of the Female Genital Tract,* 3rd ed. Springer-Verlag, 1987.

Morrow CP, Townsend DE: *Synopsis of Gynecologic Oncology,* 3rd ed. Churchill Livingstone, 1987.

29 | Gestational Trophoblastic Disease

David K. Levin, MD

Hydatidiform mole (molar pregnancy) and its malignant counterpart, choriocarcinoma, are the extremes of the spectrum of a unique neoplastic growth known as gestational trophoblastic disease (GTD). These tumors arise from proliferation of the placental trophoblast. The normal trophoblast is similar to a malignancy: it is a foreign neoplasm, it is invasive to the endometrium, and there are documented physiologic "metastases" to the maternal pulmonary circulation. Under normal conditions, defense mechanisms in the decidua prevent spread of the locally invasive fetal allograft. Our interest in GTD parallels the increase in knowledge of its biologic properties. The tumor is unique in that it arises from fetal tissue, it produces a distinct hormone marker—human chorionic gonadotropin (hCG), it is the first solid tumor to respond to chemotherapy, and the cure rate approaches 100%.

INCIDENCE

The incidence of hydatidiform mole in the USA ranges from 1 in 1500 to 1 in 2000 pregnancies, which translates to 3000 moles per year. In Taiwan, the incidence is reported to be 1 in 82. Fifteen percent of moles become invasive and 3% progress to choriocarcinoma. There are 400 new cases of choriocarcinoma per year in the USA, 1 per 40,000 pregnancies. Choriocarcinoma arises 50% of the time from an antecedent molar pregnancy, 30% from an abortion, and 20% from a term delivery.

The incidence of GTD is highest in the early and late reproductive years. There appears to be no correlation with parity or paternal age. The incidence is highest in Asia and Mexico. In the USA, it is twice as common in white women compared with black women. A familial predilection has been reported.

PATHOGENESIS & NATURAL HISTORY

The pathogenesis is that of an abnormally fertilized ovum that fails to abort. Vascular insufficiency leads to fluid collection and hydropic swelling of the villous stroma. The classic (complete) and the partial mole are discussed below.

Eighty-five percent of molar pregnancies spontaneously regress after evacuation of the uterine contents. The other 15% require therapy for persistent disease. After a patient has had one mole, the risk of GTD in a subsequent pregnancy is increased four-to fivefold. With repeat moles, the chance of malignant sequelae increases. After 2 or more moles, few patients have normal pregnancies, although normal outcomes have been reported.

CYTOGENETICS

The complete or classic mole has a 46,XX karyotype with both genes being of paternal origin as a result of duplication of a 23 chromosome haploid sperm in an empty ovum. Three to thirteen percent of complete moles are 46,XY from dispermic fertilization of an empty ovum. A 46,YY conceptus is not viable. Dispermic complete moles have a 4-fold increase in residual GTD compared with monospermic moles.

The partial mole commonly has a triploid (69-chromosome) karyotype. A normal haploid (23,X) ovum undergoes dispermic fertilization to form a 69,XXY (70%), 69,XXX (27%), 69,XYY (3%) conceptus.

SYMPTOMS & DIAGNOSIS

Patients present with amenorrhea and a positive pregnancy test. First-trimester bleeding occurs in 80–90% of patients. Hyperemesis, a result of the high hCG level, is also common. Often, the uterine size does not correlate with the gestational age: 50% of uteri affected with GTD are larger than expected for the gestational age and 25% are smaller. The presence of pregnancy-induced hypertension, including proteinuria and edema, at less than 20 weeks of gestation is virtually pathognomonic for GTD. Large theca lutein cysts of the ovary, usually bilateral, occur in 15% of patients. Rarely, a patient is seen with clinical hyperthyroidism (tachycardia, goiter, heat intolerance) resulting from the thyroid-stimulating activity of hCG. Occasionally, a patient will spontaneously expel grape-like clusters of hydropic villi.

When a patient has any of the above symptoms and when fetal heart tones are absent, pelvic ultrasonography is indicated to document the "snow-storm" appearance of the intrauterine hydropic villi (Figure 29–1).

The differential diagnosis includes threatened or missed abortion, multiple gestation, incorrect menstrual dates, ectopic pregnancy, fibroid uterus, and ovarian neoplasm. Pelvic ultrasonography is extremely useful in excluding these entities.

CLASSIFICATION & DESCRIPTION

General Classification

Both benign and malignant forms of GTD are recognized, and each group is subdivided as outlined in Table 29–1.

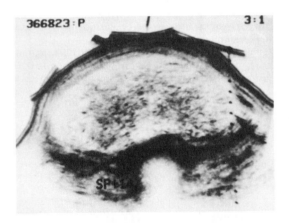

Figure 29-1. A gray-scale ultrasonogram depicting the typical intrauterine multiple-echo pattern of hydatidiform mole. *(Reproduced, with permission, from Pernoll ML [editor]:* Current Obstetric & Gynecologic Diagnosis & Treatment, *7th ed. Appleton & Lange, 1991.)*

Table 29-1. Classification of benign and malignant gestational trophoblastic disease (GTD).

Benign GTD
    Hydatidiform mole
        Complete (or classic)
        Partial
Malignant GTD
    Nonmetastatic
        Persistent mole
        Invasive mole (or chorioadenoma destruens)
        Choriocarcinoma
    Metastatic
        Good prognosis–low risk
        Poor prognosis–high risk

Benign Hydatidiform (Complete & Partial) Moles

In the complete or classic mole, embryonic death occurs before organogenesis, and no fetal parts are recognized. In contrast, the partial mole consists of both placenta and fetus. Fetal death occurs early, but in rare cases, there is a live-born fetus at term, usually with multiple anomalies. Clinically, there is little difference between the 2 entities, although malignant sequelae are less common in the partial mole. The diagnosis is based on histologic evaluation.

Complete molar pregnancy is distinct microscopically from normal pregnancy in that both trophoblastic layers proliferate in contrast to the single layer of syncytiotrophoblasts and cytotrophoblasts in a normal pregnancy. Fetal blood cells are few or absent, and hydropic degeneration of the villous stroma occurs. Frequently, there is cytologic atypia.

In the partial mole there is a mixture of both hydropic and normal villi. Scalloping and crinkling of the villi are common. Trophoblast proliferation is focal and limited to the syncytial layer. The fetus, fetal red blood cells, cord, and membranes can be seen.

Malignant Gestational Trophoblastic Disease

Malignant GTD is classified as either nonmetastatic or metastatic. Histologically, nonmetastatic malignant GTD is categorized as persistent mole, invasive mole (chorioadenoma destruens), or choriocarcinoma. Trophoblast proliferation is excessive, and distant metastases are rarely found. Histologic study of choriocarci-

Table 29-2. Metastatic malignant gestational trophoblastic disease (GTD).

Good Prognosis-Low Risk	Poor Prognosis-High Risk
Pretreatment hCG titer <40,000 mIU/mL	Pretreatment hCG titer >40,000 mIU/mL
Duration of symptoms <4 months	Duration of symptoms >4 months
No liver or brain metastases	Liver or brain metastases
	Previous failed chemotherapy
	Disease following term pregnancy

noma reveals sheets of trophoblasts, demonstrating invasion, hemorrhage, and necrosis. Hyperchromatism and anaplasia are seen, and fetal villi are not recognized.

Metastatic GTD is divided into good prognosis–low risk and poor prognosis–high risk categories (Table 29-2). There is also an International Federation of Gynecology and Obstetrics (FIGO) staging system (Table 29-3) based on anatomic spread and a World Health Organization (WHO) scoring system (Table 29-4) useful in determining the diagnosis and thus the type of therapy.

TREATMENT

Benign Gestational Trophoblastic Disease

Once a molar pregnancy is diagnosed, treatment should begin immediately. The preoperative evaluation includes a history and physical examination, complete blood cell and platelet counts, clotting parameters, thyroid function tests, blood type and crossmatch, quantitative β-hCG measurements, and a chest x-ray film.

After therapy for any medical complications, the uterine con-

Table 29-3. International Federation of Gynecology and Obstetrics (FIGO) definitions of the clinical stages in gestational trophoblastic disease (GTD).

Stage I	GTD strictly confined to the uterine corpus.
Stage II	GTD extends to the adnexa outside the uterus but is limited to the genital structures.
Stage III	GTD extends to the lungs with or without genital tract involvement.
Stage IV	All other metastatic sites.

Table 29-4. World Health Organization scoring system for gestational trophoblastic disease.

Prognostic Factors	Score[1]			
	0	1	2	4
Age (yr)	< 39	> 39		
Antecedent pregnancy	Mole	Abortion, ectopic	Term	
Months since last pregnancy	< 4	4–6	7–12	> 12
hCG (mIU/mL)	< 10^3	10^3–10^4	10^4–10^5	> 10^5
ABO blood group (female × male)		O × A A × O	B AB	
Largest tumor (cm)	< 3	3–5	> 5	
Site metastases		Spleen, Kidney	GI[2] area; Liver	Brain
Number of metastases		1–4	4–8	> 8
Prior chemotherapy			Single drug	2 or more drugs

[1] Low risk: 4 or less; middle risk: 5–7; high risk: 8 or greater.
[2] GI, gastrointestinal.

tents should be evacuated, preferably by suction curettage under general anesthesia. Hysterotomy should not be performed regardless of the uterine size because even a large uterus will rapidly involute following suction curettage. Potential complications of suction curettage include hemorrhage, perforation, sepsis, trophoblastic embolization leading to pulmonary compromise, thyroid storm, and high-output cardiac failure. Invasive monitoring may be required. Rh (D) immune globulin (RhoGAM) is recommended for the Rh-negative patient. A postoperative chest x-ray film should be obtained.

For the patient who desires sterilization, primary hysterectomy with the mole in situ is acceptable and potentially reduces the chance of malignant sequelae. Theca lutein cysts spontaneously regress after treatment and need not be surgically excised.

After treatment, serial serum quantitative β-hCG levels should be tested weekly until the levels approach normal; then the normal levels are confirmed 1 month later and every 2 months thereafter for 1 year. Qualitative urine or serum pregnancy tests are not acceptable for this purpose. Contraception, preferably birth control pills, should be used during the year of postmolar surveillance because a pregnancy would result in rising titers that could not be differentiated from persistent GTD. Few authors recommend prophylactic chemotherapy for all patients with molar pregnancy. Because there is only a 15% chance of malignancy, this measure is not practiced at most centers.

Malignant Gestational Trophoblastic Disease

A plateau or rising hCG titer demands staging and workup for malignant GTD. It is important to distinguish between metastatic and nonmetastatic GTD. In addition to routine blood studies, metastases must be excluded by physical examination (especially of the vagina); chest x-ray film; computed tomographic scan of the abdomen, pelvis, and brain; and possible lumbar puncture.

Nonmetastatic malignant GTD can be treated with single-agent chemotherapy, whether it is a persistent mole, invasive mole, or choriocarcinoma. Common regimens include methotrexate, methotrexate with folinic acid rescue, and actinomycin-D, which are equally effective as initial therapy.

Metastatic disease is found in the lungs, vagina, brain, liver, kidney, gastrointestinal tract, or other sites. The patient may present with a cerebrovascular accident, space-occupying brain lesion, hyperthyroidism, pneumonia, pulmonary embolus, metastatic lung tumor of unknown primary lesion, hepatic tumor, gastrointestinal bleeding, hematuria, vaginal bleeding or skin lesion. Whenever a symptom consistent with one of these presentations follows any gestational event (term or ectopic pregnancy, abortion), metastatic GTD should be excluded.

Patients in the good-prognosis–low risk group can be treated with any single-agent regimen. Patients who do not respond to single-agent treatment (ie, who have a rising or plateauing hCG titer) and those in the middle risk or poor prognosis–high risk groups should be treated with a multiagent regimen. The standard triple therapy has been methotrexate, actinomycin-D, and chlorambucil (MAC). Patients who do not respond to MAC therapy have been treated with Einhorn's regimen (vinblastine, bleomycin, and cisplatin). Other regimens that are more effective than MAC include Bagshawe's regimen (hydroxyurea, vincristine, methotrexate with folinic acid rescue, actinomycin-D, cyclophosphamide, and doxorubicin) and EMA-CO (etoposide, methotrexate, actinomycin-D, cyclophosphamide, and vincristine). Because of the complexity of the treatment of women with high-risk disease, they should be referred to a qualified gynecologic oncologist or to an established regional trophoblastic disease center. Radiation may be used in special situations for brain, liver, or lung metastases. Surgery is usually reserved for patients in whom foci of disease persist after chemotherapy.

PLACENTAL SITE TROPHOBLASTIC TUMOR

Formerly called the **trophoblastic pseudotumor,** the placental site trophoblastic tumor (PSTT) is now classified as a separate pathological and clinical entity that can follow any pregnancy. With this type of tumor, the placental bed trophoblast proliferates, not the villous trophoblast, and the myometrium and blood vessels are invaded. Pleomorphism, polyhedral and spindle cells in irregular nests, and cytoplasmic vacuoles are recognized histologically. The tumor fills the uterine cavity, growing in a polyploid fashion.

Clinically, the patient's initial symptom is vaginal bleeding, occasionally with virilization or nephrotic syndrome. The tumor tends to produce lower levels of hCG than other forms of GTD. Human placental lactogen is a more useful marker.

Treatment is related to the number of mitoses. Because PSTT rarely metastasizes, hysterectomy is usually the primary treatment. Response to chemotherapy is less dramatic than in other forms of GTD.

SUGGESTED READINGS

Berkowitz RS, Goldstein DP: Advances in gestational trophoblastic disease: A symposium. *J Reprod Med* 1991;**36**:1.

DiSaia PJ, Creasman WT: Gestational trophoblastic neoplasia. Chap 7, pp 214–240, in: *Clinical Gynecologic Oncology,* 3rd ed. Mosby, 1989.

Hammond CB, Lewis JL Jr, Mutch DG: Gestational trophoblastic neoplasms. Chap 48, pp 1–29, in: *Gynecology and Obstetrics.* Sciarra JJ (editor). Lippincott, 1986.

Mazur MT, Kurman RJ: Gestational trophoblastic disease. Chap 24, pp 835–875, in *Blaustein's Pathology of the Female Genital Tract,* 3rd ed. Kurman RJ (editor). Springer-Verlag, 1987.

Morrow CP, Townsend DE: Tumors of the placental trophoblast. Chap 13, pp 345–388, in: *Synopsis of Gynecologic Oncology,* 3rd ed. Churchill Livingston, 1987.

Section V: Normal Pregnancy

Physiology of Pregnancy | 30

Maureen P. Malee, MD, PhD

A discussion of the physiology of pregnancy should be undertaken with the understanding that pregnancy does not alter basic physiologic principles. Rather, pregnancy is accompanied by adaptation in every organ system, the sum of which support and maintain the maternal-fetal unit.

Pregnancy results in widely varied alterations in multiple organ systems, particularly in the reproductive system. Because marked subjective and objective variations among individuals occur and can result from physiologic and pathologic processes other than pregnancy, diagnostic criteria for pregnancy are classified as follows: (1) presumptive, (2) probable, and (3) positive.

MANIFESTATIONS OF PREGNANCY

Presumptive Manifestations

Symptoms and signs are as follows: (1) amenorrhea; (2) nausea, vomiting, and queasiness; (3) breast tenderness, engorgement, and colostrum secretion; (4) urinary frequency and urgency; (5) constipation; (6) fatigue; (7) increased skin pigmentation, including chloasma ("mask of pregnancy") and linea nigra (pigmented linea alba); (8) vaginal cyanosis (Chadwick's sign); and (9) perception of fetal movement.

Probable Manifestations

Symptoms and signs include the following: (1) abdominal enlargement; (2) uterine changes that include softening of the cervix, softening of the uterocervical junction (Hegar's sign), and corpus enlargement; (3) painless (Braxton-Hicks) contractions; (4) fetal ballottement within the amniotic fluid; (5) palpation of fetal outlines; and (6) endocrine tests, for example, a radioimmunoassay employing antibodies against the beta subunit of human chorionic gonadotropin (hCG). The increased level of hCG first becomes detectable 7–10 days after ovulation and continues to rise exponentially. The hCG doubling time estimates range from 1.2–3.5 days.

Positive Manifestations

Once the level of the hCG exceeds 1800 mIU/mL, a uterine gestational sac should be visible on ultrasonographic examination. A strong correlation between mean gestational sac size and hCG levels exists until approximately 8 weeks. At this time, the sac averages 25 mm in maximum diameter and should be readily detectable by ultrasound. In fact, well-accepted positive signs of pregnancy include (1) identification of fetal heart rate with ultrasound by 8 weeks; by Doppler instrument by 10–12 weeks; and by DeLee stethoscope by 18 weeks (not to be confused with the funic or cord souffle, which is synchronous with the fetal heart beat, and the uterine souffle, synchronous with the maternal pulse); (2) detection of fetal movement by the examiner; and (3) radiographic recognition of the fetus by 14–16 weeks.

DIFFERENTIAL DIAGNOSIS

All the presumptive and probable symptoms and signs of pregnancy can be caused by other physiologic and pathologic conditions. These include, but are not limited to, the following: endocrine dysfunction; malnutrition; peptic ulcer disease; infectious process; urinary tract disease; galactorrhea; pelvic congestion syndrome; uterine myoma, sarcoma, hematometra, or pyometra; ovarian or tubal tumor; uterine sacculation; and an intrauterine fetal demise.

PREGNANCY DATING

The average length of pregnancy is 266 days. Most patients (60%) deliver within 2 weeks of the expected day of confinement (EDC). The EDC can be calculated from Nägele's rule, that is, EDC = [(first day of the menstrual period + 7 days) − 3 months]

+ 1 year. Note that this rule is based on a 28-day cycle with ovulation on day 14. Only 4% of patients deliver on their EDC after spontaneous labor.

There is good correlation of uterine size and duration of amenorrhea between 8 and 28 weeks of pregnancy. Furthermore, ultrasound is increasingly relied on for pregnancy dating. Indeed, current criteria supported by the American College of Obstetricians and Gynecologists for determining fetal maturity include (1) documentation of fetal heart tones for up to 20 weeks by non-electronic fetoscope or up to 30 weeks by Doppler instrument; (2) elapse of 36 weeks since a positive serum urine hCG pregnancy test result; and (3) measurement of a crown-rump length between 6–11 weeks or another ultrasonographic examination before 20 weeks gestation.

PHYSIOLOGIC CHANGES

Physiologic changes that accompany pregnancy are numerous and include profound metabolic alterations. Average total weight gain is 24 pounds, 2 pounds in the first trimester and 11 pounds each in the second and third trimesters. The majority of weight gain is attributable to the uterus and its contents, the breasts, and fluid volume. A small fraction involves the deposition of new maternal fat and protein, the so-called maternal reserve. The caloric requirement exceeds that of the nonpregnant female by 300 kcal/d.

Increased water retention is normal and is minimally 6.5 L, with 3.5 L being the water content of the fetus, placenta, and amniotic fluid and 3 L being the result of increased maternal blood volume and increased size of the breasts and uterus. Eighty percent of normal pregnant women will experience lower extremity edema as a result of the increase in venous pressure below the level of the uterus. Weight loss in the early puerperium averages 5 pounds in the normal primiparous patient.

Metabolic Changes

A. Protein Metabolism: The total increase in protein normally induced by pregnancy is 1 kg. Of this amount, the term fetus and placenta, which together weigh about 4 kg, contain approximately 500 g of protein. The remaining 500 g of protein is added to the uterus as contractile protein, to the glands of the breast, and to maternal blood as hemoglobin and plasma proteins. There is also considerable alteration in the plasma protein profile. For example, the serum albumin level decreases while that of fibrinogen increases. The α-globulin, alpha-fetoprotein, synthesized by the fetus, peaks in maternal serum by week 14 and declines gradually thereafter. The concentration of this α-globulin is increased in maternal serum under conditions of fetal open neural tube defect, upper gastrointestinal tract obstruction, in multiple gestations, and with fetal death.

B. Carbohydrate Metabolism: Pregnancy is considered diabetogenic because diabetes can be aggravated by pregnancy and may appear only during pregnancy, with carbohydrate metabolism reverting to normal postpartum. Indeed, the normal pregnant woman has a very narrow euglycemic range, with a mean 24-hour plasma level of 84 ± 10 mg/dL. Early in pregnancy, carbohydrate metabolism is affected by increased levels of progesterone and estrogen, which result in beta cell hyperplasia, increased insulin secretion, and increased tissue sensitivity to insulin. These higher levels of progesterone and estrogen, in turn, result in increased glycogen deposition, increased peripheral glucose utilization, decreased hepatic glucose production, and a decrease in the fasting blood glucose by approximately 10%. However, by about 5 months gestation and thereafter, the presence of increasing concentrations of human placental lactogen synthesized by the syncytiotrophoblast, prolactin, and cortisol result in decreased glucose tolerance, insulin resistance, increased hepatic glucose production, and decreased hepatic glycogen production. Glucosuria, a frequent occurrence in healthy pregnant women, results from increased glomerular filtration rate and decreased renal tubular glucose absorption and is typically not indicative of a pathologic state.

C. Fat Metabolism: Plasma lipids increase considerably during pregnancy, involving increases in total lipids, esterified and nonesterified cholesterol, lypoproteins, phospholipids, neutral fat, and free fatty acids. Typically, fat is deposited early in pregnancy at a time of increased utilization of glucose and amino acids by the fetus, as a result of increased levels of progesterone, estrogen, and insulin, which increase fat synthesis, increase fat cell hypertrophy, and inhibit lipolysis. Later in pregnancy, increased concentrations of human placental lactogen result in lipolysis and fat mobilization.

D. Mineral Metabolism: A normal pregnancy requires approximately 1 g of elemental iron or 4–5 mg/d. Of this amount, 500 mg augments maternal hemoglobin, 300 mg is needed by the fetus and placenta, and the remainder is lost during delivery and the puerperium. Because maternal iron stores are small and absorption is limited, a daily supplement of 30–60 mg of elemental iron is recommended, more if anemia exists. Folate requirements are increased by pregnancy, given the demands of increased erythropoiesis. A dose of 0.8 mg/d is recommended, with greater daily doses being required under certain conditions, such as multiple pregnancy, anemia, and alcohol abuse.

Acid-Base Balance & Blood Electrolytes

Progesterone increases pulmonary tidal volume resulting in a decrease in the partial pressure of CO_2 (PCO_2) of 5 mm Hg. This decrease in PCO_2 is accompanied by a moderate decrease in plasma HCO_3, which partially compensates for the respiratory alkalosis such that the pH increases only minimally. Although this increase in pH shifts the O_2 dissociation curve to the left, increasing the affinity of maternal hemoglobin for oxygen, decreasing the oxygen-releasing capacity of maternal blood, and impairing release of oxygen from mother to fetus, the increase in pH also stimulates 2,3-diphosphoglyceric acid production. Increased 2,3-diphosphoglyceric acid counteracts this Bohr effect, shifting the curve back to the right and facilitating oxygen release to the fetus.

Hematologic Changes

Hematologic changes during an uncomplicated pregnancy are profound, involving both plasma and cellular elements. The increase in maternal blood volume averages almost 50%, reaching a maximum in the late third trimester and remaining fairly stable for the few weeks before delivery. The expansion begins in the first trimester but is much more rapid in the second trimester. Expansion then remains stable for 6–8 weeks before delivery. The volume increase is primarily a function of expansion of the plasma compartment, but a less dramatic increase in the total quantity of red blood cells occurs as well. These changes are anticipated in pregnant women with normal nutrition as well as adequate iron and folate supplements. These changes in plasma and red blood cell volume require a concomitant increase in production mechanisms. Indeed, there is diffuse hyperplasia of the hematopoietic system. This hyperplasia results in a normal hemoglobin concentration at term of 12–13 g/dL.

The total leukocyte count usually increases in pregnancy with a range of 10,000–14,000/mL. The white blood cell concentration can increase dramatically with the onset of labor, reaching 25,000/

mL. Several of the factors involved in blood coagulation increase during pregnancy, most notably fibrinogen, which increases about 50% to a normal pregnant value of 450 mg/dL. The increase in coagulation factors accounts for the increased sedimentation rate seen in normal pregnancy. Other factors that increase include VII, VIII, IX, and X. Platelets do not change in concentration, morphology, or function during normal pregnancy.

Endocrine System

The pituitary gland enlarges minimally during pregnancy, but there are no changes in visual fields. The production of the majority of anterior pituitary hormones remains unchanged, although the levels of growth hormone (GH) and follicle-stimulating hormone (FSH) decrease. Prolactin levels increase markedly during pregnancy. In spite of elevated prolactin levels, lactation does not occur during pregnancy because of the inhibitory effect of estrogen on prolactin and of progesterone on lactalbumin. Postpartum, prolactin levels fall, and with normal pituitary, thyroid, and adrenal function, milk production begins. Suckling stimulates pulsatile bursts of prolactin secretion. Posterior pituitary hormones remain unchanged during pregnancy. An intact posterior pituitary, capable of secreting oxytocin, is not necessary for labor. Suckling stimulates oxytocin release, resulting in contraction of breast myoepithelial cells and milk ejection. Vasopressin secretion remains the same as that in nonpregnant women.

Pregnancy stimulates an enlargement in the thyroid gland as a result of glandular hyperplasia and increased vascularity. Although the basal metabolic rate increases by about 25% with pregnancy, this increase is not due to increased thyroid activity but rather to the metabolic activity of the products of conception. A normal pregnant patient remains euthyroid. Estrogen stimulates an increase in the level of thyroxin binding globulin, with subsequent increases in total T_3 and total T_4. However, the concentration of free active hormone remains unchanged.

Parathyroid hormone (PTH) levels during pregnancy are not consistently different from nonpregnant concentrations. Of major importance in the regulation of PTH is the plasma level of ionized calcium, and this level is not altered by pregnancy. Calcitonin levels, in contrast, are considerably higher in the pregnant patient, as are those of the active form of vitamin D. These 3 hormones work in concert to maintain maternal calcium homeostasis while also supplying the demands of the fetus.

The concentration of cortisol increases but is counterbalanced by the estrogen-stimulated increase in transcortin. Thus, the concentration of free cortisol remains the same until later in pregnancy when the concentrations of corticotropin (adrenocorticotropic hormone, ACTH) and free cortisol increase, prompting the suggestion of a "resetting" of feedback controls. The secretion of aldosterone is greater during pregnancy and offsets the natriuretic effects of progesterone. The stimulus for this increased secretion remains uncertain. Although the activity of the renin-angiotensin system is increased, no correlation exists between aldosterone and angiotensin II levels. Another adrenocortical hormone is deoxycorticosterone (DOC), which is also increased, particularly late in pregnancy.

Ovarian production of progesterone and estrogen supports the corpus luteum until this function is taken over by the placenta. Progesterone concentrations reach a plateau at 36 weeks and remain stable until term. The production of 17-hydroxyprogesterone decreases as the function of the corpus luteum declines in early pregnancy but increases again near term.

Prostaglandins have many varied functions, including the regulation of blood flow and labor augmenting activity. The various component types of prostaglandins may have increased or decreased concentrations, depending on the organ system examined and the time in gestation when measured.

Changes in Skin, Hair, & Breasts

Because of their common occurrence during pregnancy, many changes in skin, hair, and nails can be considered physiologic. For example, the ratio of actively growing (anagen) hairs to resting (telogen) hairs is normally 9:1. High levels of estrogen and progesterone during pregnancy stimulate more hairs to enter the anagen phase, resulting in considerable scalp hair growth. If vellus hairs are stimulated to become terminal hairs, there will be increased facial hair growth and, at times, generalized hirsutism. After delivery, the hair cycle ratios reverse, and many scalp hairs fall out (telogen effluvium). This condition is temporary, and hair cycles normalize. The hirsutism is typically transient. Nails may become more brittle and show other dystrophic signs, such as ridging and onycholysis.

Pruritis is the most common skin complaint during pregnancy. Increased estrogen levels cause acneform lesions to clear in most patients but result in several vascular changes. Vessel distention, proliferation, and instability are common, as exemplified by palmar erythema, spider angiomas, and a mottled venous skin pattern. Marginal gingivitis, secondary to gum hyperemia and edema, occurs often. Linear, atrophic striae, or "stretch marks," commonly develop. Although the color, light red to violet, fades, the striae are permanent because of alterations in collagen. The bilaterally symmetric, lacelike facial hyperpigmentation called chloasma develops slowly and fades in the months postdelivery. The pigment deposition results from estrogen, progesterone, and melanocyte-stimulating hormone. This increase in pigmentation can be widespread, frequently involving the axillae, pudendum, and areolae as well as the linea alba, now referred to as the linea nigra.

Striking changes also occur in the breasts. Tenderness is common, and alveolar hypertrophy causes a nodular size increase. Delicate veins become apparent under the skin. The nipples become larger, more deeply pigmented, and erectile. By the second trimester, colostrum can be expressed, and the areolae become broader and more deeply pigmented with elevations called the follicles of Montgomery.

Respiratory Performance

Considerable changes in respiratory physiology accompany pregnancy. At term, the circumference of the female thoracic cage has increased 5–7 cm to compensate for the 4-cm decrease in vertical diameter caused by the gravid uterus pressing up on the diaphragm and rib cage. Capillary engorgement throughout the respiratory tract results in mucosal edema and hyperemia, and epistaxis occurs more frequently. Lung excursion is normal throughout pregnancy and on chest x-ray, increased vascular markings caused by the engorgement of the pulmonary vascular tree simulate congestive heart failure. Among the parameters that change in pregnancy, respiratory minute ventilation is one of the earliest and most obvious, increasing by 50% at term. This increase results from a progressive rise in tidal volume and is accompanied by a slight increase in respiratory rate such that, at term, alveolar ventilation has increased by about 70%. Studies have shown that oxygen consumption, maximum breathing capacity, and timed vital capacity remain unchanged. Conversely, the functional residual capacity is decreased at term by about 20% secondary to a decrease in expiratory reserve volume and residual volume. The volumetric loss of expiratory reserve is compensated for by an increase in inspiratory capacity and inspiratory reserve volume. Consequently, vital capacity is essentially unchanged. The single most common complaint associated with the respiratory tract in the first 2 trimesters is dyspnea, with as many as 60–70% of pregnant women complaining of mild dyspnea without interference with physical activity.

Cardiovascular System

Remarkable changes in the cardiovascular system accompany pregnancy. The pulse rate typically increases by 10–15 beats/min. On chest x-ray, an increase in the size of the cardiac silhouette is noted as a result of the displacement and rotation of the heart by the elevated diaphragm. Because of the variability in the size and position of the uterus, the strength of the abdominal muscles, and the configuration of the abdomen and thorax, the extent of these changes make the diagnosis of pathologic cardiomegaly difficult. During pregnancy, cardiac volume increases 10% as a result of increases in both left ventricular wall mass and end diastolic dimensions. Heart rate, stroke volume, and cardiac output also increase. Heart sounds are also altered. The first heart sound is loudly split, and a third heart sound is sometimes heard. Functional murmurs are also heard, with a systolic murmur noted in 90% of pregnant women and a transient soft diastolic murmur found in about 20%. No characteristic changes in the electrocardiogram accompany pregnancy other than a slight left axis deviation. During normal pregnancy, arterial blood pressure and peripheral vascular resistance decrease, whereas blood volume, basal metabolic rate, and weight increase. Studies have shown that cardiac output increases during the first trimester and remains elevated, being enhanced later in pregnancy in the left lateral decubitus position as venous return is optimized. Blood pressure is also affected by position, being lowest in the left lateral decubitus position. Typically, blood pressure reaches its nadir in the second trimester and rises slowly to normal nonpregnant levels by the end of gestation. Venous pressure is elevated in the lower extremities and is also affected by position. Venous return improves in the left lateral decubitus position since the pressure of the enlarged uterus is relieved from the pelvic vessels and inferior vena cava.

Musculoskeletal Effects

Pregnancy prompts significant changes in gait, posture, and stance. Balance is maintained by an increase in lumbar lordosis and neck flexion. Increased mobility of pelvic joints and weight-bearing demands are responsible for back, muscular, and, at times, nerve root pain, as well as the fatigue, that occur in pregnancy.

Progressive lordosis is characteristic of normal pregnancy, compensating for the enlarging anterior uterus by shifting the center of gravity back over the lower extremities. Increased mobility of sacroiliac, sacrococcygeal, and pubic joints result from hormonal changes and may contribute to the change in maternal posture.

Gastrointestinal Tract

The enlarging uterus displaces the stomach and bowel. The tone and motility of the gastrointestinal tract is typically decreased, prolonging gastric emptying and intestinal transit time. Pyrosis, or heartburn, is a frequent complaint and is likely the result of reflux of acidic gastric secretions into the lower esophagus. Reflux is favored for several reasons, which include the altered position of the stomach, lower intraesophageal and higher intragastric pressures, and slower and lower amplitude esophageal peristaltic waves, the latter of which are related to hormonal changes. Although less motile, absorption from the small intestine is adequate. Colonic hypotonicity results in increased water absorption and decreased bulk. Thus, constipation is common. Hemorrhoids are also a frequent occurrence and result from this constipation as well as venous engorgement of pelvic vessels.

No change in liver morphology accompanies pregnancy, although the gall bladder becomes distended as a result of hypotonicity with subsequent bile stasis. Gallstone formation is therefore more common in pregnancy. The results of most liver function tests remain within the normal nonpregnant range in uncomplicated pregnancy, including measurements of serum bilirubin, lactic dehydrogenase (LDH), aspartate transaminase (AST), and alanine transaminase (ALT). However, total serum alkaline phosphatase almost doubles, largely because of the heat stabile isoenzymes of placental origin. Conversely, plasma albumin and cholinesterase decrease.

Renal Function

Various anatomic and physiologic alterations in the renal system occur in pregnancy. An increased metabolic rate with an associated increase in renal blood flow of 30–40% results in the following changes: (1) glomerular filtration rate and creatinine clearance increases of 40–50% and blood urea nitrogen and creatinine values lower than the normal nonpregnant value; (2) a lower renal absorption threshold for glucose, resulting in glucosuria as a common occurrence; and (3) increased renal blood flow and estrogen stimulation of the renin-angiotensin-aldosterone system, resulting in changes in sodium and water homeostasis during pregnancy. The increased glomerular filtration rate results in increased filtered sodium accompanied by increased tubular reabsorption, resulting in a positive sodium balance. Proportionately, more water is retained, contributing to dependent edema. By mid first trimester, there is some dilatation of the upper urinary tract in about 90% of pregnant women, usually greater on the right than the left. This hydronephrosis is caused by several conditions. First, the fetus compresses the lower ureter, resulting in upper urinary tract dilatation, and second, the hormonal milieu decreases ureteral tone, interfering with ureteral peristalsis. Frequently encountered lower urinary tract symptoms include the following: (1) frequency, secondary to increased fluid intake and glomerular filtration rate, as well as the pressure of the gravid uterus on the bladder neck and urethra; (2) nocturia, secondary to mobilization of edema fluid and pooled venous blood, exacerbated by the recumbent position; (3) stress incontinence, in as many as 50% of pregnant women, caused by elongation of the posterior urethral angle and descent of the bladder neck; and (4) retention, especially with a retroverted gravid uterus.

SUGGESTED READINGS

Creasy RK, Resnik R (editors): *Maternal-Fetal Medicine: Principles and Practice.* 2nd ed. Saunders, 1989.

Gleicher N et al: *Principles and Practice of Medical Therapy in Pregnancy,* 2nd ed. Appleton & Lange, 1991.

Queenan JT: *Management of High-Risk Pregnancy.* Medical Economics Books, 1985.

31 | Placental & Early Fetal Development

Sarah J. Kilpatrik, MD, PhD

PLACENTA

The placenta is a plentiful, fascinating, and unique organ, yet the intricacies of its functions remain elusive. The placenta is of fetal origin and actually invades maternal tissue and vessels, but it is not perceived as foreign and is not rejected by the mother. Further, this invasive quality, which is critical for adequate development of the maternal-fetal blood supply, is time and area limited and thus rarely becomes a malignant process.

This chapter discusses the development and maintenance of the maternal-placental-fetal unit with particular emphasis on the placenta—its development, anatomy, and function. Embryonic and fetal development and basic principles of teratology are also discussed. All references to weeks of development are in postconception weeks, not the more often clinically used gestational weeks. With gestational weeks the last menstrual period (LMP) is the starting point rather than conception. Because the LMP generally begins 2 weeks before ovulation, the equivalent time estimate expressed in gestational weeks is 2 weeks greater than the estimate expressed in postconception weeks.

Implantation & Early Development

Fertilization takes place in the ampulla of the fallopian tube within 12–24 hours after ovulation. The fertilized egg or zygote then proceeds through the tube into the uterus, which it reaches in approximately 4 days. During this time mitotic divisions occur, resulting in the transition from **zygote** to **blastomere** to **morula** and finally to the formation of the **blastocyst** by 3–4 days after fertilization, coincident with entry into the uterus. The blastocyst, which is the morula after uterine fluid has entered creating a cavity, consists of an inner cell mass with a trophoblast shell. The blastocyst begins implantation into the endometrium at about day 6–7 after fertilization. This process is completed by the ninth day, when the blastocyst fully burrows into and becomes surrounded by the endometrium. Through the process of implantation, the blastocyst makes contact with the maternal blood supply by trophoblastic invasion into maternal vessels. Once the blastocyst reaches the uterus, many developmental changes occur concurrently. However, to coherently present these changes, it is necessary to discuss them separately. Thus, developmental events are not in strict chronologic order throughout this chapter.

During this first week of pregnancy the endometrium undergoes a progesterone-dependent physiologic and morphologic change called the **decidual reaction** and hence is referred to as **decidua,** from the Latin for falling off. Further, depending on its relationship to the now implanted blastocyst, the surrounding decidua has different names. The **decidua basalis** is that endometrium lying immediately inferior to the blastocyst. The **decidua capsularis** covers the blastocyst like a cap and closes over the invading blastocyst. The **decidua vera** or **parietalis** is the remaining endometrium, usually on the opposite wall of the uterine cavity from the blastocyst.

The blastocyst consists of an inner cell mass destined to become the fetus, an extraembryonic cavity, and a surrounding trophoblast shell, destined to become the chorion and placenta. As the blastocyst grows the decidua capsularis protrudes into the central cavity of the uterus. The trophoblastic shell develops into primary villi, which consist of very characteristic frond-like tissue. The villi adjacent to the decidua capsularis and the decidua capsularis atrophy and develop into the membranes called **chorion laeve.** These layers eventually expand with the growing blastocyst to close the uterine cavity and subsequently fuse with the decidua vera at about 10–12 weeks.

Where the blastocyst invades into the uterus determines the location of the placenta. Implantation of the placenta is in the uterine fundus in one-third of pregnancies, in the anterior fundus in another one-third, or in the posterior uterine wall in the remaining one-third of pregnancies. As discussed in Chapter 39, in rare cases the placenta implants over the cervix, a condition known as **placenta previa,** which is potentially a source of severe hemorrhage.

The inner cell mass during this time is composed of 3 layers: the **ectoderm, mesoderm,** and **endoderm.** Initially, these layers lie flat and parallel to each other with the ectoderm adjacent to the placenta, the endoderm closest to the extraembryonic cavity, and the mesoderm in between. However, as the inner cell mass grows, it also folds, thus changing the relationship of these layers to each other. The **amnion** is derived from the ectoderm and begins about day 8 as a small sac filled with fluid. As the embryo grows, it herniates into the amniotic cavity, and gradually the amnion covers first the entire embryo then the umbilical cord. By 12 weeks the amniotic sac has expanded to reach the chorion laeve and close the extraembryonic cavity. Thus, the membranes are composed of the **chorion** and the amnion. The chorion is the outermost layer and is predominantly derived from the trophoblast. The amnion is the avascular innermost layer and is derived from the ectoderm of the embryo. Other derivatives of the ectoderm include the brain; spinal cord; peripheral nervous system; sensory epithelia of the ear, eye, and nose; epidermis; hair; nails; mammary glands; pituitary gland; and the enamel of the teeth.

The endoderm develops into a cavity, a portion of which becomes the **yolk sac.** With embryonic folding some of the yolk sac is incorporated into the gastrointestinal tract and liver. The yolk sac is the source of fetal germ and hematopoietic cells. Also derived from the endoderm are the tonsils, the lining of the respiratory tract, thyroid, parathyroids, thymus, pancreas, lining of the bladder and urethra, tympanic antrum, auditory tube, and the lining of the tympanic cavity.

Although there is some controversy about the early development of the mesoderm, a predominant view is that it contributes to the chorion and trophoblastic villi. Emerging from the tail of the embryo, the mesoderm grows to cover the inner surface of the trophoblastic shell. Subsequently, it pushes into the trophoblast, forming the villi and providing a path for fetal vessels to follow. Adjacent to the embryo, the mesoderm condenses with fetal vessels from the yolk sac and becomes the umbilical cord. Additional derivatives of mesoderm include cartilage, bone, connective tissue, muscles, heart, kidneys, gonads, genital ducts, serous membranes lining body cavities, spleen, adrenal cortex, blood, and lymph.

Maternal-Fetal Blood Supply

Approximately on day 9 as the trophoblast invades the decidua, **lacunae** develop and eventually fuse to become the intervillous space. This space interdigitates between the tertiary villi as they invade into decidua and myometrium. By day 10–12 this space is bathed with maternal blood and becomes the beginning of uteroplacental circulation (Figure 31–1). Because the trophoblast is in

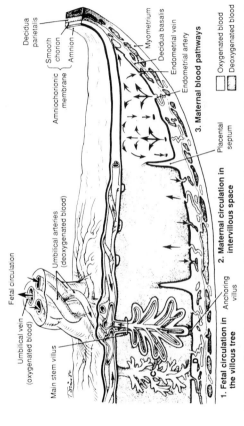

Figure 31-1. Schematic drawing of a section through a full-term placenta: **1.** The relation of the villous chorion (C) to the decidua basalis (D) and the fetal placental circulation. **2.** The maternal placental circulation. Maternal blood flows into the intervillous spaces in funnel-shaped spurts, and exchanges occur with the fetal blood as the maternal blood flows around the villi. **3.** The inflowing arterial blood pushes venous blood into the endometrial veins, which are scattered over the entire surface of the decidua basalis. Note that the umbilical arteries carry deoxygenated fetal blood to the placenta and that the umbilical vein carries oxygenated blood to the fetus. Note that the cotyledons are separated from each other by placental (decidual) septa of the maternal portion of the placenta. Each cotyledon consists of 2 or more main stem villi and their many branches. *(Based on Moore: The Developing Human, 3rd ed. Saunders, 1982.)*

Fetal circulation

Umbilical vein (oxygenated blood)

Umbilical arteries (deoxygenated blood)

Main stem villus

Decidua parietalis

Smooth chorion
Amnion

Amniochorionic membrane

Myometrium

Decidua basalis

Endometrial vein

Endometrial artery

Placental septum

Anchoring villus

☐ Oxygenated blood
▦ Deoxygenated blood

1. Fetal circulation in the villous tree

2. Maternal circulation in intervillous space

3. Maternal blood pathways

direct contact with maternal blood, the human placenta is referred to as **hemochorial.**

The maternal spiral arteries, branches of the arcuate arteries, which are branches of the uterine arteries, are invaded by cytotrophoblasts that replace the endothelium. The muscular coat is destroyed, causing the arteries to straighten and become less elastic, which results in low-resistance blood flow to the placenta. The blood flow through these arteries bathes the intervillous space. By day 14 tertiary villi each contain fetal vessels that eventually connect and become branches of the umbilical arteries and vein. Thus, in the intervillous space the maternal oxygenated blood bathes the villi; fetal veins in the villi absorb the oxygenated blood, carrying it through the umbilical vein to the fetus; and metabolic waste in the blood returning from the umbilical arteries is picked up by maternal veins. By day 22 the fetal heart begins to beat and hence the beginning of the fetal circulation through the umbilical cord into the intervillous space.

Placental & Umbilical Cord Anatomy

The average placenta is round and measures approximately 20 by 15 by 2 cm and weighs 425–550 g. This placental weight is usually one-seventh of the neonate's birth weight. The placenta reaches its maximum size at about 36 weeks and thereafter continues to mature without increasing in weight. The umbilical cord is most often centrally inserted into the placenta and is 40–60 cm long. It contains 2 umbilical arteries and 1 umbilical vein. The umbilical vein carries oxygenated blood from the intervillous space through the fetal ductus venosis and portal sinus to the fetal inferior vena cava. The umbilical arteries, branches of the fetal hypogastric arteries, return deoxygenated blood across the intervillous space from the fetus to the mother. In about 1% of deliveries, only one umbilical artery is present, a condition that may be associated with fetal anomalies.

Occasionally, there is an eccentric insertion of the cord into the placenta as a result of an abnormal position of the inner cell mass within the trophoblast shell. Marginal cord insertion with the cord attaching at the edge of the placenta is called a **Battledore placenta,** referring to its raquet appearance, and is probably the most common abnormal cord insertion. A **velamentous insertion,** or attachment of the cord directly into the membranes, infrequently occurs but is potentially dangerous because the blood vessels must travel over an area of just membranes on their way to the placenta. Thus, the cord may easily avulse at the time of delivery, in which case the placenta must be removed manually or with the aid of instruments. Rarely, the membranes containing vessels may cover the cervical os, a condition known as **vasa previa,** and necessitates a cesarean section to prevent catastrophic fetal hemorrhage if the vessels rupture. There may be an extra lobe of placenta, called a **succenturiate lobe,** connected to the main placenta by vessels. Although there is generally no danger to the pregnancy in this situation, it is important to recognize its existence because both lobes must be removed from the uterus at the time of delivery.

The maternal surface of the placenta is red and meaty in appearance. It consists of 15–20 lobes, which are separated by septae formed of decidua. Each lobe has multiple **cotyledons** on the fetal side. Each cotyledon is supplied by one branch of an umbilical vein and an umbilical artery. The fetal side of the placenta is smoother and paler than the maternal side because of the presence of the amnion and chorion. At delivery the placenta, generally with the membranes and remaining cord attached, may commonly have areas of small infarction on the maternal side, which may be firm and yellow to white.

Placental Functions

A. Endocrine Function: The placenta produces multiple hormones, including steroids, protein hormones, neuropeptides, and growth factors. The importance of many of these hormones is well described, but the role of others is still unclear.

The putative functions of progesterone include priming the endometrium for implantation, relaxation of the uterus throughout gestation to prevent uterine contractions, suppression of the maternal immune response to prevent maternal rejection of the fetus, provision of substrate for the fetal adrenal to synthesize glucocorticoids and mineralocorticoids, and, in conjunction with estrogens, promotion of maternal breast growth. Although there is some controversy about these functions for progesterone, there is no doubt that without progesterone the pregnancy will not survive. The corpus luteum is the critical source of progesterone during the first 6 weeks of gestation. Between 6 and 12 weeks both the placenta and the corpus luteum provide progesterone, and after 10–12 weeks the placental progesterone is sufficient to maintain pregnancy. Progesterone is synthesized by the syncytiotrophoblasts. They contain low-density lipoprotein receptors that bind maternal cholesterol and initiate the steroidogenic pathway to progesterone. By term, approximately 250 mg of progesterone is synthesized daily by the placenta.

The functions of estrogen include increased uterine blood flow, synergism with progesterone for endometrial preparation for implantation, and breast development. Four estrogens are present during gestation: estradiol (E2), estriol (E3), estrone (E1), and estetrol (E4). Because estradiol and estriol are the most important, the remaining discussion is primarily limited to them.

The placenta lacks the enzymes to directly synthesize estrogens from cholesterol. Specifically, it lacks 17-hydroxylase, the enzyme necessary to transform pregnenolone and progesterone to 17-hydroxypregnenolone and 17-hydroxyprogesterone, respectively. Either of these steps is necessary for estrogen synthesis. To make up for this deficit, a unique synergistic system has developed between the placenta, the mother, and the fetus. As with progesterone, the corpus luteum is the major source of estradiol during the first 6 weeks of gestation. After 6 weeks the placenta begins to secrete estradiol synthesized from initially maternal dehydroepiandrosterone sulfate (DHEAS). As the fetal adrenal begins to function at about 7–9 weeks, fetal DHEAS also contributes to the synthesis of placental estradiol. In addition, fetal DHEAS is the source of estrone.

The synthesis of estriol is somewhat different than that of estradiol and estrone because the predominant source of its precursor is the fetus. After 20 weeks, 90% of estriol secretion is accounted for by 16α-hydroxydehydroepiandrosterone sulfate (16α-OHDEAS) from the fetal liver. The fetal adrenal cortex converts pregnenolone sulfate to DHEAS, which then is converted to 16α-OHDHEAS in the fetal liver and transferred to the placenta. This dependence on a functioning fetal adrenal and liver for normal estriol output was thought to be an adequate way to assess fetal well being. In fact, before the development of surveillance techniques such as nonstress tests, biophysical profiles, and ultrasonography, maternal urinary estriol levels were used in the third trimester to assess the health of the fetus. Estriol is first detectable at approximately 9 weeks and normally increases throughout gestation.

hCG is a peptide hormone similar to luteinizing hormone (LH) synthesized by the syncytiotrophoblasts. Its alpha subunit is identical to that of LH, follicle-stimulating hormone (FSH) and thyroid-stimulating hormone (TSH). hCG is detectable as early as 8 days after conception and is what is measured in both urine and serum pregnancy tests. In a normal pregnancy, hCG doubles each 48 hours until about 8–10 weeks when it plateaus with a subsequent slow decline. The functions of hCG include stimulation of steroidogenesis in the corpus luteum, particularly estrogen and progesterone; inhibition of new follicular development; and stimulation in the male fetus of gonadal cells to produce testosterone. hCG may also play a role in immunologic protection of the blastocyst. hCG is absolutely necessary for progesterone production and hence pregnancy maintenance until approximately 6–8 weeks. There is some evidence that hCG may be related to the nausea and vomiting that are common during the first trimester when hCG is highest. Moreover, hCG levels increase in multiple gestations as does the incidence of nausea and vomiting.

Human placental lactogen (hPL), another protein hormone synthesized by the syncytiotrophoblasts, has properties similar to growth hormone and prolactin. Its functions are not fully clear, but include anti-insulin actions and lipolysis, processes that make glucose and free fatty acids available to the fetus. hPL may contribute to the normal tendency for pregnant women to have a lower fasting blood sugar but higher postprandial blood sugar than nonpregnant women. hPL may also have some growth-promoting action. However, unlike hCG and progesterone, hPL is not absolutely necessary for a successful pregnancy. It is first detected at 6 weeks gestation, rises until about 32 weeks, then plateaus. By term, approximately 2 g/d is synthesized and released. This is the highest production rate of any hormone in the human.

Interestingly, nearly all the neuropeptides or releasing hormones identified in the hypothalamus have also been found in the placenta. These neuropeptides include gonadotropin-releasing hormone (GnRH), proopiomelanocortin-derived peptides, melanocyte-stimulating hormone, inhibin, somatostatin, corticotropin-releasing hormone, and thyrotropin-releasing hormone. Generally, activity similar to that of these neuropeptides has been localized to the cytotrophoblasts, implying that this is the site of their synthesis. Little is known of their function. Speculations about GnRH have generated the most literature. It is highest in early pregnancy (< 16 weeks) and may be involved in feedback control of hCG.

Many other protein hormones have been identified in the placenta, but their roles remain obscure. Examples include human chorionic thyrotropin (which may be identical to hCG), SP1 (Schwangerschafts protein 1), PP5 (placental protein 5), PP12 (placental protein 12), and PAPP-C (pregnancy associated plasma protein C). In addition, the placenta has been the source of nearly all of the currently isolated growth factors.

B. Placental Transport: A crucial function of the placenta is to transport CO_2 and O_2 between the mother and the fetus and to thus regulate the fetal acid-base balance. Basically, the placenta assumes the function of respiration.

Oxygen delivery to the fetus depends on many factors: some are inherent in the differences between maternal and fetal physiology, some depend on placental characteristics, and others depend on maternal blood flow. The major factors are the oxygen-carrying capacity of maternal and fetal blood. Oxygen in maternal blood is dissociated from oxyhemoglobin, transferred across the placenta, and then picked up by fetal hemoglobin. This process is facilitated by the following: (1) adequate uterine blood flow (500 mL/min at term which is 10% of maternal cardiac output); (2) large surface area of the placenta for exchange; (3) short distance between maternal and fetal vessels in the intervillous space; (4) increased binding of oxygen to fetal hemoglobin compared to adult hemoglobin (hemoglobin A); (5) decreased affinity of maternal hemoglobin to oxygen secondary to the more acidic environment in the intervillous space because the oxygen dissociation curve shifts to the left, releasing more oxygen in acidic environment; (6) higher hemoglobin level in the fetus compared with that in the mother (at term the range for neonatal hematocrit is 57–68%); and (7) the diffusion capacity of the placenta.

Thus, factors that affect any of these steps could alter the partial pressure of oxygen (P_{O_2}) of fetal blood. Table 31–1 lists the normal ranges of gas concentrations in fetal blood. Anything that decreases uterine blood flow, maternal or fetal hemoglobin, placental diffusing capacity, or functioning surface area could decrease fetal oxygen transfer. Examples include uterine contractions, which temporarily decrease fetal P_{O_2}, maternal hypotension, maternal or fetal anemia, placental abruption or infarction, and umbilical cord compression.

CO_2 transport is simpler in that its diffusion constant is much larger than that of O_2, so it rapidly diffuses across the placenta

Table 31–1. Normal blood gas values for maternal and fetal blood.

	Maternal Artery	Umbilical Vein	Umbilical Artery	Fetal Scalp Sample
P_{CO_2} (mm Hg)	27–32	40–43	48–50	45
P_{O_2} (mm Hg)	100–108	27–30	15–20	22–25
pH	7.40–7.45	7.32–7.38	7.28–7.32	7.30
Base excess (mmol/L)	−3 to −5	−5	−6	−6

from fetus to mother. A large gradient must be present to maintain this direction of diffusion. During pregnancy, the normal maternal PCO_2 decreases to 30–34 mm Hg, which is much lower than the normal fetal PCO_2 of 40–50 mm Hg. The maternal acid-base status is likewise important in maintaining fetal pH and fetal PO_2 levels. For example, if the mother is hyperventilating enough to cause an alkalosis, less oxygen will be released to the fetus because the oxygen dissociation curve will be shifted to the right in the presence of relative alkalosis in the intervillous space.

Clinically, measurement of cord gases, specifically from blood in the umbilical vein (UV) and umbilical artery (UA), at the time of delivery can be important in assessing the newborn's acid-base status. In addition, sometimes during labor it becomes important to assess the fetal acid-base status, and a fetal scalp blood gas measurement is performed (Table 31–1). Note how relatively hypoxic the normal fetus is compared with the adult, and note that the fetal scalp gas results normally range between the values measured in the umbilical vein and umbilical artery. If there are low Apgar scores, decreased PO_2 levels, or acidosis at birth, differences between the UA and the UV values help delineate the likely causes. Fetal respiratory acidosis alone is usually not of long-term significance and is associated with decreased PO_2, elevated PCO_2, and mild acidosis primarily reflected in the UV. The UA remains normal. Respiratory acidosis is caused by an acute decrease in placental or umbilical blood flow, which could result from cord compression, uterine hyperstimulation, and acute placental abruption. If respiratory acidosis persists, metabolic acidosis will occur as a result of the accumulation of lactic acid. This accumulation leads to abnormal gases in both the UV and the UA blood with decreased PO_2 and pH and increased PCO_2 and base deficit. Other causes of fetal metabolic acidosis are maternal acidosis, maternal hypoventilation, chronic uteroplacental insufficiency, and fetal hypoxemia.

Table 31–2. The US Food and Drug Administration classification of drugs and associated fetal risk.

A. Controlled studies in human have demonstrated no fetal risk.
B. Either animal studies indicate there are no fetal risks and there are no human studies, or adverse effects have been demonstrated in animals but not in well-controlled human studies.
C. No adequate studies are available.
D. Evidence of fetal risk but benefits outweigh risk.
E. Proven fetal risk and contraindicated during pregnancy.

This situation is obviously potentially more serious for the neonate.

EMBRYONIC & FETAL DEVELOPMENT BY SYSTEMS

Embryonic and fetal development is a complicated subject about which entire books have been written. This section reviews only developmental milestones and critical time periods for most of the major systems of the body. The interested reader should refer to the texts on embryology listed as suggested readings.

During the first 2 weeks after fertilization, the dividing zygote migrates down the fallopian tube into the uterus, implants in the uterine wall, and develops into the bilaminar embryonic disk. The development of this disk marks the beginning of the embryonic period, which lasts until the end of the eighth week. During this time all major systems have begun organogenesis and thus the developing human is most susceptible to teratogens during this embryonic period. The fetal period begins at the onset of the ninth week and continues until delivery.

Nervous System

The template for the central nervous system (CNS) and peripheral nervous system (PNS) is the neural plate, which appears in the third week. This plate will develop into neural crest cells, the precursor of cranial, spinal, and autonomic ganglia and nerves, and the neural tube. The neural tube is apparent by the middle of the fourth week, and the cranial two-thirds will become the brain and the remainder the spinal cord. The neural tube is initially open at both ends. The cranial, or rostral end, closes about day 25, and the caudal end closes several days later. The lumen of this tube is the forerunner of the ventricular system of the brain and the central canal of the spinal cord.

When the cranial pore of the neural tube closes, 3 primary brain vesicles are formed: the forebrain, or prosencephalon; midbrain, or mesencephalon; and hindbrain, or rhombencephalon. During the fifth week, the forebrain divides into telencephalon and diencephalon, and the hindbrain divides into metencephalon and myelencephalon, creating 5 secondary brain vesicles. The characteristic shape of the brain begins as the result of the rapid growth and curvature the brain undergoes during particularly the fourth and fifth weeks when the major flexures appear. These are the midbrain, pontine, and cervical flexures.

The telencephalon is the precursor of the cerebral hemispheres, which initially have a smooth contour. As the brain grows, sulci and gyri develop, greatly expanding the surface area of the cortex. The complexity and the number of sulci and gyri increase throughout gestation, and an assessment of their development can aid in the estimation of gestational age on ultrasound in utero or in premature infants. The diencephalon develops into the thalamus, hypothalamus, and pineal gland. The midbrain remains the midbrain and includes structures such as the tectum, superior and inferior colliculi, tegmentum, substantia nigra, and cerebral peduncles. The metencephalon becomes the pons and the cerebellum. The myelencephalon develops into the medulla. Many of these changes begin approximately in the fifth week.

The pituitary gland has a unique embryology. It is derived from both the epithelium of the mouth and from the diencephalon. An outpouching, Rathke's pouch, from the roof of the primitive mouth cavity grows up to the diencephalon during the fourth week. By the sixth week the connection to the mouth has disappeared, and the pituitary gland has appeared. The significance of the 2 origins of the hypophysis is that the gland is essentially 2 glands, each composed of different tissue and hence dedicated to a different function. The anterior pituitary (adenohypophysis) is derived from the mouth, and the posterior pituitary (neurohypophysis) is the diencephalic portion of the pituitary.

Eyes & Ears

During the fourth week, the otic and optic pits and the lens are visible. The retinal pigment appears the fifth week, and the eyelids and external ear form by the end of the eighth week. The eyelids close approximately the tenth week and remain fused until about 22–24 weeks, when they open again.

Cardiovascular System (CVS)

Blood vessels derived from the mesoderm begin to form during the third week and contain blood formed by the yolk sac and the allantois. The heart begins to form with the 2 endocardial tubes and appears at the end of the third week. By day 21–22 (fourth week) the heart begins to beat, an event that can now be detected by ultrasonography, particularly with a vaginal probe. Blood formed by the embryonic liver, spleen, bone marrow, and lymph begins by the fifth week. The liver provides the majority of hematopoiesis from 5–12 weeks, the spleen from 12–28 weeks, and the bone marrow after 28 weeks. Thus, the CVS is the first system to begin to function, and the critical period for cardiac development is from day 20 to day 50 (from 3 to 8 weeks).

Lungs

The lung is unusual because its function develops relatively late compared with other organ systems. Obviously, this delay is in part due to the fetus's lack of necessity for lungs early in gestation. Lung buds and subsequently bronchial buds at the end of the laryngotracheal tube are apparent by the fifth week. Further lung development is divided into 3 phases. The pseudoglandular phase occurs from weeks 5 to 17, and during this time growth occurs but respiration cannot. The canalicular phase is from weeks 16 to 25, and from about 24 weeks onward primitive alveoli are forming. Thus, respiration is at least theoretically possible. By 24 weeks type II pneumocytes secrete surfactant (a lipid necessary for aveolar function in respiration). The third phase is the terminal sac period and refers to the remaining lung maturation. The fact that survival is very low in babies born at less than 26 weeks, despite supreme effort on the part of neonatologists, is no doubt due to the immaturity of the lung.

Gastrointestinal (GI) Tract

The GI tract begins to develop during the fourth week, when a portion of the yolk sac is incorporated into the embryo as it folds and becomes the foregut, midgut, and hindgut. Umbilical herniation of the bowel into the umbilical cord occurs at 6–7 weeks, but by 10 weeks the bowel has undergone rotation and reentry into the abdominal cavity. Between weeks 6 and 8, the foregut develops into the pharynx, lower respiratory tract, esophagus, stomach, duodenum, liver, pancreas, gallbladder, and biliary ducts. Bile formation begins at about 12 weeks, and the pancreas begins to secrete insulin and glucagon at about 20 weeks. The midgut forms the small intestine, cecum, appendix, ascending colon, and part of the transverse colon. The hindgut develops into the remainder of the transverse colon, descending colon, sigmoid colon, rectum, epithelial bladder, most of the urethra, and part of the anal canal.

Genitourinary (GU) System

The genital and urinary systems develop in close association to each other, which is why about 20% of people with an abnormality in reproductive structure have an abnormality in the urinary system as well. However, for clarity each system is discussed separately. The kidneys develop from the metanephroi, which are apparent by the fifth week. The metanephroi begin as ureteric buds near the cloaca. With growth and development, the ureters, renal pelves, calices, and collecting tubules form from the ureteric buds. Of significance the position of the kidneys is first in the pelvis, but by the ninth week they have migrated to the adult position. This change is largely due to the growth of the fetal abdomen. Urine production and thus kidney function begins at about 11–13 weeks. From then on the major component of amniotic fluid is fetal urine.

The first 6 weeks of embryogenesis is called the indifferent stage because female and male embryos are indistinguishable. They each have primordial germ cells, an undifferentiated gonad, 2 sets of genital ducts, and the primordia for the external genitalia. The primordial germ cells migrate from their source, the yolk sac, to the genital ridge at about 5 weeks. By 6 weeks the primary sex cords are present in association with the germ cells. If there is a Y chromosome, the primary sex cords will develop into seminiferous tubules, and the indifferent gonads will become the testes with Leydig cells that release testosterone, and Sertoli cells that secrete müllerian inhibiting factor (MIF). This begins to occur in the male about the seventh week. During the indifferent stage, there are 2 sets of genital ducts present: the mesonephric (wolffian) and the paramesonephric (müllerian). Under the influence of testosterone, the mesonephric ducts develop into the epididymis, vas deferens, and seminal vesicles. MIF is necessary to inhibit the growth of the paramesonephric ducts. The undifferentiated external genitalia consist of the genital tubercle, urogenital sinus, and genital swellings. In the male these become the glans penis and scrotum. By 10–12 weeks, the external genitalia distinguish female from male fetuses.

If no testosterone is present, a female genital system will develop. Note that no hormonal stimulation is necessary for this route of maturation. The female genitalia develop slightly later than the male counterparts. After the germ cells migrate to the gonadal ridge, the ovaries develop but are not identifiable until about 10 weeks. By 16 weeks primordial follicles with oogonia are present. The mesonephric ducts regress, and the paramesonephric ducts develop into the uterus, fallopian tubes, and upper one-third of the vagina. By 18 weeks a uterus is present. The external genitalia, which form from the genital tubercle, urogenital sinus, and genital swellings, are the clitoris, lower two-thirds of the vagina, and the labia, respectively.

Limbs

The embryo begins its characteristic curve during the fourth week. The appearance of the upper and lower limb buds also occur in the fourth week. By the fifth week hand plates are visible, by the seventh week the fingers and thumb are webbed, and by the eighth week they are separated. The lower limbs develop in the same fashion but a few days later than the upper limbs. The embryo initially has a tail, which completely regresses by the end of the eighth week. Thus, by the end of the eighth week the fetus is emerging with its distinct human appearance. This is the reason for the renaming of the embryo as the fetus. Fingernails are present by 24 weeks and toenails by 30 weeks. Hair appears by 20 weeks, and vernix (the cheesy material covering the fetal skin) by 18 weeks. Although the fetus is often moving, the mother usually does not appreciate these movements until 17–20 weeks.

Thyroid & Adrenal Glands

The thyroid gland is the first endocrine gland to develop at 24 days (fourth week). It begins near the tongue and then migrates down to the anterior nuchal region by seven weeks. Thyroxine is present by 11–12 weeks. The adrenal glands begin development at about 6 weeks. The cortex is derived from mesoderm, whereas the medulla is derived from neural crest cells. The fetal adrenal cortex has an important function during gestation of providing precursors to the placenta for synthesis of estrogens. Because of this function, the fetal adrenal cortex is 10–20 times larger than the adult adrenal cortex relative to weight. After birth it regresses to the small newborn size in 2–3 weeks.

TERATOLOGY

Any agent that causes a permanent defect in fetal function or structure is a teratogen. To fulfill this definition, the agent must meet 2 criteria: (1) the agent must cross the placenta and (2) the agent must reach the fetus during a susceptible time period. Basic principles of placental transport, critical time periods for fetal development, and known teratogens are discussed below.

Multiple factors are involved in chemical transport across the placenta. For the sake of discussion, it is assumed that whatever chemical or drug is involved has been adequately absorbed into the maternal circulation—obviously a necessary prerequisite for placental transfer. Important molecular characteristics are the size of the molecule, lack of ionization, and lipid solubility. Generally, chemicals cross the placenta more readily if the molecular weight is less than 1000 and if they are lipid soluble and nonionizing.

Transport mechanisms involved include simple diffusion, facilitated diffusion, active transport, pinocytocis, and bulk flow. Simple diffusion refers to transfer based solely on concentration gradients. Transfer occurs from a high to a low concentration. Examples of substances transported by this method are oxygen, carbon dioxide, sodium, potassium, immunoglobulin G (IgG), albumin, transferrin, and fibrinogen. Facilitated diffusion requires some energy to promote transport across the placenta. This type of diffusion not only depends on concentration gradients but also is characterized by saturation kinetics and competitive inhibition. Glucose is transported in this fashion. Active transport requires a carrier to transfer chemicals against a concentration gradient. Examples include amino acids, iron, calcium, magnesium, iodine, B vitamins, vitamin C, and folic acid. Pinocytosis is involved in the transport of IgG after 22 weeks and low-density lipoprotein receptors. Bulk flow transport depends on hydrostatic or osmotic gradients and is the method by which water is transported across the placenta.

Once the agent has reached the fetus, a teratogenic effect requires that the fetus be susceptible to its influence. The first 2 weeks after conception are often referred to as an "all or none" period because, if an embryo is exposed during this time to a drug, to radiation, or to an environmental agent, generally it either dies or survives intact. As is clear by the previous discussion, organogenesis occurs between 2 and 8 weeks after fertilization, and it is during this time that the embryo is most susceptible to teratogens. Specific defects depend exactly on when the exposure occurs and hence what system is developing. For example, thalidomide exposure during days 21–40 after fertilization will cause limb reduction defects.

The US Food and Drug Administration has classified drugs into categories based on what is known about their risk as a teratogen. This system is listed in Table 31–2 (see page 321) because it is in common use in the USA; however, most physicians believe that it is not fully accurate. For example, oral contraceptives are listed as category E (proven fetal risk and contraindicated during pregnancy) based on early data that suggested a relationship between first trimester use and fetal cardiac anomalies. When those data were reevaluated, no correlation was found between birth control pills and fetal cardiovascular defects. Thus, use of birth control pills during the first trimester is now not considered to be a significant risk to the fetus. Most drugs are listed as category C (no adequate studies are available), which leaves pertinent counseling up to the physician. In general, the physician should inform the patient that little is known about most drugs and most should be avoided in the first trimester and used only if medically indicated.

SUGGESTED READINGS

Benirschke K: Placental implantation and development. In: *Assessment and Care of the Fetus: Physiological, Clinical, and Medicolegal Principles.* Eden RD, Boehm FH (editors). Appleton & Lange, 1990.

Briggs GG et al: *Drugs in Pregnancy and Lactation: A Reference Guide to Fetal and Neonatal Risk,* 3rd ed. Williams & Wilkins, 1990.

Cunningham FG, McDonald PC, Gant NF: *Williams Obstetrics,* 18th ed. Appleton & Lange, 1989.

Moore KL: *The Developing Human: Clinically Oriented Embryology,* 4th ed. Saunders, 1988.

Yen SSC: Endocrinology of pregnancy. In: *Maternal-Fetal Medicine: Principles and Practice,* 2nd ed. Creasy RK, Resnik R (editors). Saunders, 1989.

Young BK: Placental regulation of fetal oxygenation and acid-base balance. In: *Assessment and Care of the Fetus: Physiological, Clinical, and Medicolegal Principles.* Eden RD, Boehm, RH (editors). Appleton & Lange, 1990.

Prenatal Care | 32

Elizabeth G. Livingston, MD

The aim of prenatal care is to reduce maternal and perinatal morbidity through a program of preventive medicine. Since 1935, maternal morbidity has fallen from more than 1 in 200 to less than 1 in 10,000. Certainly, access to antibiotics, blood products, and intravenous fluids has had tremendous impact on maternal death. In addition, the evolution of prenatal care has played a major role in preventing maternal mortality. The 1989 US National Institute of Child Health and Development conference on prenatal care noted that, even in the absence of disease, prenatal care appears to lead to healthier pregnancies. For women in countries without access to prenatal care, risk of death in pregnancy remains 200 times higher than in countries that provide prenatal care. Even in the USA, prenatal care appears to have an impact on maternal mortality. In 1983, a religious group in Indiana that refused medical care had maternal mortality rates 100 times that of other Indiana residents. Despite apparent benefit, significant numbers of pregnant American women receive no prenatal care. Both patients' lack of access to care and also patients' failure to recognize the value of care appear to play a role in these underserved pregnancies.

Although epidemiological evidence suggests that good prenatal care is effective in preserving the health of the mother, prenatal care has not been as effective in preventing perinatal mortality. We have not yet met the 1990 US Surgeon General's "Objectives for the Nation" goal of 9 deaths for every 1000 liveborn infants (no more than 12 for any county or racial or ethnic subgroup). In 1988, the overall infant mortality rate in the USA was 9.9 per 1000 live births, with the rate for blacks listed at 18 per 1000. Also, improved methods of prenatal care targeting the health of the fetus and neonate need to be developed.

THE PRECONCEPTUAL VISIT

The ideal time for a woman to initiate care for her pregnancy is before the pregnancy occurs. The teratogenic period in humans occurs before many women know they are pregnant. A preconceptual visit allows the health care provider to identify risks to the pregnancy, such as preexisting medical illness, risk for genetic disease, substance abuse, or poor social conditions. A physical examination may reveal unidentified medical problems, such as elevated blood pressure. Laboratory tests may be offered to diagnose, counsel, and possibly treat syphilis, rubella susceptibility, or infection with the human immunodeficiency virus (HIV). A preconceptual visit allows the woman to change her medications, seek social support, or change her environment before conception. The visit allows health education to begin for the patient and her partner at a time when it may have the most impact.

Diabetic control is an excellent example of the positive impact of preconceptual care. Lowering glycosylated hemoglobin levels through intensive insulin therapy before conception may decrease the fetal anomaly rate in diabetics.

THE FIRST OBSTETRIC VISIT

At the first visit, the health care provider should establish a database with a complete history, physical examination, and laboratory studies. This is a critical visit to establish a rapport with the patient and to initiate pregnancy education. If the woman has had preconceptual care, these tasks will have already been initiated. Not only can the first visit have far-reaching effects in pregnancy, but pregnancy may be one of the few times a woman may obtain any health care. Pregnancy may also be one of the few times she is motivated to change her health behaviors. It is important to include general, as well as pregnancy-specific, health advice in prenatal education.

History
A. Current Pregnancy: The most important historical data obtained at the first visit pertains to the length of gestation. During the first visit, the patient's memory is freshest and provides her best recollection of significant dates. Documenting the last menstrual period (LMP) is central to dating the pregnancy. Was the LMP of normal length? When was the previous menstrual period? Other historical features may aid in dating the pregnancy. Some patients may know the exact date of ovulation because they are familiar with the symptoms or they are using ovulation kits. Other

patients can give the date of conception as a result of specific circumstances, such as artificial insemination, travel plans, or in vitro fertilization.

Other important historical features at the first visit include a history of bleeding and pain. These symptoms may indicate impending spontaneous abortion or ectopic pregnancy. The presence of nausea, vomiting, or weight loss should be ascertained. For patients presenting later in pregnancy, data regarding fetal movement or contractions should be obtained.

B. Past Medical History: The health care provider should determine if the patient has any history of chronic medical illness. Diabetes, asthma, hypertension, and epilepsy are common and may carry a significant risk for the pregnancy. Alternatively, the pregnancy may also impact on these preexisting diseases. All current and recent medications, both prescribed and over the counter, should be recorded. Any use of vitamin A derivatives over the last few years should be noted. The patient should be queried regarding significant drug allergies or drug intolerance, especially to penicillin and its derivatives. A history of sexually transmitted diseases should be obtained as well as a history of sexual behaviors that might place the patient at risk. Previous operations and details regarding previous pelvic or abdominal procedures need review. A patient with a history of blood product administration between 1979 and 1985 should be offered HIV screening.

C. Previous Obstetric History: Previous pregnancy performance is one of the best predictors of pregnancy outcome. The dates of all previous pregnancies and their outcomes may be valuable information in determining risk factors for the current pregnancy. The gestational age, birthweight, route of delivery, necessity for labor induction, and current health status of offspring should be recorded in the obstetric database.

D. Social History: Socioeconomic status has a tremendous impact on pregnancy outcome. With questioning, many women may reveal a lack of such basics as food and shelter. A social worker is a crucial part of the health care team, assisting the patient in accessing resources in the community. A gentle inquiry should be made as to the woman's relationship with the father of the baby and his support of the pregnancy.

Unfortunately, violence against women is common in our society. Pregnant women are particularly vulnerable to violent acts. Most assaults on women are inflicted by someone they know. Supportive questions and the results of physical examination may provide clues to an abusive home or work situation.

The health care provider should inquire about details of the patient's work, both inside and outside the home. Possible hazardous exposures or behaviors for the pregnancy may be identified.

E. Habits: Every patient should be questioned about whether she uses legal (alcohol, nicotine, tranquilizers) or illicit drugs (narcotics, cocaine, amphetamines). All may have a negative effect on pregnancy. Pregnancy may be the rare time when a woman may be motivated and successful in changing her behavior, such as discontinuing smoking or use of other tobacco products. Questions should be made in a concerned but nonaccusatory fashion. For example, asking the question, ''You don't use drugs, do you?'' is not a useful way to gain information.

The patient who uses intravenous drugs needs to provide a detailed history of her injection habits, which might place her at risk of contracting bloodborne viruses. The woman whose pregnancy is complicated by drug use should be strongly advised about her personal risk and her offspring's risk. She should also be supported when she takes the first step toward improving her and her baby's health by revealing her use.

If the patient is willing and if the programs are available, the patient should be referred for counseling. The medical and legal role of toxicology screens in prenatal care has not been clearly defined. Frequently, the primary obstetric health care provider may be the only professional the patient is willing to see. Therefore, the primary responsibility in counseling the patient lies with this health care provider. Expressing concern and even just asking about these behaviors may be therapeutic for the pregnant patient with a legal or illegal drug dependency.

F. Family History: Inquiries should be made about the health of the future parents' families. A family history of genetic diseases, such as cystic fibrosis, should prompt referral to a genetic counselor. The ethnicity or country of origin of the parent's family may suggest risk for genetic diseases, such as a hemoglobinopathy or Tay-Sachs disease. Some obstetric disorders may be related to family history. A strong family history of diabetes may place the mother at higher risk of this complication. Maternal preeclampsia may place her female offspring at higher risk of this complication. Even a family history of certain infectious diseases, such as tuberculosis and hepatitis, may place the expectant mother and her fetus at risk.

Physical Examination

At the first visit, a complete physical examination should be performed. Once again, this may be the patient's only contact with a health care provider for many years. Therefore, a complete, general physical examination should be performed. At later visits, the physical examination can be tailored to the needs and complaints of the patient. A complete set of vital signs should also be obtained at the initial visit.

A. Head and Neck: Any problems with neck and jaw mobility that might interfere with airway management should be noted. The thyroid gland may be slightly symmetrically enlarged during normal pregnancy, but a visibly or irregularly enlarged gland should be evaluated. A source of lymphadenopathy should be determined. Poor dentition may prompt referral for dental care.

B. Chest and Back: Systolic ejection murmurs are common during pregnancy, but harsh systolic murmurs, diastolic murmurs, or extra sounds should be evaluated, as should the presence of wheezes, rales, or rhonchi.

More than 10% of women will develop breast cancer in their lifetimes. A thorough breast examination is important, and the patient should be educated about the value and method of self breast examination. Routine mammograms should be delayed until after pregnancy and breast feeding. The presence of a mass should be evaluated as in the nonpregnant state.

Severe scoliosis may lead to pulmonary insufficiency in later pregnancy. Previous back surgery may contraindicate conduction anesthesia.

C. Abdomen: If the top of the fundus is palpable, the fundal height should be recorded. The presence of fetal heart tones should be confirmed with an electronic or nonelectronic device. The health care provider should note scars, tenderness, or hepatic enlargement.

D. Pelvic Area: The external genitalia should be examined for presence of lesions consistent with sexually transmitted diseases, such as condylomata, venereal warts, or herpes. A scant white discharge is normal in the pregnant patient; other discharge should be evaluated with a wet mount. A Papanicolaou smear and cultures for gonorrhea and frequently for chlamydia are obtained from the cervix.

On bimanual examination the uterus should be evaluated for appropriateness of size for gestational dates. However, even with the most experienced hands, the estimate based on the bimanual examination may be 2 weeks off from the actual date. A common way to determine gestational age on bimanual examination is to compare the size of the uterus to that of various fruits. When the uterus is the size of an orange, gestational age is 6–8 weeks, a grapefruit is equivalent to 10–12 weeks, and a cantaloupe is equivalent to 14–16 weeks. Any irregularities in shape or position of the uterus should be noted. Molar or tubal pregnancy may be suspected if size is inappropriate for dates. The position of the uterus should be recorded. Rarely, the severely retroflexed uterus may become entrapped in the early second trimester. The length, dilatation, and softness of the cervix should be evaluated for any evidence of premature cervical dilatation. The adnexa should be palpated for the presence of a mass. Although frequently a physiologic cyst may be felt, occasionally a neoplasm, whether benign or malignant, may be first detected in the obstetric clinic. A tender adnexal mass may also suggest ectopic pregnancy.

E. Pelvimetry: At the time of pelvic examination, the health care provider should assess the size and shape of the bony pelvis. This assessment may help identify the woman at risk for dystocia at term. In the method of Caldwell-Moloy, the pelvis is usually described as gynecoid, anthropoid, android, platypelloid, or a combination of these types (Figure 32–1). Gynecoid is the most common female pelvic type with a rounded inlet and straight sidewalls. The anthropoid pelvis has a more oval inlet, whereas the rare platypelloid pelvis is wide and flat. The android pelvis is heart-shaped with convergent sidewalls. The patient with an android pelvis at term is at higher risk for cesarean section.

Several bony features should be evaluated in determining the pelvic type. The pubic arch is considered narrow if it is less than 90-100 degrees—more "gothic" than "romanesque." The ischial spines should be palpated and noted if prominent or sharp. The distance between the spines is narrow if less than 10 cm, and this indicates a narrow midpelvis. The inclination of the sacrum, whether average, backward, or forward should be assessed. The diagonal conjugate, the distance from the pubic arch to the sacral promontory, is an estimate of the obstetric conjugate, the inlet of the true pelvis. A diagonal conjugate of less than 11–12 cm is considered contracted and may place the mother of a normal-sized child at risk of abnormal labor.

Laboratory Studies

A. Type, Rh Factor, and Antibody Screen: A blood type, Rh factor, and antibody screen should be performed as early as possible on all pregnant women to look for the presence of antibodies that might lead to erythroblastosis fetalis. Also, it will allow identification of Rh negative patients that need Rh immune globulin

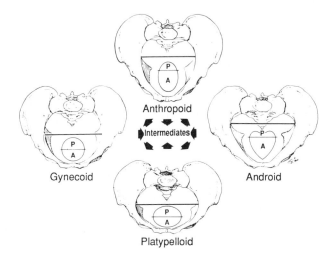

Figure 32-1. The four parent pelvic types of the Caldwell-Moloy classification. A line passing through the widest transverse diameter divides the inlet into posterior (P) and anterior (A) segments. *(Reproduced, with permission, from Cunningham FC, McDonald PC, Gant NF:* Williams Obstetrics, *18th ed. Appleton & Lange, 1989.)*

prophylaxis. The antibody screen may be repeated in the third trimester.

B. Hematocrit or Complete Blood Count: A hematocrit or complete blood count may identify the woman nutritionally at risk with iron deficiency anemia. It may also aid in identifying women who should undergo a hemoglobinopathy screen. The patient with a low mean corpuscular volume (MCV) in addition to a low hemoglobin is particularly at risk.

C. Serology for Syphilis: Serologic tests for syphilis should be performed early in pregnancy to allow treatment of infected women and possibly to avert congenital syphilis. Repeat testing in the third trimester and at delivery is justified in high-risk populations.

D. Rubella Antibodies: Screening for rubella immunity should be performed to identify patients at risk for congenital rubella syndrome and those that should be vaccinated postpartum.

If lack of immunity is identified at a preconceptual visit, consideration should be given to vaccination and avoidance of pregnancy for 3 months following inoculation.

E. Papanicolaou Smear: Because the prenatal examination may be the only recent contact with a health care provider that the patient has had, cytologic screening of the cervix should be performed. If the smear is abnormal, the patient should undergo colposcopic examination. Abnormal Papanicolaou smear results may also lead to a change in plans for an operative delivery or tubal ligation.

F. Urine Testing: All patients should be screened for the presence of underlying renal disease or urinary tract infection with a urinalysis and possible urine culture. Patients with underlying renal disease are at much higher risk of preeclampsia. Among the 10% of pregnant women with asymptomatic bacteriuria, almost one-fourth will progress to pyelonephritis.

G. Hemoglobin Electrophoresis: Patients that have a family history of hemoglobinopathy, that are of African descent, or that have low mean corpuscular volume (MCV), or other risk factors should undergo hemoglobin electrophoresis. Not only will it reveal the cause of a low hematocrit, but it will also identify the fetus at risk for inheriting a hemoglobinopathy.

H. Tuberculin Skin Test: If at risk, patients should be screened with a skin test for tuberculosis. Patients with a current positive test or previous positive test should undergo chest x-ray with abdominal shielding. If the chest x-ray is positive, consultation should be sought to determine if the patient needs therapy during or after pregnancy.

I. Cervical Cultures: Cervical cultures for gonorrhea and chlamydia are indicated in a high-risk population or in patients with evidence of other sexually transmitted diseases, such as condyloma acuminatum, *Trichomonas,* or syphilis. If the results are positive, the patient should be treated promptly. Tetracyclines should be avoided. Currently, there is controversy regarding universal screening for group B streptococcus.

J. Hepatitis Surface Antigen: Vertical transmission from mother to infant is responsible for almost 3500 cases of hepatitis B yearly in the USA. This transmission can be interrupted by prompt administration of hepatitis B immune globulin and hepatitis B vaccine to neonates of infected mothers. Antenatal screening is clearly worthwhile in high-risk mothers, such as those from Southeast Asia or intravenous drug users. Some medical groups have encouraged and some states in the USA have legislated routine screening of all pregnant women.

K. Maternal Serum Alpha-Fetoprotein: Maternal serum alpha-fetoprotein is another screening test many states require to be offered. This test is usually performed between 15 and 19 weeks. Very high values may indicate neural tube defects. An association between low values and chromosomal abnormalities has also been noted.

L. Human Immunodeficiency Virus: Infants born to HIV positive mothers have approximately a 30% chance of being infected with the virus. Pregnancy also offers the opportunity to identify infected mothers and bring them into the health care system. For these reasons, HIV screening should be offered to high-risk mothers after informed consent is obtained. It is still controversial whether the test should be offered routinely to all mothers during pregnancy.

M. Glucose Challenge Test: For mothers without known diabetes, glucose screening after a glucose load should be considered to determine the presence of gestational diabetes. This test is usually performed early in the third trimester, between 25 and 28 weeks. It may be performed earlier in mothers at high risk for gestational diabetes. The American College of Obstetricians and Gynecologists recommends screening only high-risk groups, whereas the World Health Organization recommends routine screening.

N. Ultrasonography: When the size of the fetus does not correlate with the gestational age or when the fetus is at risk for anomalies, ultrasonography can be helpful. Routine screening ultrasonography has not been strongly advocated in the USA, but has been found to be useful in other national health care systems.

O. Recording: Recording and conveying the information in the collected database may be done in several ways. Accessibility for staff in both the clinic and the hospital is essential. Gestational age, laboratory data, and risk factors should be easily identified. The record should be kept up to date. Commercial forms are frequently used, such as that provided by HOLLISTER. Computerized prenatal databases are popular because of their ready accessibility. The computer record may also assist in compiling delivery statistics.

Plan for Pregnancy

At the conclusion of the first visit, significant findings should be reviewed with the patient and her partner, and a plan for the pregnancy should be devised. The patient should be labelled high risk if concurrent medical illness, previous poor pregnancy performance, or poor psychosocial situation is identified. When appropriate, the patient should be referred to a perinatologist or other medical specialist. A plan for education, including the partner, should encompass danger signs for various points during the pregnancy, childbirth preparation, and breast feeding.

FOLLOW-UP VISITS

In general, the follow-up visits will be much more brief than the preconceptual or new obstetric patient visit. Follow-up visits should include a brief interval history that focuses on potential problems such as premature labor. An abbreviated physical examination is conducted that includes measurements of blood pressure, fundal height, and fetal heart tones; any other appropriate examinations as indicated by history should also be performed. Urinalysis may be performed at each visit. Care should be taken to not miss the appropriate dates for alpha-fetoprotein or glucose tests.

The traditional follow-up interval is based on a model to detect preeclampsia. The usual routine is infrequent visits early in the pregnancy—about every 4 weeks until 28 weeks. Between 28 and 36 weeks, the patient is seen every 2–3 weeks and weekly thereafter until delivery. If medical or obstetric complications are present, a physician should determine an appropriate follow-up interval.

NUTRITION

During prenatal care, it is important to identify the patient who is at risk nutritionally. Risk factors for undernutrition include being teenaged (13–17 years old) or being of low socioeconomic status; being underweight; having recent or frequent pregnancies; and abusing alcohol or other drugs. Food faddists and women engaging in pica (compulsive eating of nonnutritive substances, such as starch or clay) may place themselves at risk. Inquiring whether there is an adequate quantity of food in the home may identify women who need emergency aid or referral to a food assistance program, such as the Women, Infants, and Children (WIC) program.

Weight Gain

Prepregnancy weight and weight gain during pregnancy are related to birth weight. In the past, obstetricians in the USA severely limited weight gain in the unsubstantiated hope of decreasing the incidence of preeclampsia. Most current sources recommend a weight gain of 10–15 kg (20–35 lb). Certainly, the pregnant patient, even the obese patient, should not lose weight. Excessive weight gain will not benefit outcome and will be difficult to lose postpartum. Weight gain should be assessed at each visit. Poor weight gain in a pregnant patient may indicate anything from inadequate food in the home to a misguided desire to preserve her figure. Rapid weight gain in the last weeks of pregnancy may be a harbinger of fluid retention secondary to preeclampsia. Fluids should never be restricted in the normal pregnant patient.

Appropriate weight gain can usually be achieved by consuming an extra 300 kcal each day. This amount varies depending on the size and activity of the woman. For many women, the lessened activity of pregnancy may negate the need to consume more calories or "eat for two." Additional nutrients will be required if the patient elects to breast feed postpartum.

Protein

The fetus, placenta, uterus, and breasts require a steady supply of protein to grow during pregnancy. Sources recommend as little as 10 extra grams to as much as 30 extra grams of protein. Protein is most easily obtained from animal sources.

Vitamins & Minerals

The requirements for most vitamins and minerals increase slightly during pregnancy. Vitamin and mineral supplements are no substitute for a well-balanced diet. The roles of selected vitamins and minerals are summarized below.

A. Folic Acid: Folic acid is necessary whenever cells are dividing. Because the fetus and placenta are growing rapidly, the folate requirement during pregnancy increases to twice the nonpregnant requirement. Folate deficiency is common in women in the USA. In animal studies, folic acid deficiency may cause congenital defects. In humans, there is some evidence that folate supplementation may decrease the risk of neural tube defects. Folate remains the one vitamin for which supplementation, in addition to dietary intake, may be useful.

B. Vitamin B$_{12}$: Vitamin B$_{12}$ deficiency is uncommon. Occasionally, it can be found in the strict vegetarian (consuming no animal products) or in the presence of pernicious anemia. Its deficiency should be considered in the patient with megaloblastic anemia before treatment with folate.

C. Vitamin A: The requirements for Vitamin A do not increase during pregnancy. Very high doses and certain vitamin A derivatives may be teratogenic. The patient on very high doses should delay conception.

D. Vitamins C and D: While both vitamin C and vitamin D are necessary for fetal growth and maternal health, megadoses may be hazardous. High doses of vitamin C in the mother may result in scurvy after birth in the offspring. High doses of vitamin D in animals is teratogenic and may be in humans as well.

E. Iron: Iron deficiency is the most common nutritional deficiency in the US diet, affecting 5–20% of American women. Iron requirements double during pregnancy to provide the gram of iron required by the fetus and expanding blood volume. It is very difficult for pregnant women to consume adequate iron without consuming excessive calories. Therefore, as with folate, supplementation of 30–60 mg of elemental iron during pregnancy is warranted. Dietary iron is most easily absorbed from animal sources.

F. Calcium: Calcium requirements in pregnancy and lactation are more than 1 g/d. Consumption of food rich in calcium, such as a quart of low-fat milk per day, may obviate the need for supplementation. Many adults of African or Asian heritage may be lactose intolerant and develop diarrhea, cramps, and flatulence with milk. These people may tolerate an alternative diary source, such as cheese.

G. Zinc, Iodine, and Potassium: While zinc deficiency may produce congenital defects in animals, almost all humans obtain adequate zinc in their diets. Adequate iodine can be obtained in iodized salt. Some products contain high levels of iodine (eg, older expectorants), and excessive ingestion may result in fetal goiter. Potassium levels should be monitored in women with excessive nausea and vomiting.

OTHER CONCERNS

Work

Most pregnant women continue to work throughout pregnancy. Unless medical or obstetric problems complicate the pregnancy, it may be in the patient's and her offspring's socioeconomic interest to support her decision to continue working. A work history should be obtained to evaluate for exposure to potential hazards or teratogens, such as radionucleides or x-rays. Heavy lifting should be avoided, as should long periods of sitting or standing. There is little evidence to suggest that sitting at a data terminal is hazardous. Operating rooms are now equipped with efficient scavenging systems for anesthetic gases that should protect pregnant care providers from that hazard.

Sex

Most sexual activity is not dangerous during pregnancy. The woman's libido may increase or decrease. The enlarging uterus may necessitate experimentation with different positions for intercourse during pregnancy. There are a few precautions for sex during pregnancy. Oral sex with vaginal insufflation has been implicated in deaths from air emboli. Certainly, intercourse should be avoided in patients with placenta previa. Nipple stimulation in the third trimester may potentially lead to tetanic contractions. Many physicians discourage their patients with premature labor from intercourse and orgasm for fear of worsening contractions. The patient who is treated for a sexually transmitted disease should insist her partner be treated and counseled as well before resuming sexual activity.

Travel

Cautious travel may be undertaken during pregnancy. Seat belts should be worn by the pregnant woman. However, the patient should be careful to place the lap belt low over her pelvis, not over her fundus. The pregnant patient should walk at frequent intervals while traveling because of her increased risk of deep venous thrombosis. Air travel in a pressurized cabin is acceptable. Many airlines discourage women in the late third trimester from flying. If a prolonged trip must be undertaken, the patient should consider carrying some of her medical records with her.

Exercise

With the current emphasis on fitness, many women are now exercising throughout pregnancy. Most evidence shows that exercise is safe in the uncomplicated pregnancy. If there are no medical or obstetric complications, the obstetric health care provider can be supportive of continued athletic activity in pregnancy.

A few guidelines can be offered to the pregnant woman. One rule of thumb is that most activities the woman did before pregnancy can be done during pregnancy, but no new or more vigorous programs should be undertaken. The patient should avoid sports in which balance is important or the risk of injury is great. Sky diving, horse jumping, springboard diving, or downhill skiing are not advisable during pregnancy. Scuba diving is also not recommended. The pregnant woman should avoid hyperthermia and should keep her exertion in a submaximal range. She should avoid prolonged exercise flat on her back. For any person, it is never advisable to walk, jog, bike, or swim alone. Many cities now have prenatal exercise classes, and many videotapes are now available with low impact aerobic programs geared to the pregnant female.

Clothing

Clothing should be loose and comfortable during pregnancy. Some companies now specialize in maternity clothes appropriate for the workplace. Some women find maternity support hosiery helpful for leg discomforts during pregnancy. No stockings or garters that might inhibit venous return should be worn. Frequently, larger shoes may be required. High heels may further disrupt unsteady balance.

Personal Hygiene

Both tub baths and showers are safe during pregnancy. Care should be taken to avoid falling in the bathroom as a result of unsteady balance. Hyperthermia, as might be induced in a jacuzzi, should be avoided. Most cosmetics are safe. Although there is little evidence to suggest danger, some health care providers discourage their patients from having hair dyes or permanents in the first trimester.

Immunizations

Ideally, the need for immunization was identified and remedied at the preconceptual visit. During pregnancy all live virus vaccines, such as rubella, should be avoided, although the risk is mainly theoretical. Polio and yellow fever vaccines may be used if necessary. Certainly, other vaccines should be given if a clear-cut indication exists, such as in a patient with a puncture wound who has had no tetanus toxoid in 10 years.

Dental Care

The pregnant patient should continue to receive her regular dental care. Frequently, at the new obstetric patient examination, caries are identified. If asymptomatic, treatment can be deferred until the first trimester is completed. If abscess appears likely, care should be undertaken immediately. Dental x-rays with abdominal shielding may be performed. Local anesthesia is not contraindicated. Inhalation agents should not be used in pregnant women because of the risk of aspiration. If indicated, antibiotics may be used, but tetracycline should be avoided. If the patient usually receives bacterial endocarditis prophylaxis, it should be given.

Recreational Drugs & Smoking

Recreational drugs, including alcohol and tobacco, should be avoided during pregnancy. Alcohol may lead to fetal alcohol syndrome. A safe level of consumption has not been defined. Other recreational drugs are not safe alternatives to alcohol and should be avoided. Cocaine has been implicated in abruption, premature labor, and learning disabilities. Heroin has been associated with intrauterine growth restriction and may result in neonatal withdrawal. Tobacco products have also been associated with lowered birth weights. Pregnancy may motivate women to discontinue self-destructive habits. Substance abuse by the patient's partner may place the family at risk not only for HIV and hepatitis, but also for poverty and abuse.

DISCOMFORTS OF PREGNANCY

Cardiovascular Problems

A. Syncope: Lightheadedness or fainting caused by postural hypotension may occur in pregnancy. Encouraging a patient to rise to her feet slowly may prevent these episodes. Lightheadedness may be due to hypoglycemia from fetal glucose consumption. The symptoms may respond to small frequent meals. If the patient experiences loss of consciousness or a fall, she deserves a full medical evaluation for syncope.

B. Ankle Edema and Varicose Veins: Third spacing of fluid in the lower extremities and varicosities are common during pregnancy because of increased venous pressure. Frequent elevation of the lower extremities or support hosiery may be useful. The patient should be discouraged from fluid restriction for edema. Hand or face edema may herald impending preeclampsia. The patient with varicosities should be observed for development of superficial thrombophlebitis or deep venous thrombosis.

Respiratory Problems

Breathlessness is a common symptom in pregnancy. Higher levels of progesterone may increase respiratory drive. Also, the increased maternal metabolic rate and oxygen consumption by fetal tissues increase maternal respiratory drive. When this increased drive is combined with an expanding fundus, many pregnant women feel that they cannot "catch their breath." Nasal congestion, common during pregnancy, may worsen this sensation. Frequently, measurements of arterial blood gas reveal a respiratory alkalosis with adequate oxygenation. For these women, reassurance and relaxation may aid their distress. For patients who present with shortness of breath and a rapid respiratory rate, serious causes should be excluded. Pregnancy occasionally exacerbates asthma, and pregnant women may be at higher risk for pulmonary embolus.

Gastrointestinal Problems

A. Nausea and Vomiting: Nausea and vomiting are common in early pregnancy. The so-called "morning sickness" may occur at any time in the day. For most women, small, frequent meals, soda crackers at the bedside, and avoidance of spicy, aromatic foods may be the only therapy needed. For the ketotic, dehydrated patient, more aggressive intervention with intravenous fluids and possibly antiemetics may be indicated. Behavioral therapies, such as psychotherapy, hypnosis, and biofeedback, may be useful to treat vomiting during pregnancy. Acupuncture has even been used. The patient can be reassured that, for almost all women, the problem resolves by 20 weeks. Serious causes of gastrointestinal distress, such as appendicitis, cholecystitis, and pancreatitis should be excluded as causes of vomiting.

B. Ptyalism: One problem that may worsen nausea and vomiting during pregnancy is ptyalism, or the hypersalivation that some women experience with pregnancy. Occasionally, these patients may be identified by the cups or piles of tissue that they carry to accommodate their saliva. Not only nauseating and inconvenient, this condition may lead to loss of fluids and electrolytes. Although anticholinergic drugs are frequently effective, they should be used with caution during early pregnancy.

C. Heartburn and Reflux: In the third trimester, patients will frequently complain of symptoms of reflux. Small frequent meals, remaining upright after eating, avoidance of spicy foods, and use of antacids usually afford relief.

D. Constipation and Hemorrhoids: Smooth muscle relaxation, decreased activity, and oral iron makes constipation a frequent complaint during pregnancy. Dietary measures, such as increased fiber, fruits, vegetables, and fluids, may be adequate to correct constipation. Docusate and Milk of Magnesia are frequently prescribed to correct this problem.

The combination of constipation and increased venous pressure frequently leads to hemorrhoids. Avoiding long periods of standing and correcting constipation should be attempted. Witch hazel pads, a doughnut cushion, and hydrocortisone cream may also afford relief.

Pelvic Symptoms

A. Urgency and Frequency: Decreased bladder capacity and edema of the trigone may lead to urgency and frequency. Urinary tract infection is common in pregnancy and needs to be excluded in the patient with these complaints.

B. Leukorrhea: A whitish vaginal discharge occurs in most pregnant women. It is rarely so heavy as to require a perineal pad. Other causes of discharge, such as cervicitis, vaginitis, and ruptured membranes, should be investigated.

C. Round Ligament Pain: Occasionally, during the second trimester the pregnant woman will complain of a unilateral or bilateral pulling pain. Traditionally, this pain has been ascribed to rapid growth of the uterus, leading to tension on the round ligaments. This is a diagnosis of exclusion, and all serious causes of abdominal pain should be ruled out.

SUGGESTED READINGS

Cunningham FG, McDonald PC, Gant NF: Prenatal care. In: *Williams Obstetrics,* 18th ed. Appleton & Lange, 1989.

Frigoletto FD, Little GA (editors): *Guidelines for Prenatal Care.* American Academy of Pediatrics; American College of Obstetricians and Gynecologists, 1988.

33 | Genetic Screening, Counseling, & Prenatal Diagnosis

Thomas L. Pinckert, MD

Few experiences are as devastating to a parent as the birth of an infant with a major, sometimes life-threatening, congenital anomaly. Of the 3.5 million live births in the USA in 1990, 2–5% of infants were born with major congenital anomalies. Unfortunately, this small percentage of births accounted for 20–30% of the perinatal deaths. Of those infants with a genetic disease who survive, many suffer from significant morbidity, which requires extensive physical and medical therapy. Estimates and hospital records suggest that approximately 20–30% of pediatric inpatient admissions are directly related to complications of a genetic disease.

The role of prenatal diagnosis is to determine which couples are at risk for conceiving a fetus with a genetic abnormality and to screen the developing fetus for the presence of the anomaly. In many cases, the results of prenatal diagnosis will indicate that the fetus is unaffected, allaying the fears of parents with a high-risk pregnancy. If the fetus is affected, couples may then use the information ascertained by prenatal diagnosis to make choices regarding the pregnancy. These options may include pregnancy termination to allow the birthing of only unaffected offspring, psychological and medical anticipation for the birth of an abnormal child, or diagnostic tests to permit prenatal treatment of a few selected genetic diseases.

TYPES OF GENETIC ABNORMALITIES

Before undertaking the task of prenatal screening, it is essential that the clinician understand the different types of genetic diseases that exist. This understanding will enable the clinician to make an accurate risk assessment of each pregnancy in question and will facilitate the appropriate choice of diagnostic tests for screening a fetus at risk. Genetic diseases can be classified into

4 different categories: (1) chromosomal abnormalities, (2) single gene disorders, (3) multifactorial inheritance disorders, and (4) environmental factors.

Chromosomal Abnormalities

The category of chromosomal abnormalities refers to abnormalities of the chromosome number or structure. The normal chromosome complement is 46,XX (female) or 46,XY (male). Each person has 23 pairs of chromosomes for a total of 46 chromosomes. Individuals receive one-half of their chromosomes from their father and one-half from their mother. The number of chromosomes normally received from each parent is called the **haploid number** or n. The total complement of 46 chromosomes is called the **diploid number** or 2n. **Aneuploidy** is the general term used to describe chromosome abnormalities with fewer or greater numbers of chromosomes than 46. These abnormalities of number are further described as **trisomies** (2n + 1) when one chromosome more than 46 is present, and **monosomies** (2n − 1) when one fewer is present. Occasionally, entire duplications of the haploid contribution from one parent may be seen, which is referred to as **polyploidy** (although these abnormalities are usually lethal). **Triploidy** (3n) probably results from failure of one of the maturation divisions (sperm or egg), and **tetraploidy** (4n) results from failure of completion of the first cleavage division of the fertilized egg.

In addition to numerical aberrations of the chromosomes, structural changes within the individual chromosomes also occur. **Translocations** of chromosomes involve an exchange of material from one chromosome to another. Both chromosomes break, and the genetic material is rearranged abnormally. Translocations are described as balanced if the genetic material is mutually exchanged and no loss of chromosomal material occurs. An unbalanced translocation occurs when there is a nonreciprocal exchange of material between chromosomes with a net loss or gain of genetic material.

Deletions of portions of chromosomes are also encountered. These deletions may be from the terminal end of a chromosome requiring a single break or from the interstitial portion of the chromosome, occurring between 2 breaks. Deletions cause serious consequences because of the loss of the genetic material contained in the deleted portions. If a large amount of material is lost or if the deleted portion codes for a critical element, death or severe morbidity are the usual result.

Chromosomal **inversions** result in a rearrangement of the order of the genes. Inversions result from 2 breaks in the chromosome with an inversion of the portion of chromosome between the breaks. If the breaks occur on the same side of the centromere, they are described as **paracentric.** If the inverted section of chromosome involves the centromere, then it is called a **pericentric inversion.** Inversions may be a cause of frequent spontaneous abortions because of unbalanced gametes that form with crossovers. Paracentric inversions may cause **acentric** or **dicentric** chromosome fragments that lead to the loss of a large amount of genetic material; these anomalies are usually lethal. Pericentric inversions cause duplications and deletions of chromosomal material at the time of gamete formation. These changes may result not only in spontaneous abortions but also in the birth of anomalous live-born infants.

Major chromosomal abnormalities are seen in only 0.56% of live births but are found in more than 50% of first trimester abortuses. Twelve to fifteen percent of clinically recognized pregnancies end in a first-trimester spontaneous abortion, many of which are due to chromosomal abnormalities. Autosomal trisomies represent the largest category of chromosomal abnormalities in spontaneous abortions with trisomy 16 (7%), trisomy 22 (2%), and trisomy 21 (2%) as the most common. Monosomy X (45,X) is found in approximately 8–9% of spontaneous abortions and is the leading single cause of first trimester spontaneous abortion. It is common for a couple with a history of a prior pregnancy loss as a result of a chromosomal abnormality to be referred for prenatal diagnosis.

Not all chromosomal abnormalities result in spontaneous abortion. Trisomies 21 (1:650), 18 (1:5000–7000), and 13 (1:12,000–24,000) have been associated with live-born infants. Trisomies 13 and 18 are almost always lethal, but such infants may survive several months. All these trisomies have been associated with severe cardiac anomalies, serious central nervous system (CNS) malformations, and dysmorphic physical features. Those infants who live are all moderately to severely retarded. With proper medical care, trisomy 21 individuals may live into their fifth or sixth decade. Structural chromosomal rearrangements that occur de novo in the fetus are believed to carry a 10–15% risk of associated anomalies in the fetus. Because of the significant morbidity associated with chromosomal abnormalities, it is imperative that these conditions be diagnosed prenatally to offer couples the best possible counseling regarding their options.

Single Gene Disorders

Single gene disorders occur in about 1.5% of all infants and are estimated to account for 8% of congenital anomalies noted at birth. Mendelian inheritance, as this category is also known, is thought to arise from a defect in a single gene on a chromosome. There are many more disorders in this category than in the chromosomal abnormalities group. Thus far, more than 2200 disorders have been clearly identified as mendelian, and approximately 2100 others have been suspected of following mendelian inheritance. Because genes are found on every chromosome, both autosomal and sex chromosome (sex-linked) abnormalities may be found.

A normal genetic complement consists of 23 pairs of chromosomes. Some disorders are seen when the mutant gene is present on only one chromosome of the chromosomal pair and are called dominant disorders. Other disorders are manifested only when both chromosomes of the pair carry the mutant gene. Disorders that necessitate 2 doses of the same mutant gene are called recessive disorders. Thus, the 4 patterns of mendelian inheritance encountered are as follows: (1) autosomal dominant, (2) autosomal recessive, (3) sex-linked dominant, and (4) sex-linked recessive.

Autosomal dominant disorders can occur if the trait is inherited from an affected parent or if it arises as a new mutation. In the heterozygous state, the affected individual has a 50:50 chance of passing the trait on to an offspring, male or female. Males and females usually have an equal chance of having an autosomal dominant trait. Unaffected individuals (those not carrying the trait) have no chance of passing on the trait to their offspring.

Autosomal recessive traits occur when the individual is homozygous for the mutant allele. An autosomal recessive trait is usually the product of 2 heterozygotes mating. Here, the likelihood of having an affected offspring is 25%.

X-linked recessive traits are manifested in all males that carry the abnormal X chromosome. Usually, a heterozygous female transmits the abnormal X chromosome to 50% of her male or female offspring. Males receiving the abnormal X chromosome will be affected. Females receiving the allele will be heterozygous carriers and will generally be unaffected. Heterozygous female carriers may express manifestations of an X-linked disorder because the random inactivation of the X chromosome (Lyon hypothesis) may leave a variable number of normal X chromosomes inactivated.

X-linked dominant traits are rare. In this method of inheritance, female heterozygotes for mutations on the X chromosome do express the disorder. The frequency of affected females is twice that of affected males, and females are usually less severely affected (again due to the random inactivation of mutant and normal X chromosomes in females). An affected male will have all affected female offspring but no affected male offspring. Heterozygous females will transmit the disorder to one-half of their offspring of either sex. Homozygous females will transmit the disorder to all their offspring; thus, homozygous transmission resembles autosomal dominant transmission. Autosomal dominant transmission can be distinguished by the pattern of inheritance in the progeny of affected males.

Prenatal diagnosis of mendelian inherited disorders is difficult, but possible, for some of the disorders. Many of these disorders have phenotypic manifestations that can be detected with prenatal sonography (eg, intrauterine growth retardation, skeletal dysplasias, cardiovascular or CNS manifestations) if the presence of a disorder is suspected. Other conditions, with enzyme deficiencies, immunological changes, or skin changes such as ichthyosis may be ascertained by direct tissue sampling. However, there are too many disorders to screen for without a goal or suspected diagnosis in mind. Mendelian disorders are most often investigated after an affected family member has been diagnosed, and a recurrence risk is requested for a current pregnancy. Unfortunately, many of these disorders still have no readily identifiable marker, and prenatal diagnosis is not possible.

Multifactorial Inheritance

Multifactorial inheritance is most often associated with those conditions that are a combination of genetic and environmental factors. Diseases such as cleft lip and palate, pyloric stenosis, spina bifida, dislocations of the hip, clubfoot, and congenital heart disease fall into this category. Unlike single defects, which should have the same recurrence risk for each pregnancy at risk, the recurrence rate for diseases with multifactorial inheritance may vary. There appears to be a relationship between recurrence risk and population frequency, with a greater risk for a given defect occurring in a population with a high frequency than in one with a low frequency of the disorder. Also of note in multifactorial inheritance is an increased risk of recurrence (RR) of the condition after 2 affected children, an increased recurrence risk with increased severity of the defect (RR after unilateral cleft lip is 2.5%, RR is 5.6% for bilateral cleft lip and palate), and a different recurrence risk depending on the sex of the studied individual (RR for pyloric stenosis is 20% for sons of affected females, RR is 5% for daughters of affected females). Fortunately, many of these diseases may be diagnosed prenatally with the use of ultrasound.

Environmental Factors

Environmental factors that alter genetic inheritance may be classified as either mutagens or teratogens. Mutagens are agents that change the genetic material of the germ cells and are thus perpetuated in subsequent generations. Teratogens alter the somatic tissues of the embryo to produce malformations; thus, the effect of the teratogen is usually limited to the affected individual. Most mutagens arc also teratogens, but not all teratogens are capable of changing the germ cells (ie, mutagens).

Whether a particular environmental factor is teratogenic or not depends on the physical and chemical makeup of the agent, the developmental stage of the embryo, and interaction with other environmental agents (eg, combination of agents, presence of an agent with radiation, heat, virus, or nutritional deficiency). Teratogens may not necessarily be exogenous. Current studies clearly show an increased risk of malformations in the offspring of diabetic mothers, suggesting that hyperglycemia or other metabolites of diabetic mothers are harmful to a developing embryo. The role of prenatal diagnosis in patients exposed to environmental factors is to determine, primarily by ultrasonography, whether the agent in question has produced effects in the fetus.

TECHNIQUES FOR PRENATAL DIAGNOSIS

History

Once a couple has been identified as a candidate for prenatal diagnosis, the most important task for the geneticist is to obtain a thorough family history. This history should include information on at least 3 generations for each partner. The family history forms the foundation for making an accurate genetic risk assessment.

Frequently, a skilled genetic counselor will uncover potential genetic diseases that neither member of the couple or the referring health professional had considered. Diagnostic tests may need to be performed for other family members to help confirm the diagnosis of an abnormality or to elucidate its mode of transmission. An example of such testing is the use of hemoglobin electrophoresis to evaluate a family with a hemoglobinopathy. Alternatively, creatine phosphokinase levels can be measured and used as a marker for muscular dystrophy. Once the information regarding family history and the diagnostic test results are obtained, a genetic disease can be assessed for its prevalence, mode of inheritance, and the potential manifestations of the disease in the fetus.

The family history and genetic data should be summarized in a family pedigree. This chart uses standard abbreviations and symbols to identify the family members and those affected with the disease. The family member in question (usually the fetus in prenatal diagnosis) is called the proband or propositus. Examples of the symbols used are shown in Figure 33–1.

Alpha-Fetoprotein

At present, the only prenatal blood test designed to detect the presence of a congenital anomaly in utero is maternal serum alpha-fetoprotein. Alpha-fetoprotein (AFP) is a glycoprotein that has been discovered in fetal and maternal serum but is not normally found in the serum of nonpregnant women. AFP is initially produced in the fetal yolk sac during early gestation and is subsequently made by the fetal liver. While the highest levels of AFP remain in the fetal serum, the normal fetus excretes small amounts of AFP into the amniotic fluid as a normal constituent of fetal urine. Small amounts of AFP also pass through the fetal skin into the amniotic fluid. During normal gestation, the peak ratio of fetal serum AFP to amniotic fluid AFP levels is about 200:1.

Although the exact mechanism of transfer from the fetal compartment to the maternal compartment is unclear, low levels of AFP can be measured in maternal serum during normal gestation. At the middle of the second trimester, the normal ratio of maternal serum AFP to fetal serum AFP levels is 1:100,000.

The role of fetal AFP in normal pregnancy is unclear, although 2 possible options for this protein have been postulated. AFP may serve as an anti-immune protein to help prevent rejection of the fetus by the mother. Alternatively, it may act as a carrier protein for the fetus, becoming the principal oncotic substance and binding to bilirubin, fatty acids, and estrogen.

Maternal serum AFP is useful as a prenatal diagnostic tool because any fetal anomaly that causes a break in the usual dermal integument results in a markedly elevated amniotic fluid AFP level and subsequently an elevated maternal serum AFP level. The most common causes for elevated levels of AFP are neural tube defects, such as anencephaly, spina bifida, and encephalocele, or ventral wall defects, such as omphalocele or gastroschisis. Disorders that interfere with fetal swallowing may also be associated with a rise in AFP levels. Most studies suggest that approximately 80–85% of all neural tube defects can be detected by screening maternal serum between 15–20 weeks gestation. This estimate includes about 80% of all open spina bifida cases and 90% of anencephaly cases. Un-

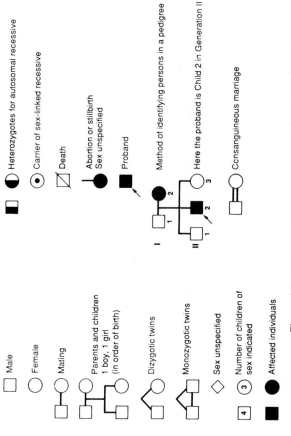

Figure 33-1. Symbols commonly used in pedigree charts.

Male

Female

Mating

Parents and children
1 boy, 1 girl
(in order of birth)

Dizygotic twins

Monozygotic twins

Sex unspecified

4 (3) Number of children of
sex indicated

Affected individuals

Heterozygotes for autosomal recessive

Carrier of sex-linked recessive

Death

Abortion or stillbirth
Sex unspecified

Proband

Method of identifying persons in a pedigree

Here the proband is Child 2 in Generation II

Consanguineous marriage

353

fortunately, closed spina bifida (10% of cases) is often not diagnosed with maternal serum AFP screening because there is no break in the integrity of the fetal skin. A more recently identified benefit of maternal serum AFP screening is the detection of trisomy 21 fetuses that are associated with low maternal serum AFP values. It is estimated that 20% of Down syndrome fetuses may be identified in this manner. It is possible that other aneuploidies may also be detected as a result of low maternal serum AFP levels. Thus, current recommendations are that all pregnant women undergo maternal serum AFP testing between 15 and 19 weeks of gestation.

Once obtained, maternal serum or amniotic fluid AFP test results are expressed as multiples of the median (MOMs) AFP levels so that values may be compared from laboratory to laboratory. Cutoff levels for normal maternal serum AFP values generally range between 0.5 and 2.5 MOMs in most laboratories. The MOM is calculated by dividing the test sample value for AFP, in nanograms per milliliter, by the laboratory's median value for that gestational age. Thus, a correct gestational age is crucial in determining whether a maternal serum AFP level is abnormally elevated or not. Serum levels must also be correlated with race and multiple gestations. If an abnormally elevated AFP value is discovered, sonography is important to confirm accurate dating and to exclude other possible causes of AFP elevations, such as sacrococcygeal teratoma, cystic hygroma, skin defects, or placental hemangioma.

Ultrasonography

The ability to diagnose genetic disorders prenatally has expanded dramatically as a result of the advancement of ultrasonography. Not only has this tool allowed a "view into the womb," to assess fetal number, position, and improved gestational dating, but it has also permitted the use of more invasive diagnostic procedures, such as amniocentesis, chorionic villus sampling, fetal blood sampling, and fetal tissue biopsy. Furthermore, since many genetic conditions are associated with abnormalities that can be detected by ultrasonography, such as intrauterine growth retardation, abnormal amniotic fluid volumes (oligohydramnios or polyhydramnios), and abnormal structural development, the expanded use of routine ultrasonography has improved the clinician's ability to detect many fetuses who may be candidates for prenatal diagnosis.

Amniocentesis

Amniocentesis is the simplest and most commonly used invasive procedure in the field of prenatal diagnosis with estimates of more than 200,000 procedures performed in 1990. During the procedure, amniotic fluid and amniocytes are obtained from the amniotic cavity for subsequent genetic analysis. Amniocentesis is also used to assess fetal lung maturity, detect intra-amniotic infection or chorioamnionitis, determine fetal status in patients with isoimmunization, and evaluate elevated maternal serum alpha-fetoprotein. For example, once a fetus is potentially viable, amniotic fluid may be analyzed to determine the lecithin:sphingomyelin ratio and the presence of phosphatidyl glycerol to establish fetal lung maturity before delivery by repeat cesarean section at term or in patients in preterm labor. Alternatively, bilirubin may be measured by the change in the optical density of the amniotic fluid at 450 nm ($\triangle$OD 450) after 20 weeks gestation in patients with suspected isoimmunization to determine the extent of fetal compromise due to hemolysis. Additionally, amniotic fluid may be assessed for acetylcholinesterase and alpha-fetoprotein in patients at risk for neural tube defects as evidenced by an elevated maternal serum alpha-fetoprotein. Any of these tests of the amniotic fluid itself may be performed rapidly at any time during pregnancy, depending on the indication.

The primary indication for sampling amniocytes is to obtain fetal cells for fetal karyotype and DNA analysis in patients at risk for genetic anomalies. The most common risk factor is advanced maternal age. The age-related risk for chromosome abnormalities rises slowly until age 35 and then rises more rapidly thereafter. The risks of having a live-born child with any chromosomal abnormality (except 47,XXX) at maternal ages 35, 40, and 45 are 1 in 178, 1 in 63, and 1 in 18, respectively (Table 33–1). Thus, age 35 is generally accepted as the standard age for offering prenatal diagnosis by amniocentesis since at this age the risk of having an infant affected with a chromosomal anomaly roughly equals the risk of complication from the procedure itself.

Other indications for fetal karyotyping include a positive family history of aneuploidy or chromosomal rearrangement, a history of a previously affected child, or a maternal serum alpha-fetoprotein that is less than 0.5 MOMs (multiples of the median), indicating an increased risk of trisomy 21. In parents with a history of a child with aneuploidy, but who themselves have no evidence of chromosomal translocation, the empiric risk for recurrent aneu-

Table 33-1. Estimates of rates per thousand of chromosome abnormalities in live births by single-year interval.[1]

Maternal Age	Down Syndrome	Edwards' Syndrome (Trisomy 18)	(Patau's Syndrome (Trisomy 13)	XXY	XYY	Turner's Syndrome Genotype	Other Clinically Significant Abnormality[2]	Total[3]
<15	1.0[4]	<0.1[4]	<0.1-0.1	0.4	0.5	<0.1	0.2	2.2
15	1.0[4]	<0.1[4]	<0.1-0.1	0.4	0.5	<0.1	0.2	2.2
16	0.9[4]	<0.1[4]	<0.1-0.1	0.4	0.5	<0.1	0.2	2.1
17	0.8[4]	<0.1[4]	<0.1-0.1	0.4	0.5	<0.1	0.2	2.0
18	0.7[4]	<0.1[4]	<0.1-0.1	0.4	0.5	<0.1	0.2	1.9
19	0.6[4]	<0.1[4]	<0.1-0.1	0.4	0.5	<0.1	0.2	1.8
20	0.5-0.7	<0.1-0.1	<0.1-0.1	0.4	0.5	<0.1	0.2	1.9
21	0.5-0.7	<0.1-0.1	<0.1-0.1	0.4	0.5	<0.1	0.2	1.9
22	0.6-0.8	<0.1-0.1	<0.1-0.1	0.4	0.5	<0.1	0.2	2.0
23	0.6-0.8	<0.1-0.1	<0.1-0.1	0.4	0.5	<0.1	0.2	2.0
24	0.7-0.9	0.1-0.1	<0.1-0.1	0.4	0.5	<0.1	0.2	2.1
25	0.7-0.9	0.1-0.1	<0.1-0.1	0.4	0.5	<0.1	0.2	2.1
26	0.7-1.0	0.1-0.1	<0.1-0.1	0.4	0.5	<0.1	0.2	2.1
27	0.8-1.0	0.1-0.2	<0.1-0.1	0.4	0.5	<0.1	0.2	2.2
28	0.8-1.1	0.1-0.2	<0.1-0.2	0.4	0.5	<0.1	0.2	2.3
29	0.8-1.2	0.1-0.2	<0.1-0.2	0.5	0.5	<0.1	0.2	2.4
30	0.9-1.2	0.1-0.2	<0.1-0.2	0.5	0.5	<0.1	0.2	2.6
31	0.9-1.3	0.1-0.2	<0.1-0.2	0.5	0.5	<0.1	0.2	2.6
32	1.1-1.5	0.1-0.2	0.1-0.2	0.6	0.5	<0.1	0.2	3.1
33	1.4-1.9	0.1-0.3	0.1-0.2	0.7	0.5	<0.1	0.2	3.5
34	1.9-2.4	0.2-0.4	0.1-0.3	0.7	0.5	<0.1	0.2	4.1

Age								
35	2.5–3.9	0.3–0.5	0.2–0.3	0.9	0.5	<0.1	0.3	5.6
36	3.2–5.0	0.3–0.6	0.2–0.4	1.0	0.5	<0.1	0.3	6.7
37	4.1–6.4	0.4–0.7	0.2–0.5	1.1	0.5	<0.1	0.3	8.1
38	5.2–8.1	0.5–0.9	0.3–0.7	1.3	0.5	<0.1	0.3	9.5
39	6.6–10.5	0.7–1.2	0.4–0.8	1.5	0.5	<0.1	0.3	12.4
40	8.5–13.7	0.9–1.6	0.5–1.1	1.8	0.5	<0.1	0.3	15.8
41	10.8–17.9	1.1–2.1	0.6–1.4	2.2	0.5	<0.1	0.3	20.5
42	13.8–23.4	1.4–2.7	0.7–1.8	2.7	0.5	<0.1	0.3	25.5
43	17.6–30.6	1.8–3.5	0.9–2.4	3.3	0.5	<0.1	0.3	32.6
44	22.5–40.0	2.3–4.6	1.2–3.1	4.1	0.5	<0.1	0.3	41.8
45	28.7–52.3	2.9–6.0	1.5–4.1	5.1	0.5	<0.1	0.3	53.7
46	36.6–68.3	3.7–7.9	1.9–5.3	6.4	0.5	<0.1	0.3	68.9
47	46.6–89.3	4.7–10.3	2.4–6.9	8.2	0.5	<0.1	0.3	89.1
48	59.5–116.8	6.0–13.5	3.0–9.0	10.6	0.5	<0.1	0.3	115.0
49	75.8–152.7	7.6–17.6	3.8–11.8	13.8	0.5	<0.1	0.3	149.3

[1] Reproduced, with permission, from Hook EB: Rates of chromosome abnormalities at different maternal ages. *Obstet Gynecol* 1981;**58**:282.

[2] XXX is excluded.

[3] Calculation of the total at each age assumes rate for autosomal aneuploidies is at the mid points of the ranges given.

[4] No range may be constructed for those under 20 years by the same methods as for those 20 and over.

ploidy is 1%. Because the 1% recurrence risk following a previously affected child exceeds the risk of amniocentesis at all ages, mothers in this category are generally offered prenatal diagnosis regardless of their age. For patients with a positive family history for a nonchromosomal or mendelian inherited disorder, such as Tay-Sachs disease, hemophilia, or muscular dystrophy, the disease frequency and carrier status are considered in determining the need for amniocentesis.

Genetic amniocentesis is usually performed between 15 and 20 menstrual weeks of gestation, and the amniocytes cultured for 10-20 days before a karyotype can be ascertained. Thus, the major disadvantage of this approach for DNA analysis compared with other more rapid diagnostic techniques, such as chorionic villus sampling, is the delay in diagnosis until nearly 20 weeks of gestation. By this stage of pregnancy, the mother has usually detected fetal movement, which often results in a significant amount of parental bonding with the fetus. In addition, terminations of pregnancy are more involved and potentially hazardous after 14 weeks of gestation. If termination is elected, the delay in diagnosis encountered with amniocentesis may lead to both physical and emotional hardship for the mother.

The technique for amniocentesis is straightforward. Once informed consent is obtained, the pregnant woman is scanned with ultrasound to localize the placenta and fetus. Biometrics, such as biparietal diameter, head circumference, abdominal circumference, and femur length, should be performed on the fetus to confirm dates and establish adequate growth. After the biometrics are complete, the mother's abdomen is prepped with povidone iodine solution and then alcohol. A subdermal injection of 3-5 mL of 1% lidocaine is made at the predetermined site of needle insertion. A sterile ultrasound cover may be placed over the ultrasound transducer so that visualization can continue as the needle is being placed into the amniotic sac. A 20- or 22-gauge spinal needle (3.5 inches) is used for fluid removal under direct visual guidance. Once the needle is in the amniotic sac, approximately 20-25 mL of fluid is removed. If twins are present, a small amount of indigo carmine (1-2 mL) may be placed in the first sac at the end of fluid withdrawal before the second sac is tapped. If clear fluid is obtained from the second sac, one can be assured that the first sac was not inadvertently sampled twice. Samples of fluid are then sent for the appropriate evaluation, depending on the indications for the procedure.

The risk to the patient of a complication following amniocentesis that threatens the outcome of the pregnancy ranges from 1:200 to 1:500 procedures. The major complications include rupture of the membranes, chorioamnionitis, and preterm labor. Minor complications, such as temporary leakage of amniotic fluid, cramping, or localized pain at the needle insertion site, are reported in less than 5–10% of patients. Injury to the fetus is extremely uncommon, and may be minimized by performing the procedure under direct ultrasonographic guidance.

Chorionic Villus Sampling

Chorionic villus sampling is another technique that has been developed more recently. It provides the same karyotypic information as amniocentesis in patients undergoing prenatal diagnosis to rule out the presence of a genetic abnormality. Unlike amniocentesis, in which the amniotic cavity is entered and amniotic fluid with amniocytes is withdrawn, chorionic villus sampling (CVS) is accomplished as an extra-amniotic procedure between 10 and 12 menstrual weeks of gestation. Small fragments of chorion frondosum from the placenta are obtained by transcervical or transabdominal aspiration, and the villi are then used for DNA analysis.

The main advantage of chorionic villus sampling over amniocentesis is that genetic information about the fetus can be ascertained before completion of the first trimester, rather than waiting until 18–20 weeks for a diagnosis, as is usual for amniocentesis. If an abnormal karyotype is obtained after CVS, a less complicated first-trimester termination of pregnancy can be offered to the patient, should she desire it. Thus, the indications for chorionic villus sampling are similar to those for amniocentesis in patients at risk for chromosomal abnormalities. Additionally, CVS is indicated in women who desire a genetic diagnosis earlier in pregnancy.

The main disadvantage of CVS is the slightly increased fetal loss rate that is associated with this technique when compared with amniocentesis. In experienced hands, the loss rate after CVS that can be attributed to the procedure itself is 0.5–1.0%. CVS also does not allow for analysis of amniotic fluid parameters, such as alpha-fetoprotein, used in amniocentesis to evaluate for fetal neural tube defects. Patients undergoing CVS are advised to have maternal blood for alpha-fetoprotein assessment drawn at 15–20 weeks.

Depending on the location of the placenta, CVS may be performed at 10–12 weeks gestation by either a transcervical or transabdominal route. A posterior placenta is usually approached transcervically, while an anterior or fundal placenta is sampled transabdominally. The transabdominal approach is most like an amniocentesis. Here, the abdomen is sterilely prepped, local anesthesia is administered, and with a similar gauge 6-inch-long needle, the sample is obtained under direct sonographic guidance. Once the needle tip is placed in the thickest portion of the chorionic plate, negative pressure is exerted on the syringe, and the needle is moved slightly up and down, remaining within the placenta. This shearing motion dislodges the villi from the placenta and allows them to enter the syringe. The samples are flushed into tissue culture media and examined under a dissecting microscope to establish the presence of villi and to estimate the volume of cells obtained. Sample sizes generally range from 5–50 mg of villi.

Transcervical CVS requires the placement of a flexible plastic catheter with a malleable metal obturator through the cervical canal and into the chorionic plate of the placenta. With the patient in the lithotomy position, a sterile speculum is placed in the vagina. The cervix is cleansed with povidone iodine solution. Usually a gentle bend is placed in the catheter to accommodate each patient's anatomy and uterine flexion. Under direct ultrasound guidance, the catheter tip is localized within the placenta, and negative pressure is placed on the syringe as the catheter is withdrawn. Similar to the transabdominal approach, the sample is flushed into tissue culture media and examined under the dissecting microscope. The volume of villi obtained is similar to that obtained by the transabdominal approach.

If either technique fails to obtain villi or if the quantity is less than 5 mg, a second attempt is undertaken. However, more than 3 attempts have been associated with a higher fetal loss rate. A large collaborative study of more than 2200 patients found odds ratios of 2.2 and 4.1 for fetal losses following 2 and 3 attempts at chorionic villus sampling, respectively.

The sampled villi may be studied immediately with a direct preparation for karyotypic information within 24–48 hours, or alternatively, the cells may be cultured for 5–10 days. The disadvantage of a direct preparation is that the karyotypic spreads are sometimes more difficult to interpret for an accurate genetic diagnosis. Long-term cultures result in a more easily interpretable karyotype but take longer. The karyotypes obtained by culture may also be contaminated with maternal cells if careful laboratory technique is not followed. Finally, long-term cultures allow for harvesting of fetal cells for DNA extraction and analysis for specific gene markers of genetic diseases. This technique has been particularly valuable in the prenatal diagnosis of sickle cell disease in utero.

The complications of a CVS procedure are similar to those encountered with amniocentesis. Rupture of membranes, chorioamnionitis, bleeding or spotting, pain at needle insertion site, and fever have all been reported. Even if gross rupture of the membranes is not observed, a small percentage of patients ($< 1\%$) will be found to have oligohydramnios at subsequent ultrasound examinations at 16–18 weeks. The prognosis for these pregnancies is very poor because of the occurrence of pulmonary hypoplasia and severe deformative changes in the fetus.

Fetal Tissue & Blood Sampling

After 20 weeks of gestation, other techniques to assess fetal status become available to the geneticist. With the use of high-resolution ultrasound for guidance, it is now possible to directly sample fetal blood or tissue to determine whether a fetus is afflicted with a particular genetic disease. Biopsies of fetal skin may be used to establish the diagnosis of lethal forms of epidermolysis bullosa or ichthyosis in the fetus. A fetal liver biopsy will exclude lethal deficiencies of a urea cycle enzyme, such as carbamoyl phosphate synthetase or ornithine carbamoyltransferase.

Fetal blood sampling, or percutaneous umbilical blood sampling (PUBS) is indicated in several circumstances. In patients who present with a possible chromosomal abnormality late in pregnancy, it may be necessary to perform rapid karyotyping of the fetus in 48–72 hours to assist in obstetrical management. Neither amniocentesis nor CVS is helpful in these cases. Fetal blood sampling is also useful in suspected cases of parvovirus or toxoplasmosis infection of the fetus. Analysis of fetal blood elements may be indicated in fetuses at risk for immunodeficiency states, such as severe combined immune deficiency, in fetuses of mothers with thrombocytopenia to determine the fetal platelet count before delivery, or to establish the extent of fetal anemia in women with a history of isoimmunization. The presence of fetal coagulopathies, such as hemophilia, or inborn errors of metabolism may also be detected by fetal blood sampling. Finally, direct testing of the fetal blood may aid in determining fetal acid-base status or blood grouping and may assist in the workup of potentially lethal conditions, such as fetal hydrops.

Once fetal blood or tissue samples are obtained, they are analyzed using a variety of current DNA techniques. One technique incorporates the use of restriction endonucleases, which are bacterial enzymes that recognize specific sequences of 4–7 nucleic acids and cleave the DNA at these specific sites. After DNA has been treated with a restriction endonuclease, DNA fragments of varying lengths are produced. These fragments are then separated by gel electrophoresis. Identification of a mutation in the DNA under study is possible because a single nucleotide change in a recognition site of the restriction endonuclease leads to cleavage of a different-sized fragment of DNA at the time of enzymatic digestion. This cleavage, in turn, produces a DNA fragment that migrates to a different location on the gel electrophoresis. The DNA fragment under consideration is then compared with control fragments of specific disease entities to establish a final diagnosis.

Another technique for DNA analysis is the use of the Southern blot test in which different-sized fragments of DNA, which have been separated by gel electrophoresis after having been "cut" with restriction endonucleases, are transferred to a nitrocellulose filter. The fragments are then treated with radiolabeled probes and undergo autoradiography. DNA sequences that hybridize with the radioactive probe are seen as dark bands on the film. The patient's DNA fragments are compared once again to established control samples.

Finally, recent advances in polymerase chain reaction DNA amplification technology have been applied to the analysis of fetal samples. Polymerase chain reaction enables small samples of DNA to be amplified up to a billion-fold for subsequent DNA analysis. Thus, only a few fetal cells are required to make a prenatal diagnosis of a genetic anomaly. Rapid fetal sexing, diagnosis of some hemoglobinopathies, prenatal assessment of muscular dystrophy, and the diagnosis of hemophilia A are some of the indications for this technique.

SUGGESTED READINGS

Filkons K, Russo J: *Human Prenatal Diagnosis,* Marcel Dekker, 1990.

Simpson J et al: *Genetics in Obstetrics and Gynecology,* Grune & Stratton, 1982.

Thompson J, Thompson M: *Genetics in Medicine,* 4th ed. Saunders, 1986.

Obstetric & Surgical Complications of Pregnancy | 34

Bonnie A. Coyne, MD

Most pregnancies proceed normally to the safe delivery of a healthy infant at term. However, some gestations can be threatened by complications peculiar to the gravid state that may pose significant risk to the mother, fetus, or both. This chapter reviews the more common of these complications, focusing on their presentation and management, and includes acute surgical conditions.

PRETERM LABOR

Low birth weight (< 2500 g) is the most significant contributor to infant mortality in the USA. By far the greatest contributor to low birth weight is delivery occurring before 37 weeks. Preterm labor occurs in approximately 10% of all pregnancies, accounting for 250,000 births a year in the USA.

Preterm labor is defined in clinical studies as regular uterine contractions with a frequency of 6–7 per hour or greater, resulting in documented cervical change, occurring before 37 weeks gestation. Many patients who present preterm with regular contractions respond to treatment with bedrest, intravenous hydration, and sedation and do not actually progress to developing cervical dilation. It is difficult to distinguish these patients with excessive uterine activity from those with true preterm labor. Because successful therapy of preterm labor is more likely with early treatment, it is probable that many more patients are treated than actually have the complication. Patients who present with advanced cervical dilation ($\geq$ 4 cm) are unlikely to respond to pharmacologic intervention and go on to deliver prematurely.

The initiating factors of labor are not understood in the term or preterm woman. Changes in cervical maturation, myometrial activity, and rupture of membranes herald the onset of labor. Because the mechanism of labor has not been identified, patients at risk for preterm labor are identified by risk factors based on epidemiologic data. Assessment of a variety of medical and socioeconomic factors, daily habits, and aspects of the current pregnancy are used to predict which patients are at high risk for preterm labor. One system used to identify patients at risk is outlined in Table 34-1.

Symptoms

The symptoms of preterm labor may be subtle or overt. Patients may complain of painful, regular contractions. Less obvious symptoms include an increase in vaginal discharge, low-back pain, pelvic pressure, diarrhea, anterior thigh pain, malaise, or vaginal bleeding. Patients with infections that cause preterm labor may have a fever as well.

Table 34-1. System for determining risk of preterm delivery.

Major risk factors	Minor risk factors
Multiple gestation	Febrile illness
Previous preterm delivery	Bleeding after 12 weeks
Previous preterm labor, term delivery	History of pyelonephritis
Abdominal surgery during pregnancy	Cigarette smoking (> 10 day/d)
Exposure to diethylstilbestrol (DES)	One second-trimester abortion
Hydramnios	More than 2 first-trimester abortions
Uterine anomaly	**Controversial risk factors**
History of cone biopsy	Age less than 18 years or more than 34 years
Uterine irritability	Unusual physical or mental stress
More than one second-trimester abortion	Strenuous physical work
Cervical dilation (> 1 cm) at 32 weeks	
Cervical effacement (< 1 cm long at 32 weeks)	

Differential Diagnosis

The differential diagnosis of preterm labor includes obstetric complications that cause premature contractions, as well as other causes of abdominal pain or uterine irritability. Obstetric factors that need to be excluded include abruption, placenta previa with bleeding, and chorioamnionitis. Systemic infection, trauma, or intra-abdominal surgery may also trigger preterm labor. Intra-abdominal inflammation (eg, appendicitis) may cause a patient to present with pain and contractions.

Treatment

Initial treatment of patients with suspected preterm labor consists of bedrest with uterine and fetal monitoring, complete general examination, cervical examination with cultures for group B streptococcus and possibly for chlamydia (if this has not been done during the pregnancy), and ultrasonography to evaluate fetal age and presentation and to exclude placental or uterine anomalies. Patients with a definite diagnosis of preterm labor should be treated with tocolytic agents with no delay.

Absolute contraindications to tocolysis are documented chorioamnionitis, life-threatening maternal hemorrhage, severe preeclampsia, fetal distress, or fetal anomalies incompatible with life. Relative contraindications to tocolysis include ruptured membranes and maternal disease, such as diabetes or heart disease that increase the risk of complications from tocolysis.

In many cases, amniocentesis is used to determine fetal lung maturity. Especially in cases in which there is little risk for other complications of prematurity, a fetal lung profile that indicates maturity (ie, a lecithin:sphingomyelin ratio of > 2 or the presence of phosphatidylglycerol) may preclude the need for tocolysis.

Before tocolytic therapy is initiated, the patient should have intravenous access established, and baseline vital signs and weight should be measured. Admission laboratory studies should include complete blood count, electrolytes, glucose, urinalysis, and electrocardiogram. Total intravenous fluid should be restricted to less than 2500 mL every 24 hours to minimize the risk of pulmonary edema with tocolytic therapy.

A variety of tocolytic agents are used in the USA, but the mainstay of therapy is treatment with a β-adrenergic agonist. Indeed, the beta agonist ritodrine is the only medication currently approved for tocolysis by the US Food and Drug Administration. Other categories of tocolytics include calcium channel blockers (magnesium sulfate, nifedipine) and prostaglandin synthetase in-

hibitors (indomethacin). Maintenance tocolytic therapy is continued until 36–37 weeks, when the risk of severe neonatal respiratory
distress syndrome is virtually eliminated.

A. β-Adrenergic Agonists: These drugs work by activating
adenylate cyclase. This causes an increase in cyclic adenosine
monophosphate (cAMP), which decreases myosin light-chain kinase activity, inhibiting actin-myosin interaction. Intravenous ritodrine is the most commonly used agent for initial tocolysis. Dosing
is started at 50 μg/min and gradually increased by 50 μg/min every
15 minutes to a maximum of 350 μg/min. After tocolysis is
achieved, intravenous therapy is continued for 12–24 hours before
switching to maintenance therapy.

Maintenance therapy with β-adrenergic agonists is usually
oral (terbutaline, 2.5–5 mg every 3–4 hours). In some centers, a
terbutaline pump is used to administer the medication subcutaneously, but efficacy of this route is still under study. Dosage of
maintenance therapy is adjusted according to uterine activity and
maternal pulse rate.

Serious complications can result from the use of these agents.
Pulmonary edema may result from intravenous administration and
occurs more often in women with twin gestations. Fluids should
be limited to less than 2.5 L in 24 hours. Other side effects include
hypokalemia, hyperglycemia (of concern in diabetic patients),
tachycardia, arrhythmias, tremor, and jitteriness.

B. Magnesium Sulfate: Magnesium sulfate acts as a calcium
channel blocker to relax the myometrium. It is an effective agent
when given early in labor with an intravenous loading dose of 4–6 g
followed by a maintenance dose of 2–3.5 g/h. Serial magnesium
levels should be followed in these patients.

Side effects of magnesium sulfate include pulmonary edema,
flushing, nausea, and vomiting. With overdose, a decrease in peripheral reflexes, respiratory depression, and cardiac arrest can occur. Magnesium sulfate is often used for tocolysis in diabetic patients in whom beta agonists cause hyperglycemia. After successful
tocolysis with intravenous magnesium sulfate, most patients are
treated with oral terbutaline maintenance therapy.

C. Prostaglandin Synthetase Inhibitors: Prostaglandin release causes myometrial contraction, and therefore administration
of these agents should be useful in stopping labor. Indomethacin,
given as a 50-mg rectal suppository or an oral dose followed by
25–50 mg every 6 hours may suppress preterm labor. Concerns
with this agent are possible serious fetal side effects. Premature
closure of the ductus arteriosis is a theoretic risk; decrease in blood

flow has been suggested based on the results of Doppler studies. Decreased fetal urine production has also been shown to result from indomethacin administration. For these reasons, chronic indomethacin therapy should be considered only after other treatments have failed and only with close ultrasonographic monitoring of the fetus. Maternal side effects include nausea, vomiting, diarrhea, and peptic ulceration.

D. Calcium Channel Blockers: These agents block calcium influx into the cell and thus prevent or diminish myometrial cell contractility. Nifedipine is given sublingually (10 mg every 10 minutes) until contractions decrease (maximum 4 doses) and then orally 20 mg every 6 hours. Maternal side effects include dizziness, flushing, headache, nausea, and hypotension. Information on fetal side effects is limited.

E. Combination Therapy: Patients who do not respond to a single therapeutic agent are sometimes given combinations of tocolytic agents. One must be careful of synergistic actions that may increase side effects; for example, combined magnesium sulfate and nifedipine may result in profound hypotension or cardiac arrythmias.

F. Corticosteroid Therapy: An important adjuvant in the treatment of women with preterm labor is corticosteroid therapy. Antenatal dexamethasone administration has been shown to prevent respiratory distress syndrome in selected groups of patients. Steroids given to mothers at least 24 hours before delivery can accelerate lung maturity in the fetus. Betamethasone, 12 mg every 12 hours for 2 doses is the most widely used regimen. It has been established that the singleton fetus at 27–32 weeks with intact membranes is most likely to benefit from steroid therapy. It is less clear whether patients with multiple fetuses or those with preterm premature rupture of membranes (PROM) benefit from this treatment. Studies of the use of steroids in women with preterm PROM show conflicting results, and there seems to be no consensus about the management of these patients. Steroids seem to cause no long-term adverse effects in the fetus. Patients with ruptured membranes are at increased risk for chorioamnionitis, and for that reason many obstetricians will not give antenatal steroids to these patients. Documented chorioamnionitis is an absolute contraindication to steroid use.

As with any disease for which treatment is not always effective, it would be better to be able to prevent preterm labor. Targeting public health measures toward women who are at high risk for preterm labor may decrease its incidence. Certainly patients who obtain regular prenatal care are less likely to develop preterm labor. More frequent prenatal visits for high-risk patients, serial pelvic examinations, patient education, and modification of certain habits (eg, drug use) all seem to decrease the incidence of preterm labor. Home monitoring, with a portable tocodynamometer to detect increased uterine activity, is now being used to detect threatened preterm labor. Whether such monitoring will have efficacy and widespread application has yet to be determined.

PREMATURE RUPTURE OF MEMBRANES

Premature rupture of membranes is the spontaneous rupture of membranes before the onset of labor; if this rupture occurs before 37 weeks of gestation, it is called preterm premature rupture of membranes. Preterm PROM complicates 1–2% of all pregnancies and accounts for 30% of preterm deliveries. Patients presenting with preterm PROM are much more likely to deliver prematurely than those women who present with preterm labor and intact membranes. The cause of PROM is not known. Women at risk for preterm PROM have many clinical similarities to those at risk for preterm labor. Some experts think that PROM is caused by subclinical chorioamnionitis. Whatever the cause, it is clear that the risk of maternal and fetal infection is greatly increased. The neonate is also at risk for complications of prematurity (eg, respiratory distress syndrome, intraventricular hemorrhage). When the membranes rupture before 25 weeks of gestation, the fetus is also at risk for lung hypoplasia and skeletal deformities.

Patients with PROM complain of leaking vaginal fluid, which may be clear, blood-tinged, or meconium-stained. Patients may also have contractions at the time of presentation. The diagnosis of PROM may be confirmed with a sterile speculum examination. Pooling of amniotic fluid may be seen in the vaginal fornix and may be confirmed with positive nitrazine or ferning tests. Ultrasonography may demonstrate oligohydramnios in these patients.

Optimal management for patients with preterm PROM has not been established. As in preterm labor, infants of patients with evidence of chorioamnionitis or fetal distress should be delivered as quickly and safely as possible, with antibiotic treatment for patients with chorioamnionitis. In women with no evidence of chorioamnionitis, options for management depend on gestational age and presence or absence of labor. Overwhelmingly, these patients are managed expectantly, that is, they are closely monitored for evidence of impending infection or fetal distress. Monitoring may include obtaining a complete blood count every 12–24 hours, daily biophysical profiles, and serial ultrasonograms. For patients who have prematurely ruptured membranes and who are also in labor, expectant management involves careful monitoring but no tocolysis. The presence of labor is thought to indicate chorioamnionitis. However, with a very immature fetus, tocolysis is sometimes used in an effort to prolong pregnancy. As mentioned earlier, the use of antenatal steroids in these patients continues to be controversial. Antibiotic prophylaxis is indicated for patients with PROM who have culture-proven group B streptococcus vaginal colonization.

INTRAUTERINE GROWTH RETARDATION

Infants with low birth weight are at higher risk for perinatal morbidity and mortality. These infants may be small because of prematurity, poor growth, or both. Identifying fetuses with problems of growth in utero allows for more optimal management. For example, some fetuses may benefit from delivery, whereas others can be followed with serial ultrasonography.

Intrauterine growth retardation (IUGR) is defined as weight below the 10th percentile for age. There is some ambiguity in this definition, as norms for populations vary by geography, race, sex, and birth order. These small fetuses can be either genetically small (ie, the offspring of small parents and thus appropriately small) or they can be truly growth retarded.

Various disorders may cause IUGR and may be the result of maternal, fetal, or uteroplacental conditions (Table 34–2). IUGR

Table 34-2. Causes of intrauterine growth retardation.

Maternal	Fetal	Uteroplacental
Smoking	Infection (TORCH syn-	Uterine septae
Drugs, substance abuse	dromes,[1] protozoal)	Uterine myoma
Vascular disease	Genetic disorders	Placental abruption
Severe anemia	Congenital anomalies	Cord abnormalities
Other chronic disease		

[1] TORCH syndromes include toxoplasmosis, other (eg, syphilis, hepatitis) rubella, cytomegalovirus, and herpes simplex (see Chapter 37).

can be diagnosed only when the gestational age is accurately estimated. The best estimates of gestational age include a history of
ovulation induction, in vitro fertilization, single intercourse, and
ultrasonography performed before 20 weeks of gestation. Clinically, fetal growth is monitored by measuring the fundal height
after the 20th gestational week. When clinical growth is inadequate
or when the patient has specific risk factors for IUGR, serial ultrasonography may be used to diagnose growth retardation.

A variety of sonographic measurements have been used to
evaluate fetal growth. None can be said to definitively diagnose
IUGR. The simplest measurement to predict IUGR is fetal abdominal circumference. Fetal weight, estimated by using formulae employing head, abdomen, and femur measurements, may also be
used to identify fetuses in the lowest percentiles for growth. Because most IUGR occurs in the third trimester and affects soft tissue growth more than bone and neural tissue growth, comparison
of head and abdominal measurements can be used as a diagnostic
tool. Asymmetric IUGR is suggested when the ratio of head circumference to abdominal circumference becomes abnormally
large.

Patients who carry a diagnosis of IUGR or who are suspected
to be at high risk for IUGR should undergo close antenatal monitoring. They should have serial ultrasonograms to follow growth
and amniotic fluid volume. Antenatal testing should be performed
at least weekly once the diagnosis is made. Amniocentesis may be
used in selected cases to evaluate fetal chromosomes or fetal lung
maturity. Early delivery of the fetus with IUGR is indicated when
there is evidence of fetal distress or oligohydramnios, when fetal
lung maturity is confirmed, or when deteriorating maternal health
makes prolongation of pregnancy dangerous for mother or fetus.

POSTTERM PREGNANCY

Postterm pregnancy occurs when gestation continues longer
than 42 weeks (294 days) after the last normal menstrual period.
Perinatal outcome is not as favorable in these cases as in term pregnancy, and for this reason these women are considered high-risk
patients. About 10% of pregnancies continue after 42 weeks, and
about 4% continue past 43 weeks. Anencephalic and abdominal
pregnancies continue to postterm, but the cause of postterm pregnancy in an otherwise normal pregnancy is not known. Perinatal

mortality doubles from 40 to 42 weeks and almost quadruples by 44 weeks. Although most fetuses do well, this increase in mortality is largely preventable with proper management.

The risks to the fetus in a postterm pregnancy are multiple. The fetus can continue to grow and, because of its large size, may undergo a difficult delivery. Alternatively, if placental function is insufficient, the fetus may become growth retarded. When postterm, placental dysfunction occurs, the amniotic fluid volume usually decreases and the incidence of meconium increases, leading to greater chances of cord compression and meconium aspiration, respectively, before and during labor, which may result in fetal asphyxia or meconium aspiration pneumonitis.

Management of postterm pregnancy depends on accurate knowledge of gestational age. In addition, the condition of the cervix is important in determining how to manage postterm pregnancy. The cervix is considered "favorable" when adequate dilatation and effacement have occurred (ie, a Bishop's score of more than 5, Table 34–3). At 42 weeks, if the cervix is favorable, most obstetricians induce labor with oxytocin. If the cervix is not adequately dilated and effaced ("unfavorable" cervix), antenatal surveillance is performed twice a week and should consist of at least a nonstress test and amniotic fluid volume assessment or a complete biophysical profile. Oligohydramnios presents a threat to the fetus, and induction is begun if oligohydramnios is found, if fetal distress is detected, or when the cervix becomes favorable.

Alternative management of postterm pregnancy consists of induction of all patients at 42 weeks. In this situation, when the cervix is not sufficiently effaced or dilated, patients are treated with intravaginal or intracervical prostaglandin E_2 gel and then given oxytocin to induce labor. Proponents of this approach claim that

Table 34-3. Bishop's score of cervical maturity.[1]

	Score		
	0	**1**	**2**
Dilatation (cm)	0	1–2	3–4
Effacement (%)	0–30	40–50	60–70
Station	−3	−2	−1/0
Consistency	Firm	Medium	Soft
Position of cervix	Posterior	Middle	Anterior

[1]The cervix is considered to be favorable for labor induction when the score is 5 or more.

the cesarean section rate is lower and neonatal outcome better than when patients are managed with antenatal surveillance as outlined above.

RH ISOIMMUNIZATION

Most cases of hemolytic disease of the newborn have been prevented by using prophylactic Rh immunoglobulin during pregnancy in women who are Rh negative. The Rh (D) antigen is highly immunogenic, and because it causes production of an immunoglobulin G (IgG) antibody, which crosses the placenta, it may cause hemolysis in the fetus. Before the introduction of Rh immune globulin, Rh-negative women developed antibody to Rh-positive red blood cells. This development occurred most often during a first pregnancy (if the fetus was Rh-positive). During subsequent pregnancies, because of maternal anti-D antibodies, the Rh-positive fetus of a sensitized mother could develop varying degrees of hemolytic disease, ranging from anemia to hydrops fetalis.

Rh (D) immunoglobulin is given to Rh-negative women who are not sensitized when there is a chance that fetal red blood cells may gain access to the maternal circulation. During a normal pregnancy, prophylaxis is given at 28 weeks, and again after delivery if the infant is Rh-positive. Rh immunoglobulin is also given at the time of spontaneous or therapeutic abortion, ectopic pregnancy, amniocentesis, or external cephalic version. When any potentially large fetal-to-maternal transfusion can occur (as in an abruption), a larger amount of globulin might need to be given to prevent sensitization.

Sensitization of Rh-negative women continues to occur, primarily because they are not given immunoglobulin. Sensitization to other antigens may also cause hemolytic disease of the newborn. Such sensitization is identified by the use of bloodtyping and antibody screening performed as part of routine prenatal care. Sensitized women should be referred for expert care. Management of sensitized women includes determination of antibody titers. Indicated procedures may include amniocentesis (to determine severity of hemolytic disease), percutaneous umbilical blood sampling (to determine fetal hematocrit or perform fetal blood transfusion), in utero intraperitoneal fetal blood transfusion, antenatal surveillance, and early delivery. Neonatal mortality may thus be decreased from 30% (in untreated cases) to less than 10% with treatment.

CHOLESTASIS OF PREGNANCY

Cholestasis of pregnancy is a disorder unique to pregnancy. It occurs in the third trimester, and patients with cholestasis complain of pruritis. Mild jaundice, nausea, and vomiting may occur later in the course. For the mother, the disease is an irritating but benign one. Laboratory findings include elevated bile acids and alkaline phosphatase. Levels of aspartate aminotransferase (AST, formerly known as serum glutamic-oxaloacetic transaminase, SGOT) and alanine aminotransferase (ALT, formerly known as serum glutamicpyruvic transaminase, SGPT) are elevated (up to 500 IU/mL), but total bilirubin does not exceed 10 mg/dL. Differential diagnosis includes viral hepatitis, biliary tract obstruction, and acute fatty liver of pregnancy. There is evidence that women with cholestasis of pregnancy have an increased risk of stillbirth. For this reason, antenatal testing should begin when the diagnosis is made.

ACUTE FATTY LIVER OF PREGNANCY

Acute fatty liver of pregnancy (AFLP) is also a disorder limited to the gravid state. It occurs in the third trimester of pregnancy and involves acute hepatic failure. Mortality has been reported to be as high as 85%, but with improved recognition and immediate delivery, the mortality range is 20–30%. The disorder is usually seen after the 35th week of gestation and is more common in primigravidas and those with twins. The incidence is about 1:14,000 deliveries.

The cause of acute fatty liver of pregnancy is not known. Pathologic findings are unique to the disorder, with fatty engorgement of hepatocytes. Clinical onset is gradual, with flu-like symptoms that progress to the development of abdominal pain, jaundice, encephalopathy, disseminated intravascular coagulation, and death. On examination, the patients show signs of hepatic failure.

Laboratory findings show marked elevation of alkaline phosphatase but only moderate elevations of ALT and AST. Prothrombin time and bilirubin are also elevated. White blood cell count is elevated, and the platelet count is depressed. Hypoglycemia may be profound.

The differential diagnosis is that of fulminant hepatitis. However, liver function test results for fulminant hepatitis are higher

(> 1000 IU/mL) than those for acute fatty liver of pregnancy (usually less than 500 IU/mL). It is also important to review the appropriate history and perform the appropriate tests for toxins that cause liver failure. Preeclampsia may involve the liver but typically does not cause jaundice. The elevations in liver function tests in patients with preeclampsia usually do not reach the levels seen in patients with acute fatty liver of pregnancy.

Diagnosis of acute fatty liver of pregnancy mandates immediate delivery. Supportive care during labor includes administration of glucose, platelets, and fresh-frozen plasma, as needed. Vaginal delivery is preferred. Resolution of encephalopathy occurs over days, and supportive care with a low protein diet is needed.

Recurrence rates for this liver disorder are unclear. Most authorities advise against subsequent pregnancy, but there have been reported cases of successful outcomes in later pregnancies.

CHOLECYSTITIS

Although up to 3–5% of pregnant women have gallstones on routine ultrasound examination, they less frequently develop symptoms during gestation. Symptoms of cholelithiasis occur with obstruction or inflammation and may mandate cholecystectomy.

Acute cholecystitis results from ductal obstruction, with subsequent inflammation. Patients complain of right upper quadrant pain, nausea, and vomiting. They have fever and right upper quadrant tenderness. Laboratory findings show mild leukocytosis and slight elevation in bilirubin and liver function tests, and ultrasonography may show calculi. The differential diagnosis includes pancreatitis, appendicitis, pyelonephritis, peptic ulcer disease, and hepatitis. Treatment includes gastrointestinal rest, nasogastric suction, analgesics, antibiotics, and intravenous hydration. Definitive surgical therapy may need to be undertaken for failure to respond to medical management within 48–72 hours.

Chronic cholecystitis is characterized by recurrent nonspecific symptoms: dyspepsia, fatty food intolerance, and upper abdominal and epigastric pain. Laboratory studies are unremarkable with the exception of gallstones seen on ultrasound examination. The differential diagnosis includes peptic ulcer disease, esophagitis, and irritable bowel disease. Most cases of chronic cholecystitis that complicate pregnancy may be managed conservatively. When complications occur (acute cholecystitis, obstructive jaundice, pancreatitis), surgery may be necessary.

PANCREATITIS

Pregnancy may be a predisposing factor to pancreatitis, and acute pancreatitis occurs in 1:1,000 to 1:10,000 pregnancies. Ninety percent of cases in pregnancy are caused by cholelithiasis. Other causes include alcohol, abdominal surgery, trauma, drugs, peptic ulcer perforation, hyperparathyroidism, preeclampsia, hyperlipidemia, and viral infection.

Patients present with midepigastric pain, nausea, vomiting, and low-grade fever. Signs include tachycardia, hypotension, bibasilar rales, and abdominal tenderness. Serum amylase is usually elevated, and leukocytosis, hypocalcemia, and elevated serum lipase are seen. The differential diagnosis includes cholecystitis, peptic ulcer disease, intestinal obstruction or perforation, preeclampsia, appendicitis, myocardial infarction, and aortic dissection.

Treatment is the same during pregnancy as at other times: intravenous hydration, nasogastric suction, enteric rest, analgesics, correction of symptomatic hypocalcemia, and treatment with antacids to prevent stress ulcers.

APPENDICITIS

Appendicitis occurs no more often during pregnancy than at other times. However, it may be more difficult to diagnose because the symptoms of appendicitis are the same as the more common gastrointestinal upsets that occur during pregnancy. The location of the appendix changes as pregnancy progresses. As the uterus enlarges the appendix is pushed upward, so that by the middle of the second trimester it is at the level of the umbilicus, and by the end of pregnancy may be in the right upper quadrant. If appendectomy is done at term, elective cesarean section should not be performed at the same time because of the increased chance of endomyometritis.

TRAUMA

Accidental injury is a leading cause of death and disability among young people. Trauma is the leading nonobstetric cause of death during pregnancy. It is difficult to estimate the incidence of trauma during pregnancy, but it is probably no less common than at other times.

The nature of injuries sustained by the mother and the effects on the fetus are a function of the type and severity of the accident. Motor vehicle accidents are the most common cause of injury during pregnancy, and account for 50% of blunt abdominal injuries. Falls and assaults are other common causes of blunt abdominal trauma. Penetrating abdominal trauma is usually caused by gunshot wounds. Stabbing is seen less often. Suicide attempts during pregnancy result in death far less often than in nonpregnant patients. Most suicidal gravidas have a history of psychiatric disorders and about half are primigravidas.

The severity of injury to the mother as a result of any trauma predicts outcome for mother and fetus. The most common cause of fetal death is maternal death, and the second most common cause of fetal death is placental abruption. Other threats to the fetus that may result from maternal trauma include preterm labor, premature rupture of membranes, anoxic damage, fetomaternal transfusion, and direct penetrating injury to the fetus.

Management of the pregnant patient with multiple trauma is initially the same as that for the nonpregnant patient: cardiopulmonary resuscitation and stabilization are performed while the extent of injuries is determined. Usual trauma protocols should be followed, with the possible exception of the use of a MAST suit (military antishock trousers), which may impede uteroplacental blood flow. Diagnostic x-rays should be used fully to evaluate the extent of injury. In the case of blunt abdominal injury, diagnostic peritoneal lavage may be used to rule out intra-abdominal bleeding or ruptured viscera. However, it has a high false-negative rate during pregnancy and exploratory laparotomy may be necessary.

Once the mother has been stabilized in the emergency room (and ideally soon after her arrival to the hospital), fetal evaluation should begin. The gestational age should be estimated using portable ultrasound equipment, and continuous fetal monitoring should be initiated if the fetus is of viable gestational age. If the viable fetus shows signs of persistent fetal distress, emergency cesarean section should be performed. In most cases, this procedure should be done only after the mother has been stabilized. However, in extreme conditions, delivery may improve maternal condition by increasing cardiac return. If resuscitation of the mother is unsuccessful and maternal death is anticipated, an immediate antemortem cesarean section should be performed. Fetal survival after this type of emergency delivery depends on prompt action, with no chance of survival when more than 25 minutes have elapsed since maternal death. Continued maternal cardiopulmonary resuscitation should be performed throughout the procedure.

In the seriously injured pregnant patient whose condition is initially stable, the likelihood of obstetric complication resulting from the accident may be estimated by the presence of obstetric signs and symptoms at the time of presentation. When abdominal or back pain, contractions, vaginal bleeding, or premature rupture of membranes occur, the chance of delivery precipitated by trauma is increased. Abruption may be difficult to diagnose in this setting: vaginal bleeding and pain may be absent, and the first indication of abruption may be fetal distress. Patients who have suffered blunt abdominal trauma should undergo continuous fetal monitoring for 24 hours.

SUBSTANCE ABUSE

Illicit drug and alcohol use is widespread in the USA. Use of these substances among pregnant women is also common. The overall prevalence of alcohol and drug use among pregnant women ranges from 8–18% and does not vary with race or class. However, the pattern of specific drug or alcohol use does vary with patient population. Drug and alcohol use during pregnancy has far-reaching consequences for society, and limited resources are available for detection and treatment of drug abuse. The following discussion is limited to immediate medical, obstetric, and fetal effects of substance abuse.

Heavy alcohol use during pregnancy is associated with both obstetric and fetal complications. Alcohol consumption of 2 or more drinks per day throughout pregnancy has been shown to be associated with these complications. However, no minimum amount of alcohol use during pregnancy has been shown to be safe. Drinking during pregnancy is usually underreported by patients. One study showed that 9% of a large metropolitan population reported heavy drinking during pregnancy, 37% moderate drinking, and 53% little or no drinking. Detection of heavy alcohol use requires more than the quick history usually taken during the initial visit. More extensive questioning about alcohol use and how it affects the patient's life will yield more accurate information.

Alcohol consumption of more than 6 drinks per day (90 mL [3 oz] of absolute alcohol) may result in fetal alcohol syndrome

(FAS). FAS is the leading cause of known mental retardation, occurring in 1.9 of 1,000 births worldwide. Its diagnosis requires evidence of the following: (1) intrauterine growth retardation, (2) central nervous system abnormalities, and (3) characteristic facies. Facial abnormalities include a long philtrum, thin vermillion border, short palpebral fissures, short upturned nose, flattened nasal bridge, small mandible, and abnormally shaped or positioned ears.

Alcohol consumption of more than 1–2 drinks per day may result in isolated congenital anomalies, including facial abnormalities (any of the FAS-associated features), growth deficiency, or mental retardation. This level of consumption is also associated with a 7- to 10-fold increase in perinatal mortality, an 8-fold increase in stillbirths, and a 3-fold increase in preterm delivery. The incidence of spontaneous abortion is higher in women who are chronic drinkers.

The use of cocaine has increased dramatically in the USA in the last decade. Estimates of use among pregnant women range from 10–17%. Cocaine blocks catecholamine uptake at adrenergic nerve terminals, potentiating peripheral sympathetic responses and causing vasoconstriction, tachycardia, and hypertension. It freely crosses the placenta and blood-brain barrier and is a central nervous system stimulant. Acute complications of cocaine ingestion include severe hypertension, seizure, cerebrovascular accident, and myocardial infarction.

Obstetric complications of cocaine use include a severalfold increase in the rate of spontaneous abortion, preterm labor, preterm delivery, low birth weight, intrauterine growth retardation, placental abruption, and stillbirth. An increased use of cocaine is noted in women who do not seek prenatal care. Newborns exposed to cocaine in utero exhibit decreased interactive behavior, can be tremulous, irritable, and may sleep and feed poorly. Whether these infants continue to have developmental and learning problems is unclear but has been suggested by some experts. Anomalies seen in these infants are usually due to ischemic events that lead to permanent structural damage and may include bowel and limb defects, hypospadias, and central nervous system hemorrhage. Early studies have suggested an increased incidence of sudden infant death syndrome (SIDS) in these infants.

Although cocaine is used far more often than heroin and other opioids, 150,000–200,000 women are addicted to narcotics in the USA. These women give birth to about 5,000 infants per year. Women addicted to heroin or who are on methadone maintenance are at increased risk for medical complications, including hepatitis, cellulitis, thrombophlebitis, pulmonary infections (including tuberculosis), urinary tract infections, sexually transmitted diseases, and human immunodeficiency virus (HIV) infection.

Obstetric complications that occur more often in these patients include preterm premature rupture of membranes, preeclampsia, preterm delivery, intrauterine growth retardation, and low birth weight. The incidence of low birth weight is decreased with methadone maintenance treatment.

There are no characteristic congenital malformations associated with opioid use, and the incidence of congenital malformations is not increased. Withdrawal symptoms from opioids (including methadone) may be seen in these neonates anywhere from hours to 2 weeks after birth, but usually occurs at about 48–72 hours after birth. Symptoms include central nervous system excitability (irritability, tremor, seizure), gastrointestinal problems (vomiting, poor feeding), respiratory distress, and diaphoresis.

SUGGESTED READINGS

Burrow GN, Ferris TR (editors): *Medical Complications During Pregnancy,* 3rd ed. Saunders, 1988.

Creasy R, Resnik R (editors): *Maternal-Fetal Medicine: Principles and Practice,* 2nd ed. Saunders, 1989.

Cunningham FG, MacDonald P, Gant N: *Williams Obstetrics,* 18th ed. Appleton & Lange, 1989.

Gabbe S, Niebyl J, Simpson JL (editors): *Obstetrics: Normal and Problem Pregnancies,* 2nd ed. Churchill Livingstone, 1991.

Gleicher N et al: *Principles and Practice of Medical Therapy in Pregnancy,* 2nd ed. Appleton & Lange, 1991.

Bonnie A. Coyne, MD

Pregnancy is a time of dramatic alteration of maternal physiology, with the most striking changes occurring in the cardiovascular, hematologic, gastrointestinal, and endocrine systems. Obstetricians must be able to differentiate their patients' common complaints attributable to normal pregnancy from more serious symptoms that may herald obstetric, surgical, or medical complications. Not only are we challenged by young, healthy women who develop unexpected complications, but there has also been a great increase in the number of women with underlying medical complications who are bearing children. Medical problems may adversely affect the outcome of pregnancy and, conversely, pregnancy may alter the course of a given disease. This chapter examines the more common medical complications of pregnancy. Treatment of these complications involves consideration of both patients under care: mother and fetus. Altered maternal physiology dictates, in many cases, alteration in standard medical therapy, and any drugs used must be safe for the fetus. Appropriate consultations with internists, surgeons, anesthesiologists, neonatologists, and subspecialists will ensure optimal outcome for both mother and baby.

CARDIOVASCULAR DISORDERS

The spectrum of cardiac disease that can complicate pregnancy ranges from benign mitral valve prolapse to diseases such as pulmonary hypertension, Marfan syndrome, and cardiomyopathy that carry such a high mortality rate that pregnancy may be contraindicated. In the past, rheumatic heart disease accounted for most valvular disease seen in pregnancy. Today it is congenital heart disease that is the most common cause. Congenital heart disease occurs in about 1% of births in the USA, and most of these children live to reproductive age. Early consultation with a cardiologist, preferably before pregnancy, is necessary to achieve optimal perinatal outcome in the woman with cardiac disease. The goals of care for these women include achieving maximum hemodynamic capacity, preventing bacterial endocarditis and thromboemboli, and ensuring an optimal intrauterine environment for the fetus. Fetal evaluation should, in many cases, include ultrasound evaluations of cardiac anatomy, and serial ultrasonograms to evaluate fetal growth.

General Prognosis

Outcome of pregnancy for the woman with heart disease may be predicted by her functional cardiac capacity. In general, women with fewer physical limitations imposed by heart disease have better outcomes than those who have greater limitations. The New York Heart Association Classification (Table 35–1) may be used as a guide to outcome: patients in classes I and II in general do well; those in class III require close management, including prolonged hospitalization, to optimize outcome; those in class IV have significant complications and an increased mortality risk.

The inheritance pattern of most congenital cardiac lesions is not clear, but the question of risk of recurrence for the fetus when one parent has congenital heart disease is of concern. Estimates of risk vary but, in general, range from 2–4%. The risk of inheritance of Marfan syndrome is 50% (autosomal dominant inheritance). Patients should receive appropriate genetic counseling and have fetal echocardiography performed when indicated.

General Management

Patients with certain cardiac lesions require prophylaxis against bacterial endocarditis when undergoing genitourinary pro-

Table 35-1. New York Heart Association classification of cardiac status.

Class I:	Uncompromised. Patients with cardiac disease and no symptoms with any level of activity.
Class II:	Slightly compromised. Patients are asymptomatic at rest but symptomatic with ordinary activity.
Class III:	Moderately compromised. Patients are symptomatic with only slight activity.
Class IV:	Severely compromised. Patients may be symptomatic at rest and are unable to perform any activity without symptoms.

cedures, including vaginal delivery. Prophylaxis is recommended for patients with most congenital cardiac malformations, prosthetic va¹ ₂s, acquired valvular disease, including mitral valve prolapse with insufficiency, idiopathic hypertrophic subaortic stenosis, and for patients with a history of bacterial endocarditis. Patients with mitral valve prolapse and no insufficiency do not require prophylaxis. The recommended antibiotic regimen is as follows: ampicillin, 2 g intravenously, plus gentamicin, 1.5 mg/kg intramuscularly or intravenously, given 30–60 minutes before delivery. A repeat dose of both antibiotics is given 8 hours after the initial dose. For patients allergic to ampicillin, vancomycin, 1 g intravenously over 1 hour, is recommended as an alternative, combined with gentamicin as described above. Patients with mechanical heart valves or those with a history of thromboemboli also require treatment with an anticoagulant drug (heparin) during pregnancy.

Management of the cardiac patient during labor and delivery and during the postpartum period is governed by the cardiac lesion. During labor, cardiac output increases. Venous return may be impeded if the patient is allowed to lie on her back. Immediately after delivery, venous return increases with the loss of the uteroplacental shunt. These hemodynamic changes must be kept in mind, and the patient must be appropriately monitored during labor and delivery and especially during the first 24–48 hours postpartum, when fluid shifts are greatest. In general, a shortened second stage by assisted vaginal delivery with forceps is safer than cesarean section for the cardiac patient, and epidural anesthesia is preferred for pain relief.

Specific Cardiovascular Disorders

A. Congenital Heart Disease: Patients with corrected congenital heart disease usually tolerate pregnancy well. The exception is the patient who has pulmonary hypertension superimposed on the underlying defect. For these patients, mortality during pregnancy may be as high as 50%.

1. Atrial septal defect–This defect is the most common congenital cardiac anomaly recognized in adults. The shunt causes overload of the right side of the heart and increased pulmonary flow. Not until midlife do patients develop serious complications, including arrhythmias, pulmonary hypertension, or reversal of direction of the shunt.

Physical findings include a normal first heart sound, midsystolic murmur (from increased flow across the pulmonic valve), and a split second heart sound. An electrocardiogram may show right axis deviation and right ventricular hypertrophy. Conduction defects are also seen. Chest x-ray shows an enlarged right atrium and ventricle and increased pulmonary vascular markings. Diagnosis is confirmed by cardiac catheterization.

If the atrial septal defect (ASD) is not associated with other cardiac anomalies or pulmonary hypertension, pregnancy outcome is good. The threat posed by delivery in these patients is the occurrence of hypotension caused by either hemorrhage or anesthesia. This hypotension may cause reversal of shunt flow with accompanying hypoxia. Treatment may require vasopressors or blood transfusion.

2. Ventricular septal defect–This defect is the most common congenital anomaly in newborns. However, by adulthood the ventricular septal defect (VSD) has usually either closed spontaneously or been surgically corrected. This defect is also seen in combination with other cardiac anomalies. Clinically, functional capacity depends on the size of the defect and the degree of pulmonary vascular resistance.

On physical examination, patients may exhibit signs of cardiomegaly, with a holosystolic murmur from flow across the defect. They may also have a diastolic murmur because of increased flow across the mitral valve. The electrocardiogram may be normal or show left or right ventricular hypertrophy. Chest x-ray may reveal an enlarged left atrium, ventricular hypertrophy, and increased pulmonary markings. Echocardiography and cardiac catheterization will delineate the extent of the shunt. Patients with a small or repaired ventricular septal defect tolerate pregnancy well. However, with a large defect, heart failure may ensue. Patients with ventricular septal defects are susceptible to bacterial endocarditis and require antibiotic prophylaxis. Like women with atrial septal defects, women with ventricular septal defects may experience shunt reversal if they are hypotensive. This complication must be avoided during labor and delivery.

B. Valvular Heart Disease: Valvular heart disease may be either congenital or acquired. In either case, pathophysiology and management during pregnancy are the same with the exception of prophylaxis against recurrent rheumatic fever. Patients with a history of rheumatic heart disease or recurrent rheumatic fever should also receive 1.2 million units of benzathine penicillin monthly.

1. Mitral stenosis–Rheumatic fever causes the vast majority of cases of mitral stenosis. With obstruction of the mitral valve, left atrial pressure rises to maintain cardiac output. Pulmonary pressure may eventually rise and cause dyspnea, hemoptysis, and fatigue. Patients with mild mitral stenosis are asymptomatic, but with increased blood flow across the valve, as occurs during pregnancy, symptoms may be precipitated.

Physical findings include a loud S_1, diastolic rumble, and left parasternal heave. Chest x-ray and electrocardiogram show left atrial enlargement. Atrial arrythmias are also found. The degree of valve obstruction may be estimated by the extent of symptoms. Cardiac catheterization or echocardiogram may be necessary to quantify the impairment. Surgery is recommended when the valve area is less than 1 cm^2.

Mitral stenosis during pregnancy carries a mortality risk of approximately 1%. Death is usually caused by acute pulmonary edema, which may be precipitated by onset of atrial fibrillation or the sudden increase in venous return that occurs immediately after delivery. Pulmonary edema must be aggressively treated, and underlying causes corrected. Mitral valve dilatation by percutaneous balloon valvuloplasty or surgical commissurotomy may be necessary in women with severe mitral stenosis who do not respond to medical management. Patients who continue to be symptomatic or those with moderate to severe disease should have Swan-Ganz catheterization at the time of delivery. Patients with mitral stenosis should have bacterial endocarditis prophylaxis at delivery.

2. Mitral regurgitation–With mitral regurgitation and blood flow back across the mitral valve during systole, effective cardiac output may be reduced. Initially, left ventricular function may maintain adequate output, but eventually the ventricle will decompensate. Mitral regurgitation is caused by rheumatic fever in 50% of cases. It may also be congenital or secondary to cardiomyopathy.

Patients present with fatigue and later dyspnea. Signs of mitral regurgitation include cardiomegaly and a holosystolic murmur at the apex. Electrocardiogram shows left atrial enlargement. Chest x-ray also shows cardiomegaly.

Medical management of mitral regurgitation may include restriction of physical activity, diuretic therapy, and digitalis for left ventricular failure. Most women with mitral regurgitation who become pregnant are asymptomatic and require no treatment. Patients who develop symptoms require therapy at delivery as outlined above for mitral stenosis.

3. Aortic stenosis–Aortic stenosis may be congenital, rheumatic, or secondary to calcification of the valve. A variety of pathologic changes may be seen in these patients: left ventricular hypertrophy, elevated left atrial and pulmonary pressures, and arrythmias. Syncope and myocardial ischemia may result from a sudden decrease in cardiac output.

Symptoms of aortic stenosis develop late in the course of disease because of the ability of the left ventricle to compensate for the obstruction. Symptoms include chest pain, syncope, dyspnea, and fatigue. Patients exhibit a systolic ejection murmur radiating to the carotid arteries. An electrocardiogram shows left ventricular hypertrophy. Chest x-ray may show calcification of the valve, dilation of the aortic root, and initially a normal heart size.

Affected women of childbearing age seldom have symptomatic aortic stenosis, and usually tolerate pregnancy well. In rare cases, patients may need to be treated for pulmonary edema because of left ventricular failure. Delivery poses a special danger to these patients. If venous return decreases suddenly (as with hemorrhage), cardiac output cannot be maintained, and death may ensue. Hypovolemia and compression of the vena cava by the uterus must therefore be avoided.

4. Pulmonic stenosis–Pulmonic stenosis is congenital in origin. With obstruction to right ventricular outflow, hypertrophy occurs. With progression of disease, right atrial enlargement and atrial arrhythmias may result. Most cases of pulmonic stenosis are recognized and surgically treated during childhood.

Symptoms of pulmonic stenosis are syncope, fatigue, chest pain, and dyspnea. Patients have a left parasternal heave and a systolic murmur in the pulmonic area. The electrocardiogram shows right ventricular hypertrophy, and chest x-ray shows an enlarged pulmonary artery.

Patients with pulmonic stenosis usually do well during pregnancy. Ventricular failure should be treated with usual medical measures: rest and digitalis. Decreased venous return must be avoided during labor and delivery because it will cause sudden decline in the high right ventricular filling pressure necessary to maintain cardiac output. Antibiotic prophylaxis against endocarditis is needed.

C. Peripartum Cardiomyopathy: Cardiac failure that develops during pregnancy or during the first 6 months postpartum in a woman without a history of heart disease and with no cause for heart failure other than pregnancy is termed peripartum cardiomyopathy. The incidence varies from 1:1000 to 1:4000. It is higher in Africa. It occurs more often in older women, those with twins, and in patients with pregnancy-induced hypertension. The cause of peripartum cardiomyopathy is unknown. In patients who continue to have signs and symptoms of disease for more than 6 months postpartum, mortality is high, and subsequent pregnancy especially dangerous.

Symptoms of peripartum cardiomyopathy are those of congestive heart failure: dyspnea, chest pain, fatigue, orthopnea, palpitations, and syncope. Examination will reveal jugular venous distension, rales, edema, and a third heart sound. Chest x-ray shows cardiomegaly and may show pulmonary edema. An electrocardiogram may reveal tachycardia, and atrial or ventricular arrhythmias. Death may occur as a result of arrhythmia or embolus. Autopsy usually reveals an enlarged, dilated heart, and often mural thrombi (the source of pulmonary and systemic emboli) are found.

The treatment of peripartum cardiomyopathy includes bedrest, sodium restriction, diuresis, and digitalis. Patients may also require afterload reduction. Patients with atrial fibrillation should undergo cardioversion. Patients with persistent cardiomegaly or mural thrombi on echocardiogram require anticoagulant therapy. Long-term prognosis in these patients depends on whether cardiomegaly resolves within 6 months of the onset of symptoms. If it does not resolve, the 5-year mortality rate is 85%. If it does resolve, the mortality rate is still about 15%. If cardiomegaly does not resolve and another pregnancy intervenes, cardiomyopathy recurs in 50% of cases, with an almost 100% mortality.

D. Thromboembolic Diseases: These disorders include **superficial thrombophlebitis, deep vein thrombosis** (DVT), and **pulmonary embolus** (PE). Although superficial thrombophlebitis is common, occurring in 1% of pregnancies, it is benign if not associated with deep vein thrombosis. Deep vein thrombosis and pulmonary embolus are more threatening. Embolism is the leading cause of maternal death in the USA. Recognition of these disorders is clinically difficult, and a variety of tests are used to substantiate the diagnosis.

1. Superficial thrombophlebitis–Superficial thrombophlebitis alone does not predispose a patient to emboli. The presenting symptom is usually pain. Tenderness and swelling may also be found in the affected area. Diagnosis is aimed at excluding deep vein thrombosis. Directional Doppler flow studies, impedence plethysmography, and compressive ultrasonography may be used to confirm the diagnosis. Treatment is conservative, with bedrest, application of heat, and use of aspirin advised.

2. Deep vein thrombosis–This disorder predisposes patients to pulmonary emboli and chronic venous stasis. Diagnosis is difficult, with a clinical impression confirmed by venogram in only

50% of suspected cases. Patients present with pain and swelling and, on examination, may have edema and a positive Homans' sign. Deep vein thrombosis tends to occur later in pregnancy and in the puerperium. Other conditions that cause similar symptoms are superficial thrombophlebitis and cellulitis.

During pregnancy, noninvasive testing is the best means of diagnosing deep vein thrombosis. Directional Doppler ultrasound and compressive ultrasound have become the most used modalities in this area. If the diagnosis cannot be confirmed using noninvasive testing, venography with shielding of the maternal abdomen may be used.

Nonpregnant patients with deep vein thrombosis below the popliteal fossa are not usually given heparin but are observed for progression of thrombus. In pregnancy, this approach has not yet been shown to be safe. Treatment of deep vein thrombosis during pregnancy mandates the use of heparin, because warfarin crosses the placenta and is teratogenic. Heparin does not cross the placenta and will not lead to anticoagulation in the fetus. In addition, its effects may be rapidly reversed using protamine sulfate. Intravenous heparin may be given in a variety of regimens to achieve full anticoagulation, with the aim of a prolonged partial thromboplastin time 1.5 times normal. After 7–10 days of initial therapy, subcutaneous heparin may then be given every 8–12 hours to prolong the partial thromboplastin time to a similar degree. Patients with a history of deep vein thrombosis during pregnancy need subcutaneous heparin prophylaxis during subsequent pregnancies to prevent recurrence.

3. Pulmonary embolus–Pulmonary embolus is the potentially fatal consequence of a deep vein thrombosis. Dyspnea is the most common symptom and may be accompanied by chest pain, cough, and apprehension. Examination may reveal tachycardia, tachypnea, and low-grade fever, and patients may have the symptoms and signs of deep vein thrombosis. Patients with massive pulmonary embolus may present with hypotension, syncope, or sudden death. Findings in the patient with massive pulmonary embolus may include acute right ventricular failure, pulmonary hypertension, and decreased cardiac output.

Pulmonary embolus should be differentiated from myocardial infarction, amniotic fluid embolus, pneumonia, and other pulmonic processes. Initial workup includes a chest x-ray (which may be normal), an electrocardiogram, and measurement of arterial blood gas levels. Some experts advocate full anticoagulation with heparin while definitive testing is being arranged. The approach to diagnosis is changing. A ventilation-perfusion scan, studies to document a deep vein thrombosis, or a pulmonary angiogram may be necessary to confirm a clinical suspicion of embolus.

As with deep vein thrombosis, treatment for pulmonary embolus involves full heparin anticoagulation for 10–14 days, followed by subcutaneous heparin to achieve prolongation of the partial thromboplastin time to 1.5 times normal. Treatment should continue into the postpartum period for a total of 3–6 months. Prophylactic heparin therapy is indicated in subsequent pregnancies. Surgical interruption of the inferior vena cava is used in patients with recurrent pulmonary emboli despite anticoagulation, or in those unable to tolerate anticoagulation.

PULMONARY DISORDERS

Asthma

Chronic asthma involves both bronchoconstriction of the lower airways as well as inflammation of the submucosa. Airway obstruction is reversible and episodic. Hyperresponsiveness of the airways may be intrinsic or may be triggered by allergy, exercise, cold, or upper respiratory infection.

Most patients have a documented history of asthma. They present with wheezing, dyspnea, cough, or fever. On examination, patients appear tachypneic and may be using accessory muscles of respiration. Wheezing is found on lung examination. Differential diagnosis includes infection, upper airway obstruction, congestive heart failure, and pulmonary emboli.

In the early phase, laboratory findings include hypoxia and hypocarbia on arterial blood gas. Chest x-ray may be normal, and complete blood count may show eosinophilia. Pulmonary function tests delineate the degree of obstruction.

Pregnancy probably has little effect on the course of asthma. Patients tend to have the same severity of asthma during successive pregnancies. Severe asthma that is not well-controlled medically may result in low-birth-weight infants and increased fetal mortality.

Drugs used in the treatment of asthma include bronchodilators and anti-inflammatory agents. Bronchodilators that may safely be used in pregnancy include β-adrenergic agonists (terbutaline, albuterol), and theophylline (aminophyllin). Corticosteroids, given orally, intravenously, or by inhalation, combat inflammation and are used in conjunction with bronchodilators when the latter alone do not work. Patients who are steroid-dependent require stress doses at the time of delivery; hydrocortisone, 100 mg intravenously every 8 hours, should be given until 24 hours after delivery.

Amniotic Fluid Embolism

Amniotic fluid embolism is a rare, catastrophic event that occurs most often during labor or delivery. It is a rare complication of amniocentesis. Mortality rates range from 70% to 85% during the acute episode, and fetal loss is high.

Initially, intense pulmonary vasospasm occurs, resulting in right ventricular failure and profound hypoxia. If the patient survives this phase, left heart failure and increased pulmonary capillary wedge pressures ensue. Disseminated intravascular coagulation (DIC) develops early, and exsanguination may result. Some patients may require hypogastric artery ligation or hysterectomy to control uterine bleeding. Fetal squamous cells may be seen in maternal blood drawn from the pulmonary circulation, which is consistent with a diagnosis of amniotic fluid embolism. Treatment of amniotic fluid embolism is supportive. Mechanical ventilation with positive pressure, volume replacement, and vasopressors are required. Prompt treatment of DIC with red cell and platelet transfusion and cryoprecipitate is important.

RENAL & URINARY TRACT DISORDERS

Acute Glomerulonephritis

A variety of illnesses can cause acute glomerulonephritis: poststreptococcal pharyngitis, systemic lupus erythematous, hepatitis B, and several immune disorders. Its course is marked by rapid onset of hypertension, azotemia, edema, hematuria, and proteinuria. Examination of the urinary sediment shows red blood cell casts.

Acute glomerulonephritis occurs no more often in pregnancy than at other times. Its significance is that it may be confused with preeclampsia. Definitive diagnosis may be difficult, and the risks associated with renal biopsy may be increased in pregnancy. Treatment is the same as for the nonpregnant patient.

Nephrolithiasis

Renal and ureteral stones complicate 0.1–0.3% of pregnancies. Patients present with colicky pain, infection (including pyelonephritis), hematuria, and dysuria. Diagnosis may be confirmed by ultrasonography of the maternal collecting system. Occasionally, a limited-study intravenous pyelogram is needed.

Treatment involves bedrest, hydration, antibiotics for infection, and pain relief. A continuous epidural may permit lower narcotic doses. If symptoms persist, a ureteral stent placed from below may alleviate symptoms until postpartum, when definitive management may be undertaken.

Chronic Renal Disease

Chronic renal disease, the permanent loss of renal function, is the result of a variety of disorders, including glomerulonephritis, diabetes, hypertension, systemic lupus erythematosus, and chronic interstitial nephritis.

Patients with mild to moderate renal impairment maintain fertility, whereas those with a serum creatinine of more than 3 mg/dL have markedly decreased conception rates and poor pregnancy outcome. Pregnancy does not cause permanent decreases in renal function. Mild to moderate renal dysfunction does not adversely affect pregnancy outcome. However, if hypertension complicates renal disease, maternal and fetal outcome is worse. It has been suggested that patients with chronic renal disease are at increased risk for pregnancy-induced hypertension.

Prenatal care in these patients requires close monitoring of blood pressure, with aggressive treatment of hypertension. Monthly determination of renal function is indicated. If deterioration of renal function ensues, reversible causes (infection, dehydration, or obstruction) should be corrected. Fetal growth should be documented by serial ultrasonograms, and antenatal testing begun at 28 weeks.

Hemodialysis has been used in pregnancy to treat both acute and chronic renal failure. Patients on chronic dialysis have decreased fertility and often have pregnancy complications, including preterm labor and delivery, intrauterine growth retardation, oligo-hydramnios, and further loss of renal function.

After renal transplant, the patient with chronic renal failure has improved fertility. These women then face a variety of complications of pregnancy: pregnancy-induced hypertension, preterm labor and delivery, and intrauterine growth retardation. Rejection episodes are no more common during pregnancy; however, pregnancy outcome is better when it occurs between 2 and 5 years after transplantation. Vaginal delivery is possible in these patients as long as the transplanted kidney does not obstruct labor.

GASTROINTESTINAL TRACT DISORDERS

Hyperemesis Gravidarum

Nausea and vomiting during early pregnancy is extremely common, occurring in 50–70% of pregnancies. Most cases are mild and require no specific therapy. However, a small number of women will have persistent, severe nausea and vomiting that require hospitalization. In these women it is important to consider other causes of nausea and vomiting and to maintain hydration and provide nutrition.

The differential diagnosis of severe nausea and vomiting in early pregnancy includes gastritis, hepatitis, appendicitis, partial intestinal obstruction, diabetic ketoacidosis, molar pregnancy, and hyperthyroidism. These disorders may be excluded on the basis of history and selected laboratory tests. Patients who have no other cause for severe nausea and vomiting have hyperemesis gravidarum.

Hyperemesis gravidarum may result in severe electrolyte imbalances, ketosis, and acidosis. Longstanding disease may result in renal and hepatic abnormalities, and the fetus may be exposed to detrimental ketones. For these reasons, the patient who does not respond to simple outpatient therapy (bland food, fluid supplements, antiemetics) should be hospitalized. Treatment mandates correction of electrolyte imbalances; hydration; nutritional support, including hyperalimentation if indicated; and antiemetic therapy.

Peptic Ulcer Disease

Peptic ulcer disease is uncommon during pregnancy. The diagnosis is suggested by epigastric burning relieved by eating. It may be mistaken for reflux esophagitis, which is much more common during pregnancy. Once the diagnosis is suspected, the patient should undergo endoscopic examination. Treatment consists of antacids and dietary modification. Sucralfate, which is not systemically absorbed, is a good choice for treatment of these patients. H_2-receptor blockers should not be a first-line choice for treatment. Cimetidine, for example, has anti-androgen effects that have been demonstrated in animal studies and should be used with caution during pregnancy.

Inflammatory Bowel Disease

Crohn's disease and ulcerative colitis are chronic episodic disorders of the gastrointestinal tract of unknown etiology. They are characterized by diarrhea, fever, abdominal pain, and weight loss. Crohn's disease is also complicated by the formation of fistulas and anorectal fissures. The diagnosis is made using biopsies performed under colonoscopy. Both disorders manifest extraintestinal complications involving joints, skin, eye, and liver. Treatment involves sulfasalazine, corticosteroids, immunosuppressive agents, and supportive measures, such as antidiarrheal agents, hydration, and parenteral nutrition. Surgery is sometimes indicated in ulcerative colitis for toxic megacolon, cancer, or intractable disease. In Crohn's disease, surgery is reserved for repair of fistulas, abscesses, or obstruction.

Women with Crohn's disease have decreased fertility rates, whereas those with ulcerative colitis have normal fertility rates. The course of disease does not seem to be altered by pregnancy. Outcome of pregnancy is good in these patients except for those who first develop the disease during pregnancy. These women have a higher fetal loss rate. Treatment during pregnancy is similar to that of nonpregnant patients. Sulfasalazine should be stopped at term, because, like other sulfa drugs, it can cross the placenta and displace bilirubin from albumin in the neonate.

HEMATOLOGIC DISORDERS

Anemia

Because of an increase in plasma volume, out of proportion to the increase in red blood cell mass, hemoglobin and hematocrit levels normally decrease during pregnancy. This is referred to as physiologic anemia. However, true anemia is also a common finding during pregnancy. Anemia may affect both fetus and mother during pregnancy: the fetus may not grow well, and the mother is more vulnerable to the blood loss that occurs at delivery. It is important to establish the cause of anemia during pregnancy, treat it, and, in cases of hereditary anemia, offer genetic counseling.

The symptoms of anemia are nonspecific and, in chronic cases, often absent. These symptoms include fatigue, exercise intolerance, and pallor. The approach to evaluation involves laboratory analysis: reticulocyte index, red blood cell indices, and review of the peripheral blood smear. When the reticulocyte count is less than 2%, inadequate production of red blood cells is assumed; when it is more than 2%, increased destruction or loss of red blood cells has occurred.

The following anemias are due to inadequate red blood cell production: **iron deficiency, thalassemia, sideroblastic anemia, anemia of chronic disorders, megaloblastic anemias,** and **marrow failure.**

Iron deficiency is the most common anemia seen during pregnancy. Most women have poor iron stores because of menstrual blood loss and poor nutrition. Pregnancy requires an additional 700–1000 mg of elemental iron for fetal and maternal needs, and iron supplementation is vital during pregnancy. Diagnosis of iron deficiency is confirmed in the laboratory. Microcytic, hypochromic red blood cell indices are seen, with decreased serum iron and ferritin, and an increased iron-binding capacity. Treatment involves oral iron supplementation. It is seldom necessary to prescribe parenteral iron therapy.

The thalassemias are also hypochromic and microcytic. This inherited group of disorders vary in severity and are named by the affected hemoglobin chain. Laboratory examination shows normal serum iron, ferritin, and iron-binding capacity. Diagnosis is made using hemoglobin electrophoresis, which shows increases of usually minor forms of hemoglobin. Both alpha thalassemia and beta thalassemia mandate folate supplementation during pregnancy. Careful genetic counseling with identification of paternal hemoglobin status is mandated and should ideally be performed before pregnancy.

Macrocytic anemias can occur during pregnancy, and folate deficiency is usually the cause. Dietary inadequacy, multiparity, sickle cell anemia, and twin pregnancy predispose patients to folate deficiency. The mean corpuscular volume is elevated in these patients. It is necessary to also consider vitamin B_{12} deficiency in the patient with macrocytic anemia, but vitamin B_{12} deficiency is rare during pregnancy. Folate deficiency is treated with oral folic acid, and women at risk for folate deficiency should be given prophylactic supplements.

Many disorders cause increased destruction of red blood cells, including hypersplenism, hemolytic anemia, mechanical trauma, toxin exposure, and hemoglobinopathies. Sickle cell disease is the most common hemoglobinopathy seen during pregnancy. In the past, outcome of pregnancy in women with sickle cell disease was poor. With improved medical care, more of these patients live longer, achieve pregnancy, and have better pregnancy outcomes than in the past. Still, the perinatal loss rate can be as high as 10% in those with sickle cell disease. Painful crises are common during pregnancy, as are urinary tract infections. Management during pregnancy should include frequent prenatal visits, folate (not iron) supplementation, regular urine cultures, and antenatal surveillance. Prophylactic red blood cell transfusion has been performed during pregnancy in the past but can no longer be recommended. Treatment of crises is the same as in the nonpregnant patient. Genetic counseling should be offered to these patients, preferably in the prepregnancy period, for paternal hemoglobin screening and discussion of possible fetal prenatal diagnosis.

Thrombocytopenia

Thrombocytopenia may be seen with infection, drugs, disseminated intravascular coagulation, immunologic problems, and marrow disorders. Of special concern, because it occurs in young women in the child-bearing years, is immune thrombocytopenia (ITP). In this disorder, IgG antibodies directed against platelets are produced. Immune thrombocytopenia is diagnosed through exclusion: platelet count is less than 150,000; other causes of thrombocytopenia, especially drugs, are not present; results of coagulation studies are normal; antiplatelet antibodies are present; and megakaryocytes in the bone marrow are increased. Immune thrombocytopenia is often first recognized during pregnancy because its onset is usually during the second and third decades of life.

Maternal mortality during pregnancy due to immune thrombocytopenia is not increased over other times. Because the IgG antibodies cross the placenta, thrombocytopenia can occur in up to 70% of fetuses. However, neonatal hemorrhage has been reported in less than 5% of cases.

Treatment during pregnancy includes corticosteroids, intravenous γ-globulin, plasmapheresis, splenectomy (in those who fail to respond to steroid administration), and platelet transfusion in cases of hemorrhage. There is debate about the mode of delivery in these patients. Because the fetus is at risk for intracranial hemorrhage, it may be best to avoid head compression during labor in the thrombocytopenic fetus. For this reason, some authors recommend antenatal percutaneous umbilical blood sampling (PUBS) or an early intrapartum fetal scalp platelet count and cesarean delivery of the fetus with a platelet count less than 50,000. A few investigators believe that cesarean delivery does not decrease the chance of intracranial bleeding, and reserve cesarean delivery for obstetric indications only.

Leukemia

More children with acute leukemia are surviving to reproductive age. Those who have been treated before puberty usually maintain fertility. Case reports of pregnancy in women treated for leukemia during childhood show a normal perinatal outcome.

Women who develop acute leukemia during pregnancy are rare. Diagnosis mandates immediate treatment in most cases. The immediate and long-term effects of chemotherapy on the fetus are not clear, and the threat of teratogenesis is probably greater earlier in pregnancy. Most of these women will experience good outcomes with expert management.

Lymphoma

As with leukemia, young women treated in the past for Hodgkin's disease are surviving and are able to become pregnant, and they may have a successful outcome.

When Hodgkin's disease develops during pregnancy, optimal surgical staging may not be possible. Concerns about the effects of chemotherapy on the fetus are valid, and management of these patients requires expert care and consultation.

ENDOCRINE DISORDERS

Diabetes Mellitus

Advances in the care of the pregnant diabetic in the last 20 years have resulted in vastly improved outcomes for both mother and fetus. Effects of pregnancy on diabetes and of diabetes on pregnancy are complex and profound. The severity of diabetes will greatly influence perinatal outcome. White's classification of diabetes during pregnancy (Table 35–2) may be used as a guide to the particular problems faced by diabetic parturients. Prognosis differs with the diagnosis: gestational diabetes, insulin-dependent diabetes without vascular disease, and insulin-dependent diabetes with vascular disease have very different implications for pregnancy outcome.

A. Gestational Diabetes Mellitus: Gestational diabetes mellitus (GDM) is diagnosed on the basis of 2 or more abnormal values on a 3-hour glucose tolerance test (GTT). Gestational diabetes is common, occurring in up to 5% of pregnancies. The principal risk of gestational diabetes in pregnancy is that of macrosomia, with

Table 35-2. White's classification of diabetes during pregnancy.

Class	Definition
A	Abnormal glucose tolerance test.
B	Onset after age 20 and duration less than 10 years.
C	Onset at age 10-20 years or duration of 10-20 years.
D	Onset before age 10 or duration of 20 or more years; benign retinopathy.
F	Renal disease.
H	Coronary artery disease.
R	Proliferative retinopathy.
T	Renal transplant.

potential injury to fetus and mother at the time of delivery. Women with gestational diabetes have a high risk (up to 50%) of developing overt diabetes later in life.

1. Diagnosis–The diagnosis of gestational diabetes is made only when sought with laboratory testing. Half of women found to have gestational diabetes do not have traditional risk factors for diabetes, that is, family history of diabetes mellitus, previous stillbirth or macrosomic infant, or glycosuria. It is important that all pregnant women be screened for gestational diabetes between 24–26 weeks. Testing earlier in pregnancy is suggested for patients with risk factors. Screening is done using a 50-g glucose challenge, with measurement of serum glucose 1 hour later, which should be less than 140 mg/dL. Overall, 10–15% of women who have abnormal results after the 50-g glucose screening test have abnormal results after the 3-hour glucose tolerance test, which confirm the diagnosis (Table 35-3).

2. Management–Management of gestational diabetes is usually achieved with diet alone, but some women require insulin ther-

Table 35-3. Normal values for oral glucose tolerance test.

Time (hours)	Glucose Level (mg/dL)	
	Venous Plasma[1]	Venous Whole Blood[1]
Fasting	105	90
1	190	165
2	165	145
3	145	125

[1] If 2 or more of the glucose levels are equal to or higher than the values listed, gestational diabetes is diagnosed.

apy. Professional nutritional guidance is recommended to maintain normoglycemia, that is, a 2-hour postprandial capillary blood glucose level of less than 120 mg/dL. Women whose blood glucose levels are consistently high despite diet therapy require insulin treatment. Unfortunately, many of these women are obese and insulin resistant, and normoglycemia may be difficult to achieve. Diagnosis and initiation of therapy before 30 weeks gestation is necessary to avoid the hazards of macrosomia.

Women with well-controlled gestational diabetes do not require antenatal testing before 40 weeks unless they have other complications of pregnancy or require insulin therapy. If macrosomia is suspected, sound clinical judgement and ultrasonography may be used to assess the possibility of shoulder dystocia. A decision to elect primary cesarean section to avoid birth injury is a difficult one.

B. Insulin-Dependent Diabetes Mellitus (Type I): Obstetric complications seen in diabetic women are multiple. A high rate of spontaneous abortion and fetal anomalies (cardiac, neurologic, and renal abnormalities and caudal regression syndrome) occur in diabetics with poor glucose control and elevated glycosylated hemoglobin (Hgb A_{1C}) early in pregnancy. Hgb A_{1C} is often measured serially during pregnancy to evaluate overall glucose control.

The risk of hydramnios in the diabetic patient is double that of the nondiabetic patient, as is the risk of preterm labor. The reason for these increased risks are unclear. Women with diabetes are twice as likely to develop pregnancy-induced hypertension. However, those with vascular disease may have a 25% incidence of pregnancy-induced hypertension.

Fetal growth is affected by the presence of maternal diabetes. As in gestational diabetes, the woman with insulin-dependent diabetes mellitus (IDDM) and no vascular disease carries a fetus at risk to develop macrosomia. The macrosomia is due to fetal hyperglycemia with resultant hyperinsulinemia and alterations in fat metabolism.

Fetal lung maturity may be delayed in women with diabetes. This condition presents a particular challenge when these women experience preterm labor. A lecithin:sphingomyelin (L:S) ratio that usually connotes maturity in the nondiabetic patient may not be reliable in the diabetic patient. Additional evidence of pulmonary maturity by the presence of phosphatidylglycerol in the amniotic fluid should also be sought.

Management of the pregnant diabetic requires the efforts of obstetrician, nutritionist, diabetic educators, and at times, consultation with endocrinologists, ophthalmologists, and other medical subspecialists. Because of insulin resistance in pregnancy, insulin requirements typically rise dramatically. Home blood glucose monitoring, with determination of daily fasting (< 100 mg/dL) and postprandial (< 120 mg/dL) glucose levels, will aid adjusting insulin dosage. Regular consultation with a nutritionist will help achieve normoglycemia and optimal weight gain during the pregnancy.

Renal function should be monitored in each trimester in patients with nephropathy with measurement of creatinine clearance and 24-hour urinary protein levels. Retinal examination should also be performed early in pregnancy, and follow-up examinations performed as necessary. Fetal surveillance should include alphafetoprotein measurements at 16–20 weeks and a fetal ultrasound survey with a fetal echocardiogram at 22 weeks, as indicated, to identify congenital anomalies. Antenatal testing should begin at 32–34 weeks or earlier (28 weeks) in women with vascular disease.

Timing of delivery in the diabetic patient depends on the course of pregnancy. Because of an increased incidence of preterm labor and preeclampsia, many diabetics will deliver preterm. For pregnant diabetic women who reach term, elective induction at 37 weeks (after documentation of fetal lung maturity) is advocated by many, because of the risk of placental insufficiency, fetal distress, and stillbirth in these patients. Other experts recommend continued antenatal surveillance while awaiting the spontaneous onset of labor in order to decrease the incidence of cesarean section.

Management of glucose levels in the diabetic woman during labor is made easier by the use of intravenous insulin and glucose infusions, as dictated by hourly glucose tests. This regimen decreases the incidence of diabetic ketoacidosis during prolonged labor and decreases the incidence of reactive neonatal hypoglycemia. In the immediate postpartum period, insulin requirements drop dramatically because of the decrease in human placental lactogen (among other changes). Insulin dosage will have to be changed, and some women may not require insulin for 1–2 days.

C. Effects of Pregnancy on Diabetes Mellitus: Pregnancy has profound effects on carbohydrate metabolism. Both human placental lactogen and progesterone cause insulin resistance and result in hyperglycemia. Ketone production by the liver is increased. There is also a tendency toward fasting hypoglycemia because of fetal use of glucose and decreased hepatic gluconeogenesis. Pregnant women with diabetes are at increased risk to develop diabetic ketoacidosis.

Patients with diabetic retinopathy are at risk for progression of disease. Usually, such patients will have an increase in background retinopathy, which then decreases after delivery. Patients who have neovascularization during pregnancy should undergo laser photocoagulation.

Most women with diabetic nephropathy do not experience further loss of renal function because of pregnancy. However, in 20% of these women, the disease will progress to renal failure within 5 years of pregnancy, probably because of the natural course of their disease.

Thyroid Disease

After diabetes mellitus, thyroid disease is the leading cause of endocrine disorders that complicate pregnancy, occurring in 0.2% of all gestations. Evaluation of thyroid function is difficult not only because of cardiovascular and thermoregulatory changes that happen during pregnancy, but also because of natural changes that occur in thyroid function. Thyroid-binding globulin rises during pregnancy because of increased estrogen. Total serum thyroxine (T_4) rises, but free serum thyroxine remains unchanged. Resin T_3 uptake decreases during pregnancy. Thyroid-stimulating hormone (TSH) levels remain unchanged.

A. Hypothyroidism: Hypothyroidism does not occur often during pregnancy. Hypothyroid women often have relative infertility and are treated before conception. Women with untreated hypothyroidism have a higher pregnancy loss rate in the first trimester. Patients who are hypothyroid require thyroid supplementation throughout pregnancy, and TSH levels should be monitored to adjust thyroid doses. There are no adverse fetal side effects from this therapy.

B. Hyperthyroidism: Diagnosis of hyperthyroidism during pregnancy depends on laboratory analysis. Symptoms may include tachycardia, heat intolerance, restlessness, and hyperemesis gravidarum. Graves' disease is the most common cause of hyperthyroidism in pregnancy. Thioamides are used to prevent synthesis of thyroid hormone. Most commonly, propylthiouracil (PTU), 100–150 mg every 8 hours, is used to control symptoms and bring free thyroid hormone values to normal levels. Three to 4 weeks of treatment may be necessary before improvement is seen. Doses should be lowered as much as possible after therapy is successful because propylthiouracil crosses the placenta and can cause goiter and hypothyroidism in the fetus. The fetus of the patient with Graves' disease is also at risk for neonatal hyperthyroidism because of maternal thyroid-stimulating immunoglobulins that may cross the placenta.

Subtotal thyroidectomy may be required for patients who cannot or will not take antithyroid medication and for those who do not respond to other forms of medical therapy, such as beta-blockers. Surgery has been traditionally performed in the second trimester. Patients may need thyroid replacement medication after this procedure.

AUTOIMMUNE DISORDERS

Maternal autoimmune diseases are notable for their often remitting and relapsing courses and for their adverse effects on the fetus through immune mechanisms. The incidence of these disorders is not higher in pregnancy, but they are most prevalent in young women. There is little to suggest that the pregnant patient is immunologically any different than her nonpregnant counterpart, although she is at high risk for obstetric and fetal complications.

Systemic Lupus Erythematosus (SLE)

SLE may involve any organ system and may cause a wide variety of symptoms. Manifestations may include skin rash, joint abnormalities, nephritis, anemia, thrombocytopenia, serositis, and cerebritis. Autoantibodies to nuclear and phospholipid antigens are seen in a variety of combinations: antinuclear antibodies (ANA), anti-DNA antibodies (including anti-Ro, anti-La, anti-ssDNA, and anti-dsDNA), anticardiolipin antibodies, and the lupus anticoagulant may be present. Their titers may increase with disease activity. Complement (C3, C4, CH_{50}) levels may decrease with lupus flares.

When the disease is in remission at the start of pregnancy, the course of SLE is not adversely affected by pregnancy, with two-thirds of patients remaining well. However, active disease is exacerbated by pregnancy, and more than half of these patients worsen during pregnancy.

Pregnancy outcome in SLE patients with quiescent disease is usually good with appropriate management. SLE patients are at risk for recurrent pregnancy loss (both first and second trimester), intrauterine growth retardation, preeclampsia, and preterm delivery because of worsening maternal disease. Patients with nephritis and hypertension are at high risk of developing superimposed pre-eclampsia. Differentiating lupus nephritis from preeclampsia may be difficult. Nephritis may be accompanied by other signs of active disease (involvement of other organs, increase in autoantibody titers, decrease in complement levels, and the presence of an active urine sediment). Patients with SLE may develop severe preeclampsia as early as 20 weeks gestation. Patients with anti-Ro (anti SS-A) antibody may have offspring with neonatal lupus. These infants have skin rashes and may have congenital heart block.

Management of SLE in pregnancy should include baseline laboratory functions as listed above. Patients should be seen frequently, and disease flares treated with steroids. Renal function should be followed carefully. Fetal growth should be followed using ultrasonography, and antenatal testing should begin at 32 weeks or earlier, as appropriate. Diagnosis of fetal congenital heart block may be confirmed with echocardiography. Pacemaker insertion may be needed in the early neonatal period.

Lupus Anticoagulant-Anticardiolipin Antibody Syndrome

The presence of antibodies to phospholipids and a variety of clinical symptoms, including vascular thromboses, thrombocytopenia, and recurrent pregnancy loss, characterize the lupus anticoagulant-anticardiolipin antibody syndrome. Many of these patients have SLE-like symptoms but do not meet specific diagnostic criteria for that disease. The lupus anticoagulant is an antibody to phospholipid that interferes with activation of the complement cascade. Anticardiolipin antibody may also occur in these patients. Both antiphospholipid antibodies may cause arterial and venous thromboses.

Detection of these antiphospholipid antibodies may require a combination of laboratory tests. The lupus anticoagulant will prolong both the partial thromboplastin time (PTT) and the Russell's viper-venom time. The latter is a more sensitive predictor of disease. Anticardiolipin antibody may be detected using ELISA testing. Either antibody may cause a false-positive syphilis serology.

This syndrome may require treatment with immunosuppressive and anticoagulant medications. In patients with recurrent pregnancy loss and a diagnosis of lupus anticoagulant syndrome, treatment with daily high-dose prednisone and low-dose aspirin, begun before pregnancy and continuing until the postpartum period, has been shown to improve outcome in a small number of patients.

Rheumatoid Arthritis

Rheumatoid arthritis, a chronic disorder with persistent synovitis and extra-articular symptoms, is seen 2–3 times more often in women than in men. Cardiac, pulmonary, ocular, and central nervous system involvement may be seen. Many patients have characteristic subcutaneous nodules. Laboratory confirmation of diagnosis may include measurements of rheumatoid factor, erythrocyte sedimentation rate, and complement levels, as well as synovial fluid examination. Although many patients seem to experience a remission of symptoms during pregnancy, prospective studies show no difference in disease course in these women. Rheumatoid arthritis has not been shown to adversely affect pregnancy outcome. Mainstays of therapy during pregnancy are steroids and aspirin.

NEUROLOGIC DISEASE & PREGNANCY

Central Nervous System Disorders

A. Seizure Disorders: Chronic seizure disorders, both generalized and focal, complicate 1 in 200 pregnancies. These patients are at increased risk of adverse pregnancy outcome, and their medical disease requires close monitoring.

Studies of the effect of pregnancy on seizure frequency are not in agreement. Some studies show an increased frequency of seizures during pregnancy, whereas others do not. Patients taking antiseizure medication during pregnancy should have serum levels checked regularly, because dosage requirements may increase.

The choice of antiseizure medication in pregnancy is difficult because most of these medications have been shown to be teratogenic. Ideally, patients should be switched to less teratogenic therapy before conception. Phenytoin has been shown to cause dysmorphic facial features and other central nervous system abnormalities. Patients who are taking multiple agents may have a higher rate of congenital malformation. Overall, patients with seizure disorders have a 2–3 times higher risk of having a fetus with a congenital anomaly. This increased risk may not be due entirely to drug effects. Other adverse pregnancy outcomes in these patients include preterm delivery, intrauterine growth retardation, and intrauterine fetal death, and these patients should be closely monitored accordingly.

B. Multiple Sclerosis: Multiple sclerosis involves demyelination of the white matter of the central nervous system and results in recurrent, progressive neurologic impairment. The disease may be difficult to diagnose in its early stages. Magnetic resonance imaging is currently the diagnostic tool of choice. Pregnancy has not been shown to adversely affect the course of disease, although there may be an increase in relapse ratio in the postpartum period. Pregnancy outcome is good in these patients.

C. Stroke: Cerebral vascular accidents are rare during pregnancy. They are acute catastrophic events that should be managed in the same way as in the nonpregnant patient, with delivery based on obstetric indications. Ischemic strokes may be seen in patients with vasculitis, emboli, local thrombi or due to "crack" cocaine use. Prompt diagnosis, stabilization, and anticoagulation using heparin are indicated. Patients who have hemorrhagic strokes resulting from a ruptured aneurysm or an arteriovenous malformation require neurosurgical intervention. The fetus can often tolerate these procedures well. Appropriate fetal monitoring should be performed throughout the perioperative period.

Peripheral Nervous System Disorders

A. Carpal Tunnel Syndrome: Carpal tunnel syndrome, which is caused by compression of the median nerve, is fairly common during pregnancy with a reported incidence of 1–5%. Patients present with parasthesia, pain, and in some cases, difficulty with thumb opposition. This syndrome occurs more often in primigravidas, especially those with edema. More than 80% of patients will respond to therapy with wrist splinting, and most will have complete amelioration of symptoms after delivery. It is unusual for a woman to require surgical correction for this problem during pregnancy.

B. Myasthenia Gravis: Myasthenia gravis is an autoimmune disorder that involves destruction of the acetylcholine receptor at the motor end plate, resulting in ocular, bulbar, and peripheral nerve dysfunction that increases with exertion or stress. Most patients with this disorder do well during pregnancy; about one-third show some deterioration. Rarely, labor may be complicated by sudden, severe respiratory compromise. Patients with myasthenia gravis are very sensitive to neuromuscular blockade, and magnesium sulfate should not be used in these patients. Steroids and anticholinesterase agents are used to treat this disease during pregnancy. As in other autoimmune diseases, the neonate is susceptible to myasthenia gravis because of transplacental passage of antibodies. The disorder usually resolves within several months of birth but requires treatment until then.

SUGGESTED READINGS

Burrow GN, Ferris TR (editors): *Medical Complications During Pregnancy,* 3rd ed. Saunders, 1988.

Creasy R, Resnik R (editors): *Maternal-Fetal Medicine: Principles and Practice,* 2nd ed. Saunders, 1989.

Cunningham FG, MacDonald P, Gant N: *Williams Obstetrics,* 18th ed. Appleton & Lange, 1989.

Gabbe S, Niebyl J, Simpson JL (editors): *Obstetrics: Normal and Problem Pregnancies,* 2nd ed. Churchill Livingstone, 1991.

Gleicher N et al: *Principles and Practice of Medical Therapy in Pregnancy,* 2nd ed. Appleton & Lange, 1991.

Hypertensive Disorders During Pregnancy | 36

Steven A. Friedman, MD

CLASSIFICATION

The system currently used to categorize the hypertensive disorders of pregnancy was developed by the Committee on Terminology of the American College of Obstetricians and Gynecologists in 1972 and updated by the National High Blood Pressure Education Program Working Group Report on High Blood Pressure in Pregnancy in 1990. This classification recognizes 4 categories of hypertension in pregnancy: chronic hypertension, preeclampsia-eclampsia, preeclampsia superimposed on chronic hypertension, and transient hypertension.

Hypertension

Hypertension during pregnancy is defined as a blood pressure rise of 30 mm Hg systolic or 15 mm Hg diastolic over baseline values. This blood pressure elevation must be present on 2 occasions at least 6 hours apart. If baseline values are unknown, then blood pressure readings of 140/90 after 20 weeks of gestation are sufficiently elevated for the diagnosis of hypertension. Mean arterial pressure (diastolic pressure + $\frac{1}{3} \times$ pulse pressure) may also be used to define hypertension. A rise in mean arterial pressure of 20 mm Hg or an absolute mean arterial pressure of 105 mm Hg is indicative of hypertension.

Chronic Hypertension

Chronic hypertension is hypertension that is present before pregnancy or before 20 weeks of gestation, since preeclamptic hypertension usually begins after 20 weeks of gestation (except in cases of gestational trophoblastic disease). If blood pressures before or early in pregnancy are not known, then hypertension that persists beyond the sixth postpartum week is also considered chronic.

Preeclampsia-Eclampsia

Preeclampsia-eclampsia is usually defined as the occurrence of hypertension plus proteinuria, or edema, or both, after 20 weeks of gestation. Hypertension is defined as above. Proteinuria is defined as 0.3 g or more in a 24-hour specimen. This measurement may correlate with 0.3 g/L or greater (1 + or greater on dipstick) in a random urine determination. Edema is diagnosed as clinically evident swelling, especially of the hands and face (nondependent edema). However, excessive fluid retention may be manifest as rapid weight gain prior to the development of clinically apparent edema. Eclampsia is the occurrence of otherwise unexplained seizures in preeclamptic patients.

Preeclampsia Superimposed on Chronic Hypertension

Preeclampsia may occur in patients with chronic hypertension, thus making the diagnosis more difficult. Evidence suggests that preeclampsia superimposed on chronic hypertension leads to a much worse maternal and fetal prognosis than does either condition alone. The diagnosis of superimposed preeclampsia in these patients may be further confounded by preexisting proteinuria secondary to chronic hypertensive renal damage. It is recommended that the diagnosis of preeclampsia in such patients be based on an increase in blood pressure (30 mm Hg systolic, 15 mm Hg diastolic, or 20 mm Hg mean arterial pressure), along with the development of proteinuria or generalized edema. In addition, suggestive changes in laboratory values (such as increased levels of serum transaminases or uric acid or decreased platelet counts) may be helpful.

Transient Hypertension

Transient hypertension is the development of hypertension during pregnancy or in the first 24 hours postpartum, without other evidence of preeclampsia or chronic hypertension. The blood pressure must return to normal within 10 days of delivery. It is believed that this group may represent a heterogeneous mixture, consisting of patients with preexisting hypertension that has returned after a second trimester nadir, patients with unmasked future chronic hypertension, and patients with early mild preeclampsia.

PATHOPHYSIOLOGY OF PREECLAMPSIA

Preeclampsia is a complex clinical syndrome that is unique to pregnancy. Once considered primarily a hypertensive disease, preeclampsia is now known to involve potentially all organ systems, with hypertension representing but one manifestation. Recent studies have suggested that trophoblastic hypoperfusion and endothelial cell injury are important pathogenetic mechanisms to explain this perplexing disease.

It has been postulated that an early pathophysiologic event in the development of preeclampsia is placental hypoperfusion. The precise mechanism of hypoperfusion may be different in different pregnancies. The earliest known identifiable difference between preeclamptic and normal pregnant women is found by about 20 weeks of gestation in the spiral arterioles of the placental bed. In normal women, trophoblastic cells have invaded and replaced the arteriolar walls, resulting in the formation of dilated vessels incapable of vasoconstriction. Interestingly, in these vessels, trophoblastic cells (of fetal origin) come into direct contact with maternal blood. Preeclamptic women exhibit a failure of trophoblastic invasion, resulting in vessels of smaller caliber, which retain their musculoelastic elements and are thus capable of vasoconstriction. Thus, many authorities have concluded that the development of preeclampsia in otherwise healthy women is the result of a faulty immunologic interaction between fetus and mother. Other mechanisms for hypoperfusion of trophoblast, such as maternal atherosclerosis or vasculitis, may also predispose the mother to the development of preeclampsia.

Some authors have speculated that in response to hypoperfusion, the fetoplacental unit elaborates a substance that is toxic to endothelial cells, the cells that line virtually all blood vessels. Endothelial cells have several important functions, including secretion of vasodilating substances, maintenance of the integrity of the vascular compartment, and prevention of intravascular coagulation. The resulting endothelial cell dysfunction may account for most of the pathophysiologic changes seen in preeclampsia.

Endothelial cells are the primary source of prostacyclin, and platelets are the primary source of thromboxane. Prostacyclin has vasodilating properties, whereas thromboxane has vasoconstricting properties. Therefore, endothelial cell injury may result in an increase in the ratio of thromboxane to prostacyclin, leading to excessive vasospasm. In addition, endothelial cells produce various other factors, such as endothelium-derived relaxing factor, which are also vasodilators. Endothelial cell dysfunction may also reduce the production of these factors as well.

Such changes are believed to occur in preeclamptic women. It is known that preeclamptic women are more sensitive than normal pregnant women to the effects of all vasoconstrictors, the most well-studied of which is angiotensin II. It is unclear precisely why preeclamptic women are more sensitive to these vasoconstricting substances, but it has been postulated that a relative deficiency of endogenous vasodilators, such as prostacyclin, may explain this phenomenon. This increased sensitivity of the vasculature may lead to arterial and venous vasoconstriction. Excessive arterial spasm would result in increased blood pressure secondary to increased vascular resistance, which has been documented by invasive hemodynamic monitoring in preeclamptic women. Excessive venous spasm would result in decreased plasma volume, a known feature of preeclampsia, and would contribute to peripheral edema formation.

A second function of endothelial cells is the maintenance of the integrity of the vascular compartment. Endothelial cell injury may also result in loss of integrity of cell membranes, leading potentially to a widespread protein leak. In preeclamptic women, evidence for this process is seen in their propensity to develop proteinuria, peripheral edema, and pulmonary edema, even at moderate pulmonary capillary wedge pressures.

A third function of endothelial cells is the prevention of intravascular coagulation, both by serving as a barrier between blood and other tissues and by secreting factors that inhibit coagulation. Widespread damage to endothelial cells, which is postulated to occur in preeclampsia, would result in low-grade intravascular coagulation. Evidence that such a process occurs is seen in pathology specimens from preeclamptic and eclamptic women. Kidney, liver, brain, and placenta have shown endothelial cell injury, deposition of fibrin, and nonspecific deposition of complement, immunoglobulins, and other blood constituents. Such endothelial injury and intravascular coagulation, in combination with arterial spasm, produce hypoperfusion and necrosis in potentially all organs. When these changes are prominent in the blood, there is consumptive coagulopathy; in the central nervous system, seizures or coma; in the liver, right upper quadrant pain and hepatocyte necrosis; in the kidneys, proteinuria or renal failure; and in the placenta, intrauterine growth retardation and fetal distress.

The precise etiology of preeclampsia remains unknown, but the importance of immunologic interactions and endothelial cell injury are gaining wide acceptance.

CLINICAL FINDINGS IN PREECLAMPSIA

Risk Factors

Preeclampsia is usually a disease of primiparous women. The relatively low incidence of recurrence in subsequent pregnancies, as well as the increased incidence of recurrence when there is a new consort, suggests an immunologic basis. In addition to nulliparity, factors predisposing patients to the development of preeclampsia include chronic hypertension; advanced maternal age; multiple gestation; vascular diseases, such as diabetes mellitus and systemic lupus erythematosus; chronic renal disease; hydatidiform mole; and fetal abnormalities associated with hydropic placentae.

Diagnosis

The diagnosis of preeclampsia is usually based on the presence of the classic triad of hypertension, proteinuria, and edema, as described above. Note that, although most patients exhibit all 3 signs to some degree, some patients will not. In a recent series of eclamptic patients (in whom the diagnosis was relatively certain), 21% had diastolic blood pressures of less than 90 mm Hg, 21% had no proteinuria, and 39% had no edema before the onset of seizures.

Symptoms & Signs

In contrast to the signs of preeclampsia, symptoms are relatively uncommon. Most preeclamptic women are, in fact, asymptomatic. Because preeclampsia is a disease characterized by endothelial cell injury, diffuse vasospasm, increased capillary permeability, and activation of the coagulation cascade, signs and symptoms likely result from the suboptimal perfusion of involved organs (Table 36–1).

Preeclampsia may be described as mild or severe. Severe disease is characterized by the presence of one or more of the factors listed in Table 36–2. One particular variant of severe preeclampsia has been termed the HELLP syndrome and is characterized by *h*emolysis, *e*levated *l*iver enzymes, and *l*ow *p*latelet count. Maternal and perinatal outcome may be poor when this syndrome is present. The HELLP syndrome may occur in the absence of significant hypertension, proteinuria, or edema.

Eclamptic seizures, which complicate 1–4% of cases of preeclampsia, present as typical grand mal seizures that are usually self-limited. Approximately half of eclamptic seizures occur antepartum, with the other half evenly divided between the intrapartum and postpartum periods. Nearly all eclamptic seizures occur within 48 hours postpartum. Whenever the diagnosis of eclampsia is made, it is important to consider other possible causes of seizure (eg, drug intoxication or withdrawal, stroke, metabolic derange-

Table 36-1. Signs and symptoms of preeclampsia.

Vascular or endothelial
Hypertension
Edema
Activation of coagulation cascade
Intravascular hemolysis
Cerebral
Headache
Hyperreflexia
Seizure
Coma
Cortical blindness
Retinal
Blurred vision
Scotoma
Gastrointestinal or hepatic
Midepigastric pain and tenderness
Right upper quadrant pain and tenderness
Renal
Proteinuria
Oliguria or anuria
Placental
Abruptio placentae
Fetal distress

Table 36-2. Factors that constitute severe preeclampsia.

Blood pressure $\geq$ 160 mm Hg systolic or $\geq$ 110 mm Hg diastolic on 2 measurements 6 hours apart with the patient at bedrest.
Proteinuria $\geq$ 5 g in a 24-hour collection or $\geq$ 3+ persistently by dipstick.
Oliguria ($<$ 500 mL in 24 hours).
Cerebral or visual disturbances.
Pulmonary edema or cyanosis.
Epigastric or right upper quadrant pain.
Thrombocytopenia with platelet count of less than 100,000/mm^3.[1]
Hepatocellular damage.[1]
Intrauterine growth retardation.[1]

[1] These factors are controversial.

ment, or infection). The precise pathogenetic mechanisms that lead to seizure are not well understood.

Laboratory Findings

Laboratory abnormalities in preeclampsia may range from absent to striking. Hematologic changes may include thrombocytopenia (platelet count $< 150,000/\mu L$), hemoconcentration, and, less commonly, hypofibrinogenemia (< 300 mg/dL). Abnormalities that indicate renal dysfunction include proteinuria ($\geq 1+$ on dipstick or ≥ 0.3 g/d), hyperuricemia (≥ 5.5 mg/dL), and occasionally elevated serum creatinine (≥ 1.0 mg/dL). Elevated liver function tests, including serum transaminases and less often bilirubin, may also be seen.

PREVENTION OF PREECLAMPSIA

Several recent clinical trials have demonstrated the efficacy of aspirin in lowering the incidence of preeclampsia and intrauterine growth retardation in women who are at increased risk of developing the disease. The dose of aspirin used in these studies ranged from 60–150 mg per day. Aspirin prophylaxis was begun as early as 12 weeks and as late as 28 weeks, depending on the study.

The limitations of the current data regarding aspirin prophylaxis should be emphasized. First, these data involve a relatively small number of patients (less than 200 who actually received aspirin). Whereas efficacy has been demonstrated with this small number, safety has not. Although no frequent and serious adverse effects of low-dose aspirin have been reported, studies with many more patients are needed to guarantee safety. Second, the patients enrolled in these studies were judged to be at high risk for developing preeclampsia. Whether aspirin will prove beneficial in patients at low risk (eg, 5%) of developing the disease has not been determined. Resolution of the safety question will also impact on this issue. Third, aspirin was administered as prophylaxis to patients who had no current evidence of preeclampsia; it has not proved efficacious in treating established disease.

Other possible methods of preventing preeclampsia, such as nutritional alterations or pharmacologic treatment of chronic hypertension, have not been demonstrated conclusively.

TREATMENT OF HYPERTENSIVE DISORDERS

Antepartum Management

In general, the treatment of preeclampsia depends on the severity of disease, the age of the fetus, and the inducibility of the cervix. Often, compromises must be made to optimize both maternal and neonatal outcome. The only certain cure for preeclampsia is delivery of the products of conception.

Antepartum management of preeclampsia varies widely. For patients with mild preeclampsia remote from term, most clinicians choose expectant management with meticulous and frequent assessment of maternal and fetal well-being. However, some physicians prescribe hospitalization from the time of diagnosis until delivery; others treat patients on an outpatient basis as long as careful follow-up is ensured and maternal and fetal conditions remain stable. Assessment of the mother requires frequent determination of blood pressure, proteinuria, weight, and symptoms referable to preeclampsia. Less frequent determination of platelet count and levels of serum transaminases, serum creatinine, creatinine clearance, uric acid, and fibrinogen may also be useful. Assessment of the fetus may include any of the usual methods of fetal evaluation (nonstress test, biophysical profile, contraction stress test, sonography, measurement of fundal height, maternal perception of fetal activity), although the usual prognostic value of these tests is valid only when disease activity is stable. In the rapidly deteriorating patient, fetal (and maternal) assessment must be performed more frequently than in the stable patient.

During the period of maternal and fetal evaluation, the mother should be placed at modified bedrest. Mild sodium restriction may be recommended for symptoms related to edema, but strict sodium restriction and use of diuretics should play no role. Pharmacologic treatment of chronic hypertension should be continued, but the treatment of hypertension related solely to preeclampsia is controversial. This practice has been criticized because it obscures an important gauge of disease activity, although in the carefully monitored patient whose hypertension is out of proportion to other findings, antihypertensive therapy may have a role. Note that these interventions should be viewed as palliative, because they do nothing to reverse the underlying pathophysiologic process.

A. Mild Preeclampsia: Mild preeclampsia at or near term may be managed more aggressively, depending on the clinician's desire for delivery. Traditionally, the management of mild preeclampsia at term has depended on the condition of the cervix. A patient with a favorable cervix (Chapter 34, Table 34–3) at 37 weeks of gestation or beyond is a candidate for induction of labor. A patient with mild, stable disease and an unfavorable cervix may be observed until cervical change has occurred. More recently, however, with the introduction of protocols to effect cervical ripening, mild disease in the term patient with an unfavorable cervix may be managed with cervical ripening and induction of labor. The patient who shows evidence of deterioration despite conservative management is a candidate for induction of labor whether or not her cervix is favorable.

B. Severe Preeclampsia: Management of the severely preeclamptic patient with an immature fetus is somewhat controversial. Maternal stabilization, followed by delivery, is standard management. The decision to attempt vaginal delivery, versus immediate cesarean section, depends on the stability of the mother, the ability of the fetus to tolerate labor, the inducibility of the cervix, and the gestational age. Certainly, this approach (prompt delivery) usually leads to a favorable maternal and fetal outcome in gestations beyond 30 weeks. Some authorities have argued in favor of delaying delivery for 48 hours in order to administer glucocorticoids for fetal lung maturation. This approach may be considered if there is no evidence of maternal distress (eg, uncontrolled hypertension, severe thrombocytopenia, pulmonary edema, hepatocellular damage) or fetal distress. The possibility of expectant management for an indefinite time, in the face of severe preeclampsia and severe prematurity ($\leq$ 28 weeks), has been raised recently. In one series, delivery was effected only when there were signs of maternal or fetal distress. Although the results were promising, this approach is considered experimental.

In contrast, the management of the severely preeclamptic patient at term is straightforward: maternal stabilization and delivery. There is a commonly held belief among experienced clinicians that induction of labor will be more successful for term patients with unfavorable cervical examination results and severe preeclampsia than would be otherwise predicted. Consequently, a trial of induction seems warranted regardless of cervical condition.

Intrapartum Management

Intrapartum management of preeclampsia is guided by the following therapeutic goals: control and prevention of seizures, control of severe hypertension, mild fluid restriction, and preparation for delivery.

In the USA, prevention and control of seizures is usually achieved with magnesium sulfate. Magnesium sulfate may be administered as a continuous intravenous infusion or as intermittent intramuscular injections. The minimum therapeutic serum level of magnesium is often quoted as 4 mEq/L (4.8 mg/dL), although this figure appears to be based on subjective impression rather than published data. Because of the safety of magnesium sulfate and because a significant number of eclamptic patients have no proteinuria (21%) or only mild blood pressure elevations (21%), it is recommended that all patients who meet the blood pressure criteria for preeclampsia receive magnesium sulfate during the intrapartum period, and for 24 hours postpartum.

The signs of magnesium toxicity and the levels at which they occur should be familiar to anyone who orders or administers magnesium sulfate. These signs are as follows: loss of patellar reflex at 8–10 mEq/L (9.6–12 mg/dL); respiratory depression and arrest at 10–15 mEq/L (12–18 mg/dL); and cardiac arrest at 20–30 mEq/L (24–36 mg/dL).

The use of phenytoin for prevention and treatment of eclamptic seizures has been reported. Phenytoin may be an acceptable alternative to magnesium sulfate in certain patients, although experience with this drug is very limited compared with that for magnesium sulfate.

Hypertension should be treated only when it represents an immediate threat to the mother, usually at levels of 180 mm Hg systolic or 105 mm Hg diastolic (Korotkoff phase 5, disappearance of sound). Because of the vasoconstriction associated with decreased plasma volume in preeclamptic women, antihypertensive agents should be administered only after 500 mL of intravenous fluids have infused. Because uterine perfusion may decrease significantly if blood pressure is lowered excessively, the goal of antihypertensive therapy is to achieve blood pressures of 140–160 mm Hg systolic and 90–100 mm Hg diastolic. Hydralazine is currently the antihypertensive drug of choice in the USA, primarily because of its long record of safety for both mother and fetus. Hydralazine may be administered as a bolus of 5 mg over 5 minutes and repeated every 20 minutes until the desired effect is achieved. Rarely, hydralazine may prove inadequate in conventional doses (20–30 mg). In such cases, nifedipine (10 mg sublingually or orally every 15–30 minutes) or labetalol (20–80 mg intravenously every 30 minutes, beginning with the lower dose) have been used with success.

Ordinarily, intravenous fluids (eg, lactated Ringer's with 5% dextrose, or Plasma-Lyte) should be administered at approximately 75–125 mL/h. If oliguria (< 25 mL/h) is present, a single 500- to 1000-mL bolus of isotonic intravenous fluids may be administered over 1 hour. If oliguria persists, then central hemodynamic monitoring with a pulmonary artery catheter may be indicated. In addition, hypotension at delivery usually signifies major blood loss rather than a miraculous cure and necessitates increased intravenous fluid administration.

The preferred mode of delivery for the preeclamptic patient is vaginal. The stress of major abdominal surgery, while usually manageable, is best avoided if the patient remains stable while a timely vaginal delivery is attempted. The use of epidural anesthesia was once questionable for patients with preeclampsia, but now it is considered safe for both vaginal and cesarean delivery.

Postpartum Management

Although delivery of the fetus and placenta is the only known cure for preeclampsia, resolution of disease is not immediate. With the constraint of fetal well-being removed, the goal of the medical staff is supportive care until the disease resolves.

Hypertension is treated using the same parameters noted above, although additional antihypertensive agents may be substituted for hydralazine since fetal safety is no longer an issue. Whereas other indicators of disease activity may resolve in the first 24 hours postpartum, hypertension frequently does not. As a result, severe hypertension may need to be treated with an oral antihypertensive regimen for several weeks postpartum.

Seizure prophylaxis or treatment is usually continued for at least 24 hours postpartum, because most eclamptic seizures will have occurred by that time. In the rare patient in whom other aspects of the disease (eg, urine output, blood pressure, subjective symptoms) have not shown significant improvement by 24 hours postpartum, anticonvulsant therapy may be continued for a longer time.

Chronic Hypertension

The treatment of chronic hypertension during pregnancy remains controversial. Pharmacologic treatment of severe hypertension appears to benefit both mother and fetus and may be achieved with any of several drugs. Methyldopa is the drug that has been investigated most thoroughly and prescribed most frequently for this purpose. Beta-blockers and hydralazine have also been used extensively and are therefore acceptable second-line agents. Less experience has been reported for prazosin, nifedipine, and labetolol. The use or continuation of diuretics during pregnancy is discouraged by many, but not all, investigators. Angiotensin-converting enzyme inhibitors (captopril, enalapril, and lisinopril) are generally contraindicated during pregnancy because of fetal and neonatal complications including intrauterine growth retardation, oligohydramnios, and neonatal renal failure. In general, patients may continue their prepregnancy antihypertensive regimens, unless they contain angiotensin-converting enzyme inhibitors, which should be eliminated or replaced with another agent. The benefits of treating mild to moderate chronic hypertension during pregnancy remain unproved.

SUGGESTED READINGS

American College of Obstetricians and Gynecologists: Management of preeclampsia. *ACOG Technical Bulletin* No. 91, February 1986.

National High Blood Pressure Education Program Working Group Report on High Blood Pressure in Pregnancy. *Am J Obstet Gynecol* 1990; **163**:1689.

Roberts JM: Pregnancy-related hypertension. In: *Maternal-Fetal Medicine: Principles and Practice,* 2nd ed. Creasy RK, Resnik R (editors). Saunders, 1989.

Common Infections During Pregnancy | 37

Cheryl K. Walker, MD

Pregnant women may acquire a wide variety of localized and systemic infections. As in all individuals, organism virulence and host immunocompetence are primary determinants of the severity of the process. In addition, the maternal immune system undergoes subtle changes during pregnancy, which frequently alter susceptibility and response to infecting organisms. An added variable is the presence of a second host. The fetus may be exposed to infection from early in gestation through the neonatal period. Because fetal development, including the immune system, is an ongoing process, gestational age and stage of fetal development become important factors in determining the impact of any maternal infection on the fetus. While the incidence of adverse fetal outcome is low in comparison with the incidence of maternal infection, spontaneous abortion, intrauterine fetal demise, developmental anomalies, mental retardation, intrauterine growth retardation, preterm labor and delivery, and neonatal infection do occur.

Interactions between pregnancy and infection are myriad and complex. Some infections are more severe during pregnancy. Varicella can result in life-threatening pneumonia, long-dormant tuberculosis may be reactivated, and human papillomavirus lesions can blossom in unprecedented growth during pregnancy. Severe infections can deplete maternal resources usually available to the fetus, resulting in intrauterine growth retardation. Other infections, including those of the urinary tract, can encourage uterine contractility, thereby raising the incidence of preterm labor and delivery.

Finally, vertical transmission can occur by various pathways. Maternal bacteremia or viremia, as in *Listeria* or cytomegalovirus, respectively, can result in fetal bacteremia or viremia and can cause fetal death or congenital syndromes. Organisms can gain access to the uterus by direct spread, as in the case of gonorrhea, which has been associated with premature rupture of the membranes, intrauterine infection, and preterm labor and delivery. Some infections, such as group B streptococcus and other sexually transmitted diseases, can be acquired perinatally, through contact with vaginal secretions, blood, or breast milk.

This chapter addresses various specific infections. Common ones that present interesting problems during pregnancy are discussed first, including urinary tract infections, group B streptococcal infections, intra-amniotic infections, and hepatitis. Next, organisms that can cause congenital syndromes follow. Previously known as TORCH infections, *t*oxoplasmosis, *o*ther infections (such as varicella, *Listeria,* tuberculosis, and syphilis), *r*ubella, *c*ytomegalovirus, and *h*erpes simplex virus all are dangerous to the developing fetus. Finally, because there is an epidemic of sexually transmitted diseases among young reproductive-aged women, those of particular import during pregnancy (gonorrhea, syphilis, and chlamydia), are discussed.

URINARY TRACT INFECTION

Urinary tract infection is a term that encompasses a range of abnormalities, including asymptomatic bacteriuria, cystitis, and pyelonephritis. These infections are more common during pregnancy for several reasons. First, the enlarging uterus may mechanically obstruct outflow from the ureters and bladder, resulting in dilation of the upper collecting systems. This obstruction also increases bladder capacity and encourages stasis, incomplete emptying, and reflux. Second, elevated levels of progesterone slow ureteral peristalsis, further dilating the upper system. Finally, the composition of urine is often altered during pregnancy. Raised concentrations of bicarbonate elevate the pH level, urinary excretion of estrogens is increased, and women are more prone to glycosuria during pregnancy. These changes foster bacterial growth.

Pathogenesis & Pathology

Although asymptomatic bacteriuria appears to antedate pregnancy and is not more common in gestation, the chances of bacterial ascension to the upper tract and pyelonephritis increase markedly for the reasons noted above. Approximately 6% of pregnant women have this problem, and up to 50% of them have evidence of silent upper tract involvement on renal biopsy. The following markers identify women more likely to have asymptomatic bacteriuria: hemoglobin S trait, diabetes mellitus, increased parity, low socioeconomic status, and lack of prenatal care.

The overall incidence of pyelonephritis in pregnancy is less than 2%. However, 40% of women with untreated asymptomatic bacteriuria develop pyelonephritis. Of women with cystitis or pyelonephritis, an average of 17% have a recurrence during the current pregnancy. In women not taking suppressive antibiotic therapy, 60% develop another infection, whereas only 3% of those on suppression therapy experience a recurrence.

The most commonly seen organisms in all forms of urinary tract infection are as follows: *Escherichia coli* (60–90%), *Proteus mirabilis, Klebsiella pneumoniae,* enterococci, group B streptococcus, and *Staphylococcus saprophyticus.*

Symptoms & Signs

Asymptomatic bacteriuria has no clinical features, by definition. Cystitis is characterized classically by a combination of (1) urinary urgency and frequency with incomplete voiding, and (2) dysuria with or without hematuria, and (3) suprapubic pain. There are no systemic symptoms with a lower tract infection.

Nearly all women with pyelonephritis have signs of systemic involvement, such as fever, chills, nausea and vomiting, and flank pain is present in 85%. Symptoms of lower tract infection are present in 40%. In severe cases, this infection can be complicated by adult respiratory distress syndrome (ARDS) or frank sepsis with shock.

The development of pyelonephritis carries a 20–50% risk of preterm delivery, even with administration of appropriate antibiotics. Several theories exist to explain this disturbing phenomenon. Uterine irritability may be instigated by pyrogens, ureteric contractions, endotoxin release from gram-negative organisms, or prostaglandin release from infected tissues.

Strictly speaking, asymptomatic bacteriuria is defined as 10^5 or more colonies of a single organism per milliliter of urine on 2 consecutive, clean, midstream collections in the absence of signs or symptoms. However, given the high percentage of women with this condition and its rate of progression to clinically apparent infection, screening at the first antenatal visit is recommended as is treatment for any urine culture positive for a single organism. Treatment of those with positive cultures will prevent pyelonephritis in up to 80%.

Diagnosis

The diagnosis of cystitis can be made in someone with lower tract symptoms by obtaining a catheterized or clean-catch midstream urine specimen containing more than 10^5 colonies of a given bacteria per milliliter. Many have suggested loosening these criteria. Some investigators consider a finding of more than 10^2 colonies/mL in a patient with symptoms as indicative of urinary tract infection. The presence of a urinary tract infection involving either the lower or upper tracts is suspect when a woman has symptoms and a urinalysis with white blood cells and bacteria. Only 10% of women with pyelonephritis will have positive blood cultures.

Treatment

The goal of treatment is to create and maintain a sterile urinary tract for the remainder of pregnancy. Because of risk to the pregnancy, treatment of suspected infection must be instituted before culture results are available. Antibiotics that are concentrated and excreted in the urine are preferred because they limit maternal and fetal exposure. Antibiotic choice should be made with local bacterial resistance patterns in mind. Ampicillin-resistant *E coli* are prevalent in certain regions. Reasonable choices for lower tract infection include bactericidal agents such as ampicillin, sulfonamides, or cephalosporins or the bacteristatic agent nitrofurantoin in patients who do not have a glucose-6-phosphate dehydrogenase deficiency. Because sulfa-containing drugs may be associated with the development of hyperbilirubinemia in the newborn, they should be avoided in the third trimester.

The duration of treatment for lower tract infection varies. The traditional recommendation is for 7–21 days, although newer studies have shown similar efficacy with only 1–4 days of therapy. The advantages of shorter treatment regimens are cost effectiveness, less chance of developing bacterial resistance, and improved patient compliance.

Recurrent infection should be retreated based on sensitivities of the etiologic agent. Suppression is then recommended for the remainder of pregnancy until 2 weeks after delivery. The most commonly used agent is nitrofurantoin, 100 mg orally just after the evening meal.

Hospitalization is recommended for all pregnant women with pyelonephritis to facilitate vigorous fluid hydration, intravenous antibiotic administration, and early diagnosis of complications, including adult respiratory distress syndrome and shock. Effective antimicrobial agents include ampicillin, cephalosporins, and aminoglycosides. Antipyretics improve patient comfort and reduce core temperature for the fetus. Eighty five percent of patients improve in 48 hours, and more than 95% have symptom resolution by 4 days of therapy. Persistence of symptoms or clinical deterioration calls for a change in antibiotics and aggressive scrutiny for complications such as abscess formation. Careful monitoring of renal function is advised, because a transient decline in creatinine clearance is noted in 20% of women with gestational pyelonephritis. In these patients, aminoglycosides should be used with great caution.

Women treated for asymptomatic bacteriuria or cystitis should have a repeat culture performed within a month to confirm antimicrobial efficacy and then periodically during the remainder of pregnancy. If infection recurs, suppression is warranted. Similarly, all pregnant women treated for pyelonephritis should undergo suppressive antimicrobial therapy until 2 weeks postpartum.

The long-term implications of asymptomatic bacteriuria during pregnancy are debated. Controversy surrounds the possible association between asymptomatic bacteriuria and both hypertension and chronic renal failure. Approximately 15% of bacteriuric pregnant women will develop chronic pyelonephritis, and 1 in 3000 ultimately will develop renal failure. Periodic postpartum follow-up cultures and treatment may prevent or forestall development of these complications.

GROUP B STREPTOCOCCUS

Group B streptococcus (GBS) frequently colonizes the lower female genital tract, with an asymptomatic carriage rate in pregnancy of 5–30%. This rate depends on maternal age, gravidity, and geographic variation. Vaginal GBS carriage is intermittent, with spontaneous clearing in approximately 30% and recolonization in about 10% of women. The rectum serves as a natural reservoir for this organism. Normally, this organism is a nonpathogenic resident of the vagina, but premature rupture of membranes, intra-amniotic infection, preterm delivery, postpartum endometritis, and vertical transmission may complicate maternal colonization during pregnancy.

Another source for neonatal transmission is through contact with hospital nursery personnel; up to 45% of these health care workers can carry the bacteria on their skin.

Symptoms & Signs

Vaginal GBS colonization is asymptomatic, and the syndrome of postpartum endometritis is discussed in Chapter 44. Briefly, women with postpartum GBS endometritis develop fever, tachycardia, and abdominal distension usually within 24 hours of delivery. Approximately 35% of these women are bacteremic. The incidence of this infection is dramatically increased in women undergoing cesarean section.

There are 2 categories of GBS infection in the neonate. So-called **early-onset** infections appear within 7 days of birth, usually with onset of symptoms in the first 48 hours. The first sign of infection is usually unexplained apnea, and in its early stages, it is often confused with respiratory distress syndrome. The health of infected neonates usually worsens rapidly, even with appropriate antibiotic therapy. **Late-onset** infection occurs, by definition, after the first week of life. It is usually evident as meningitis, although a wide spectrum of infection has been reported, including cellulitis, septic arthritis, and osteomyelitis. Late-onset disease is usually less serious than early-onset disease, although deaths do occur and major sequelae are not rare.

Perinatal Effects

Adverse perinatal outcomes associated with GBS colonization include urinary tract infection, intrauterine infection, premature rupture of membranes, preterm delivery, and postpartum endometritis. The comparatively low incidence of these complications does not warrant treatment of the many asymptomatic GBS carriers; treatment is reserved for carriers who develop these complications.

GBS is a common cause of neonatal sepsis. Transmission rates are high, yet the rate of neonatal sepsis is surprisingly low at less than 4 in 1000 live births. Unfortunately, the mortality rate for early-onset disease can be as high as 50% in premature infants and approaches 25% even in those at term. Moreover, these infections can contribute markedly to chronic morbidity, including mental retardation and neurologic disabilities.

Laboratory Findings

Because of the intermittent nature of vaginal GBS colonization, cultures taken during gestation may not be reliable for identifying GBS-carriers at delivery. Obtaining a culture specimen during labor is difficult in that results may not be available for 24–48 hours, often long after delivery and too late to prevent vertical transmission.

There are 2 major options using cervical culture for identification of colonized women. One advocates universal screening at

26–28 weeks of gestation, and treatment of GBS-positive women who present in high-risk situations, such as preterm labor, prolonged membrane rupture, or intrapartum fever. Unfortunately, this approach misses the nearly 1 in 10 women who test negative initially but become colonized later in the third trimester, as well as those without prenatal care.

A selective approach to screening and treatment has also been proposed. In this scheme, culture specimens are obtained from pregnant women who present with preterm labor or preterm premature rupture of membranes, and the women are treated until culture results are available. However, depending on prematurity rates, this approach still exposes as many as 7.5% of pregnant women to unnecessary antibiotic treatment.

Various rapid tests using coagglutination and enzyme-linked immunosorbent assay (ELISA) have recently been advocated for rapid detection of GBS in an intrapartum setting. These tests are appealing in that they address problems posed by both universal and selective culturing schemes: they obviate the need for universal screening and restrict treatment of high-risk patients to selective screening protocols. Unfortunately, the sensitivity of these products appears to be inadequate to identify a significant proportion of the population at risk for vertical transmission.

Treatment

If universal screening is available, treatment should be reserved for colonized women who present with preterm labor, preterm membrane rupture, and membrane rupture at term. Alternatively, cultures should be obtained for a woman whose colonization status is unknown who is at high risk for vertical transmission, and appropriate treatment should follow. Therapy consists of intravenous ampicillin, a regimen which has been shown to cross the placenta, with therapeutic levels achieved in the fetus within 30 minutes. When delivery is not imminent, oral ampicillin, 500 mg every 6 hours, may be substituted.

INTRA-AMNIOTIC INFECTION

The term intra-amniotic infection (IAI), alternatively known as **intrauterine infection** and **clinical amnionitis**, refers to a clinical syndrome produced by infection of the uterine contents, which may include the membranes, placenta, amniotic fluid, and fetus.

Both chorioamnionitis and amnionitis are histologic diagnoses that require the presence of polymorphonuclear leukocytes and plasma cells in the membranes and placental tissues. It is estimated that this syndrome complicates the delivery of 1–10% of obstetrical patients, depending on the population studied. The primary acquisition route for intra-amniotic infection is ascending bacterial spread through the cervix. However, hematogenous spread has been documented in listeriosis, and iatrogenic intra-amniotic infection may develop in approximately 1% of women undergoing amniocentesis. A recent large-scale study has disproven the former suspicion that coitus is related to the development of this infection. The following factors do appear to be related: duration of labor, presence of membrane rupture, duration of membrane rupture, duration of internal fetal monitor placement, and the number of vaginal examinations.

Pathology

A variety of bacteria have been recovered from amniotic fluid and membrane cultures of infected women, leading most experts to consider this a polymicrobial process similar to other pelvic infections. Group B streptococci and *E coli,* along with a variety of anaerobes, are the most commonly isolated pathogens. The frequent detection of *Gardnerella vaginalis, Mycoplasma hominis,* and a variety of anaerobes has prompted the hypothesis that bacterial vaginosis and intra-amniotic infection may be associated.

Most patients with intra-amniotic infection present with fever, usually in association with membrane rupture. In addition, 2 of the following signs are required to make the diagnosis: maternal or fetal tachycardia, foul-smelling amniotic fluid, uterine tenderness, or maternal leukocytosis.

Pregnant women who develop the infection have a 2- to 3-fold increase in the incidence of cesarean section. Although the precise mechanisms governing this association are unclear, abnormal uterine activity and slower cervical dilation have been documented in the presence of intra-amniotic infection. As well, uterine atony is more common in these women. Vertical transmission of the infection is particularly dangerous in infants of low birth weight. Adverse outcome, in the form of increased rates of neonatal death, respiratory distress syndrome, intraventricular hemorrhage, and sepsis have been associated with this infection. Long-term mental and physical developmental deficits, perhaps the result of such complications, also have been ascribed to infants born of pregnancies complicated by intra-amniotic infection.

Diagnosis

Several laboratory abnormalities are under investigation for their use in early diagnosis of this infection. An elevated serum leukocyte count with a shift toward immature forms is frequently seen. The presence of bacteria on Gram stain of uncentrifuged amniotic fluid, obtained in a sterile manner by amniocentesis, is indicative of infection. Although leukocytes may be present in the amniotic fluid of women in normal labor, assays for amniotic fluid leukocyte esterase activity have been shown to be helpful in the early diagnosis of intra-amniotic infection. Similarly, gas-liquid chromatography has high sensitivity and specificity, but its expense and limited availability preclude its routine use. Amniotic fluid glucose screening is being studied extensively at various institutions; a value of less than 15 mg/dL is suggestive of intra-amniotic infection. Histologic evaluation of the amniotic membrane biopsies and placental tissue is useful in making the retrospective diagnosis of chorioamnionitis.

Treatment

Because intra-amniotic infection appears to be polymicrobial in nature, it is treated with broad-spectrum antibiotic regimens. Most treatment trials have used an aminoglycoside for facultative Gram-negative and Gram-positive coverage plus one of the penicillins, since their transplacental and fetal pharmacokinetics have been well-documented. Clindamycin should be added after the umbilical cord is clamped in the event that a cesarean section is performed to provide adequate anaerobic coverage. Many newer agents are being compared to this standard regimen and appear to be efficacious. These agents include synthetic penicillins, third-generation cephalosporins, and the penicillin β-lactamase inhibitors.

The timing of such therapy has been debated more hotly than the choice of regimen. Previously, proponents of intrapartum treatment warned of increased rates of maternal sepsis and morbidity in the event that antibiotic administration was delayed until the postpartum period. They were countered by others who valued the ability to obtain neonatal cultures unmarred by maternal antibiotic use and thus advised postponement of treatment until after delivery. Recent retrospective and prospective studies have provided strong evidence that intrapartum treatment is associated with a significant reduction in neonatal morbidity. Most now advocate prompt diagnosis and immediate treatment of infected patients without regard to the imminence of delivery. Because the endometrium is usually involved in a soft-tissue infection during intra-amniotic infection, it is also recommended that treatment continue postpartum until the patient has been afebrile for 48 hours.

HEPATITIS

Pathogenesis & Pathology

There are a variety of hepatitis infections. Hepatitis A virus (HAV) causes an acute, self-limited hepatitis without chronic sequelae. Non-A, non-B hepatitis, or post-transfusion hepatitis, is often caused by the newly identified hepatitis C virus (HCV). Delta hepatitis is an uncommon infection that requires hepatitis B virus (HBV) for replication and results in a severe, progressive, chronic, active hepatitis.

The most common of these viruses and the one of greatest concern for the obstetrician is HBV, which is the focus of this discussion. The seroprevalence of HBV is approximately 0.1% in the USA and Europe, but up to 25% in Southeast Asia, Africa, and the tropics. Acquisition risks include geography, drug use, low socioeconomic status, and working in the health care field. There are an estimated 1 million asymptomatic HBV carriers in the USA and 150 million worldwide. HBV may be transmitted vertically, sexually, or through intimate contact with blood or bodily secretions. The virus has been identified in semen, vaginal secretions, urine, feces, and saliva.

In the USA, 70% of reproductive-aged women are susceptible. Approximately 0.2% of these women develop overt HBV infection, while another 0.1% become chronic carriers. Of pregnant women who contract HBV infection in the third trimester or within a month of delivery, 90% will vertically transmit the infection to their infants.

Symptoms & Signs

The typical course of viral hepatitis begins with several days of prodrome, characterized by malaise, fatigue, headache, myalgias, and nausea, quickly followed by the development of jaundice. Jaundice persists for up to several weeks and then slowly subsides, along with the other systemic symptoms. Other symptoms include anorexia, right upper quadrant abdominal pain, low-grade fever, pruritis, loss of taste, and arthralgias. Hepatomegaly is common early in the icteric phase, and splenomegaly may be found in up to 20% of individuals. Fulminant hepatitis occasionally occurs in pregnant women, but no more often than in nonpregnant women.

The incidence of pregnancy wastage may be elevated during acute first-trimester infection, whereas later onset of infection may be associated with preterm delivery. No congenital syndrome has been described.

Vertical transmission typically results in asymptomatic neonatal carriage. Although only 10% of infants will become icteric at 3-4 months of life, 90% will be HBsAg positive by 6 months. These infants are at increased risk for the development of chronic active hepatitis and cirrhosis.

A confusing variety of antigens and antibodies are formed during HBV infection. HBsAg is produced in the liver and circulates in the blood stream. It appears at 30-50 days after exposure and 1-3 weeks before the onset of jaundice. Although it usually disappears during the icteric phase, it becomes chronic in about 1% of infections. HBcAg is released from infected liver cells but does not enter the circulation. HBeAg is related to HBcAg but can be detected in serum. It is present early in infection and persists for a variable length of time. Presence of the HBeAg usually identifies an infectious individual and a woman at markedly increased risk for vertical transmission.

Treatment

Exposure during pregnancy should be aggressively managed. Hepatitis B immune globulin (HBIG) (0.06 mL/kg of body weight) should be given in 2 doses, the first within 7 days of contact and the second 30 days later. If HBIG is not available, immune specific globulin (ISG) (0.12 mL/kg) should be immediately administered and repeated in a month. HBIG (0.5 mL) should be administered to neonates born to women who are HBsAg or HBeAg positive. It should be given as soon as possible within the first 12 hours of life and repeated at 3 and 6 months. If HBIG is not available, ISG should be substituted immediately and at 1 month of age. Hepatitis B vaccine (Heptavax, 10 μg, or Recombivax, 5 μg) should be administered by 7 days of age and again at 3 and 6 months. The vaccine and HBIG may be administered together without diminution of the effect of either.

TOXOPLASMOSIS

This infection is caused by the feline parasite, *Toxoplasma gondii*. Its principal modes of transmission are contact with housecat feces or ingestion of undercooked mutton or lamb. Prevalence rates in reproductive-aged women vary geographically, with higher rates in Western Europe and lower rates in the USA. More than half of women of childbearing age in the USA have already been exposed and carry lifelong immunity. The vertical transmission rate with primary maternal infection is more than 30%, and eventually 1 in 3 infected neonates becomes symptomatic.

Symptoms & Signs

Most adult toxoplasmosis infections are asymptomatic, although some infected patients experience malaise, fever, myalgias, lymphadenopathy, headache, and skin rash. It is difficult to distinguish toxoplasmosis from a number of viral infections, including cytomegalovirus.

Though vertical transmission rates increase with gestational length, severity of infection is worst during organogenesis. The resulting congenital syndrome may include chorioretinitis, hydrocephaly, microcephaly, and various neurological abnormalities.

Diagnosis

Antigen and antibody detection tests, including the ELISA, indirect fluorescent antibody, indirect hemagglutination, and complement fixation tests, are most commonly used to confirm the presence of maternal infection.

Once the diagnosis has been ascertained in a pregnant woman, it is possible to determine whether the fetus has been infected by testing amniotic fluid or cord blood, obtained by cordocentesis or at the time of delivery. Because maternal immunoglobulin M (IgM) does not normally cross the placenta, the presence of IgM antibodies on IgM fluorescent antibody testing or double-sandwich IgM ELISA is evidence of fetal infection. The best results have been obtained with cordocentesis performed between 20 and 26 weeks. Serial ultrasonographic examinations performed after documentation of fetal infection may confirm the development of the congenital syndrome by discerning abnormalities in the size of the lateral ventricles, the thickness of the placenta, or the presence of ascites, hepatosplenomegaly, or cerebral calcifications.

Outside of the USA in areas with high rates of toxoplasmosis, infected pregnant women are treated with spiramycin. This drug is reported to reduce the frequency of vertical transmission by more than 50%.

VARICELLA

Commonly known as chicken pox, varicella-zoster virus (VZV) has a fairly benign course when incurred during childhood but may result in serious illness in adults, particularly during pregnancy. Infection results in lifelong protective immunity. Approximately 95% of women born in the USA have VZV antibodies by the time they reach reproductive age. The incidence of VZV infection during pregnancy has been reported as up to 7 per 10,000 pregnancies.

Pathogenesis & Pathology

The incubation period for this infection is 10–20 days. A primary infection follows and is characterized typically by a flu-like syndrome with malaise, fever, and development of a pruritic, maculo-papular rash on the trunk, which becomes vesicular and then crusts. Pregnant women are prone to the development of VZV pneumonia, often a fulminant infection sometimes requiring respiratory support. After primary infection, the virus becomes latent, ascending to dorsal root ganglia. Subsequent reactivation can occur as zoster, often under circumstances of immunocompromise, although this is rare during pregnancy.

Two types of fetal infection have been documented. The first is congenital VZV syndrome, which typically occurs in 5% of fetuses exposed to primary VZV infection during the first trimester. Anomalies include limb and digit abnormalities, microphthalmos and microcephaly.

Infection during the latter two trimesters is less threatening. Maternal immunoglobulin G (IgG) crosses the placenta, protecting the fetus. The only infants at risk for severe infection are those born after maternal viremia but before development of maternal protective antibody. Maternal infection manifesting 5 days before or after delivery is the time period arbitrarily determined to be most hazardous for transmission to the fetus.

Diagnosis

Diagnosis is commonly made on clinical grounds. Although viral isolation techniques are excellent, laboratory verification of recent infection is made most often by antibody detection techniques, including ELISA, fluorescent antibody, and hemagglutination inhibition. Serum obtained by cordocentesis may be tested for VZV IgM to document fetal infection.

Treatment

There is no drug known to eradicate VZV. Varicella zoster immune globulin (VZIG) has been shown to prevent or modify the symptoms of infection in some women. Treatment success depends on identification of susceptible women at or just following exposure. Women with a questionable or negative history for chicken pox should be checked for antibody, since the overwhelming majority will have been exposed previously. If the antibody is negative, VZIG should be given within 96 hours. There is no known adverse effect of VZIG administration during pregnancy. Infants born within 5 days of onset of maternal infection should also receive VZIG (125 units).

Once identified, infected pregnant women should be closely observed and hospitalized at the earliest signs of pulmonary involvement. Intravenous acyclovir is recommended in the treatment of VZV pneumonia.

LISTERIOSIS

Listeria monocytogenes is a motile, gram-positive rod known to infect susceptible human hosts, including pregnant women, neonates, the elderly, and chronically ill or hemodialized patients. Seasonal variation has been noted, with most epidemics occurring in the late spring and summer months. Reservoirs of the infection include humans and a variety of animals. Human infection typically follows from ingestion of contaminated food, including cabbage, vegetables, and poorly pasteurized dairy products. Vertical transmission may occur either transplacentally or by ascension from the lower genital tract.

Symptoms & Signs

Most infected pregnant women are asymptomatic, with throat or gastrointestinal colonization. Some develop a nonspecific flu-like syndrome, characterized by malaise, fever, chills, myalgias, and headache, with or without gastrointestinal symptoms.

Placental and transplacental infection is common. Infection in the first 5 months of pregnancy may result in spontaneous abortion, while later it typically culminates in intrauterine infection in the setting of intact membranes, often well before term. Interestingly, in 70% of these pregnancies, the amniotic fluid is meconium-stained, even before 32 weeks of gestation. There is a high incidence of preterm labor and delivery with listeriosis, usually occurring within 2 weeks of symptom onset.

There is no recognized congenital syndrome. Early onset neonatal infection is characterized by respiratory distress, sometimes leading to heart failure. Sixty percent of these neonates are preterm, and the mortality has been estimated at 30%. Interestingly, only 45% of the mothers of infected infants report a history of symptomatic infection. For those who survive acute infection, long-term prognosis is excellent in the absence of meningitis. Meningitis is the clinical presentation of more than 95% of neonates with late onset infection. This syndrome has been less well studied.

Diagnosis

Diagnosis is made on clinical grounds with the aid of laboratory tests. The diagnosis should be considered in women with intrauterine infection before membrane rupture or with meconium-stained amniotic fluid in a preterm gestation. Amniotic fluid and cervical secretions may both be examined for presence of gram-positive rods. Bacteria may also be cultured from blood, amniotic fluid, and feces. Several rapid tests, including agglutination, complement fixation, and ELISA, have shown promise, but are still under investigation.

Treatment

L monocytogenes is sensitive to a variety of antibiotics, including penicillin, ampicillin, erythromycin, tetracycline, and trimethoprim-sulfamethoxazole. The pharmacokinetics of ampicillin have been studied well, with effective fetal levels reached within 30 minutes of maternal intravenous administration. For this reason, it is favored as a first-line agent. It should be given intravenously if intrauterine infection is present and orally in its absence. In women with allergy to penicillin, erythromycin may be therapeutic. Resistance to most of the cephalosporins has been demonstrated.

TUBERCULOSIS

Primary tuberculosis is a rare infection in the industrialized world, but important given the high susceptibility of the fetus and neonate. Infection is caused by *Mycobacterium tuberculosis,* an obligate aerobe. Approximately 7 million cases are identified annually throughout the world, but the prevalence rate in the USA is very low at less than 10 per 100,000 people. Nonetheless, this rate is rising, due in large part to outbreaks among HIV-infected individuals, the urban poor, and the many immigrants from endemic areas of the world. Among nonwhites including Hispanics, over 40% of tuberculosis cases occur in people less than 35 years of age. Women in their reproductive years and children are particularly susceptible.

Definitions

Two forms of maternal tuberculosis are of concern during pregnancy. The first is reactivation of **pulmonary tuberculosis,** often denoted by cavitation on chest radiograph. The second is **primary tuberculosis,** which is usually accompanied by systemic spread and may result in congenital infection.

Symptoms & Signs

The range of clinical symptomatology resulting from tuberculosis infection is enormous. Involvement of every organ system in the body has been documented. Pulmonary symptoms are by far the most common finding. Early infections are usually asymptomatic, and the diagnosis is most often made on the basis of an abnormal radiograph. Once infection progresses beyond its latent phase, systemic manifestations may arise, including lassitude, anorexia, weight loss, chills, and night sweats. Increased production of secretions and bronchial irritation may combine to cause a productive cough. Such coughing is usually minor, and the sputum produced is mucopurulent and nonspecific. Minimal amounts of hemoptysis typically represent advanced disease. Another late symptom is chest pain, which is caused by extrapulmonary extension of the inflammatory process to the parietal pleura. A large body of older literature describes enhanced progression of infection during and after pregnancy. With the advent of modern antimicrobial therapy, this problem appears to have been obviated.

Transplacental spread of tuberculosis is rare, although the possibility exists for fetal infection through ingestion of infected amniotic fluid. Infected neonates are usually born to women whose antenatal course has been complicated by primary infection with pleural effusion, miliary tuberculosis, or tuberculous meningitis.

Diagnosis

Information about prior exposure to tuberculosis, previous purified protein derivative (PPD) test results, and current respiratory symptoms should be sought in all women at the first antenatal visit. Screening should reflect the population being served. It should be universal in hospitals serving communities with a large proportion of immigrants from the developing world. In selective screening protocols, women from high-risk ethnic and racial groups (Asian or Pacific Islanders and Hispanics) should be tested, as should health care workers.

The most frequently used test is the Mantoux, a subdermal injection of purified protein derivative applied to the forearm and re-examined in 48 to 72 hours. A positive reaction is one in which erythema and induration has developed, measuring at least 10 mm in diameter. A control should be placed on the other arm to detect anergy.

In women with a positive Mantoux, a chest radiograph should be obtained to detect active pulmonary disease. Even with a negative chest x-ray, a woman may have extrapulmonary active disease.

Treatment

Various treatment options exist. Ethambutol and isoniazid have been well studied in pregnancy and appear safe. Streptomycin carries a 15% risk of eighth nerve damage to the fetus and is contraindicated. Rifampin administration in the first trimester has been associated with variable fetal manifestations and should be used only after organogenesis is complete. Likewise, there is limited first-trimester experience with pyrazinamide, although it is probably safe after 14 weeks. Ethionamide is probably teratogenic and should not be used.

Controversy exists regarding women with a positive Mantoux and normal chest x-ray. Most authorities believe that these women should be carefully followed during pregnancy and given a 6-month course of isoniazid postpartum, although some advocate institution of isoniazid therapy immediately. Under these circumstances, there is no need to isolate the neonate from its mother.

Women with primary tuberculosis or reactivation of old disease must be treated immediately, ideally with a combination of isoniazid and ethambutol. After 14 weeks of gestation, either rifampin or pyrazinamide should be added, and triple-agent therapy continued to complete a 9-month course. Many authorities believe that ethambutol may be dropped after 2 months of therapy. An alternative regimen includes isoniazid and ethambutol for 18 months.

Infants should receive antibiotic treatment to prevent infection in the neonatal period. If the maternal organism has been shown to be sensitive to isoniazid, this drug and isoniazid-resistant bacille Calmette-Guérin (BCG) vaccine should be administered to the neonate; if not, the mother should be considered infectious, and the baby should be isolated until maternal status can be clarified.

PARVOVIRUS

Human parvovirus B19 has been linked with the clinical syndrome called erythema infectiosum ("fifth disease"). It is a typical viral exanthem that commonly occurs in childhood. Approximately 50–60% of women display serologic evidence of previous infection by the time they reach reproductive age. High-risk groups for exposure include school and day-care personnel. This virus has only recently been studied in pregnancy, and most of the information currently available is inconclusive

Symptoms & Signs

Exposure is followed by viremia, after which a 17- to 18-day period of latency ensues. Then a mild viral syndrome with an erythematous rash and arthralgias develops. Many infections are asymptomatic or subclinical. Nevertheless, parvovirus has been known to precipitate aplastic anemia in individuals with hemoglobinopathies and pyruvate kinase deficiency.

The most controversial area of investigation is the fetal effects of maternal infection. Transplacental spread of infection is well accepted, but no congenital syndrome has been noted. Numerous case reports and small observational studies report an increase in spontaneous abortion and fetal death with infections that occur early in gestation. Other studies note a rise in hydrops and subsequent fetal death with later infection.

Diagnosis

The only conclusive methods for diagnosis of maternal infection are detection of IgM antibodies or a 4-fold rise in IgG titers. Cordocentesis has been advocated to document fetal infection. Some authorities favor testing of fetal blood for virus-specific IgM, although others find identification of the virus itself through DNA hybridization or electron microscopy to be more sensitive. There is an association with elevated maternal serum alpha-fetoprotein and impending fetal death from nonimmune hydrops secondary to infection. The interval between maternal infection and fetal death ranges from 1 to 16 weeks.

Treatment

No medical treatment exists for this infection. After maternal infection has been documented, many experts recommend serial ultrasonography to document the emergence of fetal ascites as a noninvasive screening test for the development of hydrops. Once this has been demonstrated, cordocentesis and fetal transfusion for a hemoglobin deficit of 7 g/dL or more can be performed to avert fetal death.

RUBELLA

Commonly known as German measles, this mild viral illness usually strikes during childhood. Once a person is infected, immunity is lifelong. More than 85% of women born in the USA have been infected or vaccinated by the time they reach reproductive age. The infection is spread by exposure to aerosolized nasopharyngeal secretions and direct contact. The last rubella epidemic occurred in 1964. Five years later, in 1969, the first protective vaccine was developed and widely distributed.

There was a steady decrease in reported cases of congenital rubella from the late 1960s until 1984. Since 1984 there has been a sharp rise, particularly in inner-city urban areas. Fetuses of women who contract rubella in the first trimester have a 20% risk of congenital rubella syndrome, with a 50% risk during the first month falling steadily to a 10% risk by the third month. Infection of the fetus during organogenesis may result either in death of the fetus or in the anomalies of the congenital syndrome, including cataracts, patent ductus arteriosis, deafness, microcephaly, and mental retardation. As well, there is an increase in the incidence of juvenile diabetes mellitis.

Symptoms & Signs

The latent period lasts 7–10 days and is followed by a 7-day period of viral shedding into the bloodstream and pharynx. The majority of rubella infections are subclinical, and in the remainder a mild viral syndrome occurs. The acute phase of this infection is characterized by malaise, fever, headache, conjunctivitis, arthralgias, a transient rash, and lymphadenopathy in the posterior auricular or suboccipital regions. The rash is erythematous and macular, appearing on the face 16–18 days after exposure and rapidly spreading over the rest of the body, sparing the palms and soles, and disappearing within a few days.

Diagnosis

Diagnosis based on clinical grounds alone is imprecise because of the close resemblance of this infection to other viral syndromes. Ideally, confirmation of infection should be sought through detection of a 4-fold rise in serum IgG titers obtained from acute (first week of infection) and convalescent (2 weeks later) samples. If the initial sample is high (> 1:256), documentation of acute infection can be confirmed with an elevated complement fixation test or rubella-specific IgM titer.

IgG levels can be ascertained by several methods, the most common of which are ELISA and hemagglutination inhibition (HI) antibody. Evidence of immunity is fairly certain with ELISA values of more than 1, and HI antibody ratio of more than 1:8.

Treatment

There is no treatment for this infection. The Centers for Disease Control (CDC) suggests administration of immunoglobulin to susceptible, exposed pregnant women might be useful, although its role in modifying maternal infection or preventing vertical transmission remains unclear.

A vaccine has been available since 1969. In 1979 a more effective, live-attenuated variation was developed, which is still in use today. An immune response is mounted in 90–95% of those to whom the vaccine has been administered. Susceptible nonpregnant women may be vaccinated at any time, including the immediate postpartum period. In such individuals, it is recommended that subsequent pregnancy be postponed for a period of 3 months. While its use during pregnancy is not advocated, inadvertent vaccination has not been known to result in congenital rubella syndrome.

CYTOMEGALOVIRUS

Cytomegalovirus (CMV) is a common human DNA infection that can have devastating effects on immunocompromised hosts and developing fetuses. Although CMV infection is widespread among adults, 40% of women of reproductive age lack immunity. Approximately 2% of these women become infected during pregnancy. Risk variables for CMV susceptibility include high socioeconomic status, youth, nulliparity, limited sexual partners, and late first pregnancy. Viral particles have been isolated from nearly every body secretion, including urine, cervical secretions, tears, saliva, and breastmilk. Thus, the infection can be transmitted both sexually and nonsexually. Day-care workers are particularly susceptible to infection.

Symptoms & Signs

Although most infections are subclinical, some patients infected with CMV will present with a flu-like syndrome including malaise, fever, chills, and myalgias. The virus then becomes latent and can become reactivated periodically.

Transmission may occur transplacentally or by direct contact at the time of delivery in women with primary or recurrent infection. The incidence of vertical transmission in women who contract primary CMV infection is 40%. The risk of severe congenital infection is inversely proportional to gestational age, with the greatest danger being transplacental transmission of primary infection before 20 weeks of gestation. The annual incidence of congenital CMV infection in the USA is approximately 10,000 cases. Of these, only 40% are symptomatic at birth; the remaining 60% appear asymptomatic at birth but subsequently develop significant handicaps, including microcephaly, intracranial calcifications, hearing loss, and learning disabilities. The mortality for congenital infection is approximately 30%. Peripartum transmission is less serious for the fetus, except in very low birth weight infants.

Diagnosis

The high proportion of previous exposure in the adult population limits the utility of serologic screening, and viral isolation fails to differentiate primary from recurrent infection or carriage. Antibody detection using hemagglutination, fluorescent antibody, or ELISA is most commonly used to make the diagnosis. A 4-fold rise in IgG demonstrates recent infection, and IgM titers are positive for 2 months following primary infection.

Treatment

Currently, there is no treatment for CMV infection during pregnancy, although a number of agents under investigation for

CMV infections in immunocompromised patients may have eventual applications in perinatal infection.

HERPES SIMPLEX VIRUS

Herpes is a common sexually transmitted infection caused by herpes simplex virus types 1 and 2 (HSV-1 and HSV-2). At least 85% of genital herpetic infections are due to HSV-2. This double-stranded DNA virus infects mucosal surfaces.

In the USA, the incidence of HSV infection rose sharply between 1966 and 1979, with a concomitant rise in the incidence of neonatal herpes infections. Among women of reproductive age, the prevalence of genital herpes has been estimated at up to 4%. Risk markers for herpes are different from those used to describe most women at risk for sexually transmitted pathogens in that this infection tends to occur in older, well educated, married, white individuals.

Course of Infection

HSV has an incubation period of 2–10 days, which is followed by a primary infection characterized by focal vesicle formation and a pronounced cellular immune response. Also common during primary infection are inguinal lymphadenopathy and flu-like symptoms including fever, malaise, nausea, headaches, and myalgias. Symptoms usually persist for about 2 weeks, and viral shedding persists for about 12 days. Approximately 4% of infected patients develop meningitis.

The infection then enters a latent phase, with the virus ascending peripheral sensory nerves and coming to rest in nerve root ganglia. Recurrent exacerbations occur intermittently, stimulated by poorly understood mechanisms. Approximately one-half of infected individuals experience a recurrence within 6 months. Most of these episodes are prefaced by a 1- or 2-day prodrome consisting of localized pruritis, pain, and paresthesias. Systemic manifestations are absent. The episode usually lasts about half as long as the primary outbreak, with only 4–5 days of viral shedding.

Symptoms & Signs

Although maternal HSV infection does not seem to adversely affect pregnancy, the infection may be vertically transmitted. Transplacental spread in primary infection can result in herpetic chorioamnionitis, leading to spontaneous abortion and preterm delivery, intrauterine growth retardation, neonatal infection, and death. Fortunately, transplacental transmission is rare. Symptoms in congenital HSV infection typically appear within 72 hours of birth. There is a characteristic triad of signs: skin vesicles or scarring, eye involvement, including microphthalmia, and central nervous system abnormalities, such as microcephaly and hydranencephaly. Death occurs in approximately one-third of infants, and neurologic sequelae are noted in most survivors.

Perinatal acquisition may ensue from contact with either vaginal secretions or contagious lesions in parents or hospital workers. Infants infected in the intrapartum or postnatal period usually develop symptoms after 4 days of life. Three different variations of this infection exist: skin, eye, and mouth involvement; encephalitis; and disseminated infection encompassing multiple organs. The majority of infants with disseminated infection have encephalitis as well as involvement of the liver and adrenals. Those with cutaneous infection have the best prognosis. It has been difficult to target infants at greatest risk for vertical transmission, because 70% of neonates with severe HSV infection are born to women with asymptomatic infection. Infectivity and the severity of perinatal morbidity both appear to be enhanced during maternal primary infection.

Diagnosis

Culture remains the gold standard for HSV diagnosis, with a sensitivity ranging from 70–90%. Results are available within 7 days, and typical cytopathic effects are evident in 3 days. Other methods exist for diagnosing HSV infection. ELISAs and monoclonal antibody tests compare well with culture in high-prevalence populations, but specificity decreases as HSV prevalence declines. Although intranuclear inclusions and multinucleated giant cells can be found on Papanicolaou smears in HSV-infected individuals, the sensitivity of this method is only about 50%.

Treatment

Although there is no known cure for this virus, acyclovir (Zovirax) has been shown to decrease the severity and duration of symptoms in primary infection. When administered prophylactically, it may reduce the frequency and intensity of recurrences. Since the safety of acyclovir during pregnancy has not been established, it should be reserved for severe primary infection, and suppressive or recurrent episode therapy during pregnancy usually should be avoided.

Weekly maternal vaginal cultures in the third trimester do not predict maternal viral shedding at the time of delivery and have not been shown to reduce the incidence of neonatal infection. Thus, they are no longer indicated. Cesarean section is indicated in the presence of genital lesions, regardless of duration of membrane rupture, in order to prevent perinatal HSV exposure. An infected mother need not be isolated from her infant, although care with good hand-washing should be taken to prevent direct or indirect contact with oral or labial lesions.

GONORRHEA

Neisseria gonorrhoeae, perhaps the oldest sexually transmitted disease known to man, has a variety of local and systemic presentations in women. Genital infection in women can manifest as endocervicitis, bartholinitis, endometritis, and salpingitis, and other sites of local infection include the urethra, anus, pharynx, and conjunctivae. Systemic spread may involve the skin, joints, liver, heart, and central nervous system. Approximately 3 million cases occur annually in the USA, with a reported incidence in pregnancy of up to 7.5%. Transmission occurs both sexually and vertically.

Complications

A wide variety of perinatal complications has been associated with gonococcal infection. There is a higher incidence of postabortal and postpartum endometritis in women with untreated gonococcal cervicitis. Gonorrhea may predispose patients to chronic intra-amniotic infection (IAI), which in turn leads to intrauterine growth retardation, premature rupture of the membranes, and preterm delivery. The incidence of preterm delivery in women with untreated cervical gonorrhea has been reported to be as high as 67%.

The role of intrapartum transmission of gonorrhea in the development of ophthalmia neonatorum has been acknowledged for over a century. Before the development of antibiotics, 10% of newborns were afflicted. After an incubation period of up to 21 days, bilateral purulent conjunctivitis develops and rapidly advances to corneal ulceration, scarring, and blindness.

Symptoms & Signs

More than 80% of pregnant women with gonorrhea may be asymptomatic. When present, the signs and symptoms of gonococcal infection are diverse. The site of inoculation, duration of infection, and degree of spread determine the clinical presentation.

Anogenital infection can produce urinary tract infection symptoms, such as dysuria and increased urinary frequency, increased or mucopurulent vaginal discharge, abnormal menstrual bleeding, or discomfort on defecation. Involvement of the Skene's or Bartholin's glands is usually unilateral. Extension of infection to the upper genital tract is rare during pregnancy.

Diagnosis

Culture of the cervix and any other symptomatic site is the preferred method of gonorrhea detection during pregnancy because Gram stain of infected tissues has poor sensitivity in women. Since the majority of women with gonococcal infection are asymptomatic, cultures should be obtained from all patients at the first prenatal visit and again in the third trimester in those at high risk for infection.

Treatment

Given the incidence in many urban areas of resistant strains of *N gonorrhoeae* and the coexistence of chlamydial infection in up to 50% of patients, infected women should be treated with an antibiotic regimen effective against both pathogens. For pregnant women, the CDC recommends ceftriaxone plus erythromycin. Alternatives to ceftriaxone include spectinomycin, cefuroxime, cefotaxime, and ceftizoxime.

Treatment failure among those treated with ceftriaxone plus erythromycin is extremely rare. Women receiving other treatment regimens should have follow-up cultures performed 1–2 weeks after completion of therapy, and all should be tested for reinfection in 2–3 months. Samples should be obtained from the rectum as well as the cervix since 25% of female treatment failures harbor organisms only in the rectum. As with any other STD, patients with gonorrhea should also be offered screening for HIV infection.

SYPHILIS

There had been a steady decline in the overall incidence of syphilis since 1960, due primarily to the fear of HIV and use of safer sexual practices in the male homosexual community. Unfortunately, since 1987 the incidence of syphilis has risen in the subgroup of inner-city heterosexuals, and this increase has caused a concomitant rise in the incidence of congenital syphilis. Risk markers for maternal infection include (1) less than 30 years of age, (2) nonwhite race, (3) poverty, (4) residence in the inner-city, and (4) inadequate prenatal care.

Course of Infection

Exposure to the causative organism, *Treponema pallidum,* is followed by a mean incubation period of 21 days, with a range of 10–90 days. Spirochetes cause a local infection, which eventually disseminates widely by way of lymphatic drainage. Syphilis may involve nearly every organ system. The degree of clinical expression is inversely proportional to the immune status of the host. Sixty percent of those with a normally functioning immune system remain in the latent phase. However, among patients co-infected with HIV, early syphilis can be devastating.

In **primary syphilis,** a single nontender lesion at the site of exposure marks the end of incubation and the beginning of primary syphilis. In the majority of women, this lesion arises on the vulva, introitus, or cervix. Extragenital sites include the oropharyngeal cavity, breasts, and fingers. The lesion begins as a painless red macule, which becomes a papule, then ulcerates. Ulcers are rounded with a well-defined margin and a rubbery, indurated, weeping base. Without treatment, the ulcers persist for 3–6 weeks. Painless inguinal lymphadenopathy often develops a week after the appearance of the lesion.

In **secondary syphilis,** spirochetes disseminate widely during the next 3–6 weeks, stimulating immune complex deposition. This phase is characterized by nonspecific systemic complaints, such as rash, fever, malaise, sore throat, headache, generalized lymphadenopathy, musculoskeletal pains, and weight loss.

The classic rash involves the trunk and extremities, including the palms and soles. Lesions are round, pink macules measuring less than 1 cm in diameter, which become first dull red and papular, then desquamate. Superficial ulcerations, called mucous patches, appear in the oropharynx in 30% of patients. Less than 10% of patients with secondary syphilis have other organ system involvement, manifested as arthritis, bursitis, osteitis, hepatitis, glomerulonephritis, gastritis, hypersplenism, and iritis.

Symptoms abate with the transition to **latent syphilis,** which by definition lacks signs and symptoms. In the early latent phase (arbitrarily set at < 1 year), contagious mucocutaneous lesions can recur. Although late latent syphilis (> 1 year) cannot be transmitted sexually, perinatal transmission persists. Latency may be life-long or may pass abruptly into **tertiary syphilis** as the result of various stimuli.

One in 3 infected women develops tertiary syphilis in the absence of appropriate treatment. The cardiovascular, central nervous, and musculoskeletal systems can all be involved.

The course of syphilis does not appear to be altered by pregnancy. Conversely, transplacental infection is common and has been associated with congenital infection, intrauterine growth retardation, premature rupture of membranes, and preterm delivery.

Congenital Syphilis

The majority of infants with congenital syphilis are born to mothers with primary or secondary infection. Fetal infection during the first and second trimesters carries significant morbidity, including stillbirth, congenital infection, and neonatal death, whereas third trimester exposure usually results in asymptomatic infection. Congenital syphilis rarely becomes symptomatic until 10–14 days of life. Manifestations are similar to those in many viral infections, with a maculopapular rash that desquamates or becomes vesicular and a copious nasal discharge, commonly referred to as "snuffles." Other symptoms include oropharyngeal mucous patches, lymphadenopathy, hepatosplenomegaly, jaundice, osteochondritis, iritis, and chorioretinitis. Untreated infants develop late congenital syphilis, characterized by Hutchinson's teeth, mulberry molars, deafness, saddle nose, saber shins, mental retardation, hydrocephalus, general paresis, and optic nerve atrophy.

Diagnosis

Darkfield examination of ulcer scrapings or tissue samples is the gold standard in syphilis diagnosis, because it is inexpensive and easy to perform and it provides immediate results. Ulcers should be cleansed thoroughly with saline and scraped firmly to collect serum. While a positive test result is diagnostic, a negative one does not preclude the possibility of infection.

The diagnosis of syphilis can be made indirectly using nontreponemal tests, such as the VDRL or rapid plasma reagin (RPR) test. Both measure anticardiolipin antibody and become positive approximately 2 weeks after development of the initial lesion.

After successful treatment, the VDRL should decrease 4-fold in 3 months and 8-fold in 6 months. In the majority of cases, it should be nonreactive 1 year after therapy for primary infection, and 2 years after treatment for secondary disease.

Treponemal tests include the fluorescent treponemal antibody absorption (FTA-ABS) test and the microhemagglutination assay for *T pallidum* (MHA-TP). They are more sensitive and specific than nontreponemal tests and are used for confirmation of a positive nontreponemal test. They become reactive at about the same time as the primary lesion develops. These tests remain positive for life.

Treatment

Since 1943, penicillin has been available to treat syphilis. There is no known resistance. The goal in therapy is to provide continuous low-level concentrations of penicillin in infected tissues. Penicillin is also used to treat neurosyphilis, despite concern about its penetration of the central nervous system. During pregnancy, penicillin is the only approved therapy; women with a history of penicillin allergy should undergo skin testing to validate the sensitivity, and then proceed with desensitization and penicillin therapy for optimal results.

Treatment may be complicated by the Jarisch-Herxheimer reaction, an acute process apparently provoked by the release of prostaglandins during the initiation of therapy for primary or secondary infection. This reaction may be confused with penicillin allergy. Symptoms, including fever, malaise, headache, musculoskeletal pain, nausea, tachycardia, and exacerbation of skin lesions, develop within 24 hours of receiving the first dose of antibiotic. The reaction is more common in primary disease, but symptoms are more severe in secondary. Supportive care with fluids and antipyretics is the mainstay of treatment. During pregnancy this reaction may provoke preterm labor, and patients should be advised to return to the hospital if such symptoms occur.

Follow-up is particularly important in syphilis, given its chronic course and long asymptomatic periods. Women should undergo physical examination and serological testing at 3 and 6 months. If signs and symptoms persist or if the results of nontreponemal antibody tests do not show a decrease after appropriate therapy, patients should undergo evaluation of their cerebrospinal fluid and be retreated as indicated. Treatment failure is difficult to distinguish from reinfection. As with any other sexually transmitted disease, patients with syphilis also should be offered screening for HIV infection.

CHLAMYDIA

In the USA, chlamydial infection is most frequently manifested as genital tract infections in the adult and inclusion conjunctivitis and pneumonia in the neonate. It has been estimated that up to 40% of sexually active women in the USA have serologic evidence of previous *Chlamydia trachomatis*. The prevalence among pregnant women, depending on the population sampled, varies from 2–37%. Risk markers for chlamydial infection in pregnant women include young age (less than 20 years old), low socioeconomic status, urban dwelling, and late presentation for prenatal care. The majority of women with cervical chlamydial infection are asymptomatic, creating a large reservoir for both horizontal and vertical transmission.

Symptoms & Signs

The incubation period for genital chlamydial infections ranges from 6–14 days. While the majority of infections are asymptomatic, a variety of clinical manifestations have been described in pregnancy. The endocervix is the most commonly infected site. Mucopurulent cervicitis is the signature presentation of symptomatic chlamydial cervicitis. The diagnosis of mucopurulent cervicitis is based on the findings of endocervical friability, erythema, or edema; yellow or green endocervical discharge; and more than 10 white blood cells per high-power field of a cervical smear gram stain. Acute urethral syndrome is another manifestation of chlamydial infection during pregnancy. Women with this disorder complain of dysuria and increased urinary frequency but have sterile urine or low-level bacteriuria. Although *C trachomatis* is occasionally cultured from the urethra, it is more frequently recovered from the endocervix of infected women.

Maternal *C trachomatis* infection has been implicated in the development of spontaneous abortion, fetal death, premature rupture of membranes, preterm delivery, and intrauterine growth retardation, although existing evidence is inconclusive.

In up to 50% of infants of untreated mothers, symptoms of inclusion conjunctivitis develop within 2 weeks of birth. Another 10–20% develop chlamydial pneumonia in the first few months of life. Erythromycin eye prophylaxis is very effective in reducing chlamydial conjunctivitis, but this topical preparation cannot prevent pneumonia.

Diagnosis

The optimal test for *C trachomatis* infection is culture. Use of the cytobrush rather than the conventional swab appears to enhance specimen collection and culture sensitivity. Isolation of this intracellular organism requires a susceptible tissue culture cell line, such as the McCoy cell. The sensitivity of this technique is proportional to laboratory experience, and performance of a second passage may improve organism recovery.

Two immunologic tests recently have become available for *C trachomatis* infection. The first uses fluorescent monoclonal antibody staining of chlamydial elementary bodies (Microtrac), and the other is an ELISA (Chlamydiazyme). Compared with culture, both tests have high sensitivity and specificity (> 90%) when used in high-prevalence populations, although their positive predictive value may decrease in proportion to prevalence of infection.

Treatment

Multiple treatment trials suggest the efficacy of erythromycin base and ethylsuccinate. Amoxicillin, which has been shown in limited trials to reduce vertical transmission, is recommended as an alternative regimen. Erythromycin estolate has been associated with maternal hepatotoxicity and is thus contraindicated during pregnancy.

The association of *C. trachomatis* with adverse perinatal outcome and vertical transmission necessitates diagnostic testing at the first prenatal visit and, for those at high risk for contracting this infection, again during the third trimester. Women with a positive test result should be treated and retested in 3–4 weeks to ensure treatment efficacy. It is important to emphasize the importance of partner screening and treatment, as well as education about safe sexual practices to avoid reinfection. Infected women should be tested for other sexually transmitted infections.

SUGGESTED READINGS

Sweet RL, Gibbs RS: *Infectious Diseases of the Female Genital Tract,* 2nd ed. Williams & Wilkins, 1990.

Holmes KK et al: *Sexually Transmitted Diseases,* 2nd ed. McGraw-Hill, 1990.

Centers for Disease Control: 1989 STD treatment guidelines. *MMWR* 1989; **38(Suppl)**:31.

Multiple Gestation | 38

David N. Marinoff, MD

Multifetal gestation is a high-risk situation with an associated increase in maternal, fetal, and neonatal morbidity and mortality. Although this chapter focuses on twins, the most common form of multiple gestation, the problems encountered with twins also apply to all multifetal gestations, the degree and frequency of complications increasing with fetal number.

The incidence of spontaneous twin gestation in the USA is approximately 1 in 89 births. The rate increases significantly when ovulation is induced: about 1 of every 8 pregnancies arising from the use of clomiphene citrate is a twin gestation, and the reported rate of twinning in pregnancies achieved through the use of gonadotropins ranges from 18–40%. In vitro fertilization carries a twinning rate of approximately 20%, and embryo transfer is also associated with an increased incidence of twinning.

FETAL GROWTH

Twins follow a similar growth pattern as singletons until 30–34 weeks of gestation, at which point they grow less rapidly than singletons. More than 50% of twins weigh less than 2500 g at birth. The average weight of the first twin is 2390 g, and the average weight of the second twin is 2310 g. The mean length of gestation in twin pregnancies is 37 weeks.

MATERNAL PHYSIOLOGY

In addition to the usual maternal physiologic changes of pregnancy that occur with singletons, twinning causes further increases in maternal blood and plasma volume. As a result of the expanded plasma volume, the physiologic anemia of pregnancy is exaggerated in twin gestations. Iron supplementation is often needed. Folate concentration also decreases secondary to expanded plasma volume, and folate supplementation of 1 mg daily is often prescribed, although, even in twin gestations, a diet containing adequate protein content should provide sufficient folate. Women pregnant with twins need 300 kcal/d more than women pregnant with singletons. (Optimal maternal weight gain in twin pregnancies is 15.75–20.25 kg [35–45 lb].) Maternal cardiac output is also increased in twin gestations, and uterine volume expands to a greater degree in twin gestations than in singleton gestations.

ETIOLOGY

Twins can arise either through the fertilization of a single egg by a single sperm with subsequent division (**monozygotic** or "identical" twins) or through the fertilization of two eggs by two sperm (**dizygotic** or "fraternal" twins).

Monozygotic Twins

Monozygotic twins account for 30% of all twins. The rate of monozygosity is relatively constant between populations (3.5–4 per 1000 births) and is not related to age. Monozygotic twinning is unrelated to heredity and is thought to be a chance event. Possible causes are a delay in implantation secondary to poor nutritional status, hypoxia, or other stresses. Monozygotic twins are of the same sex (except for rare instances of XO/XY mosaic).

The fetal membranes are composed of the amnion and the chorion. The timing of division of the zygote determines the number of fetal membranes in monozygotic twins (Figure 38–1) and is summarized below:

(1) 0–3 days = diamniotic, dichorionic. When the fertilized egg divides within 72 hours after ovulation, the cells destined to become amnion and chorion have not yet differentiated; thus, 2 embryos, 2 amnions, and 2 chorions will develop. Each embryo is within its own amnion and chorion. Thirty percent of monozygotic twins are diamniotic-dichorionic.

(2) 4–8 days = diamniotic, monochorionic. By 4–8 days the cells destined to become the chorion have already differentiated, but the amnion has not; thus, 2 embryos in separate amniotic sacs but with a single chorion will develop. Two-thirds of monozygotic twins are diamniotic-monochorionic.

(3) 8–13 days = monoamniotic, monochorionic. The amnion

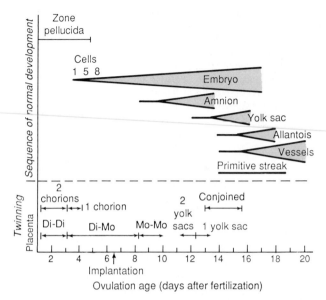

Figure 38-1. The timing of the monozygotic twinning process. The types of placenta expected from embryonic events are: Di-Di, diamniotic-dichorionic; Di-Mo, diamniotic-monochorionic; Mo-Mo, monoamniotic-monochorionic. *(Reproduced, with permission, from Benirschke K:* N Engl J Med *1973:288:1276.)*

is established by 8 days; thus, if division occurs at this stage, there will be 2 embryos within a single amnion and chorion. One to two percent of monozygotic twins are monoamniotic-monochorionic.

(4) More than 13 days = conjoined twins. Division after 13 days of gestation results in conjoined twins. This type of gestation occurs in approximately 1 in 60,000 births.

Dizygotic Twins

Dizygotic twins account for approximately 70% of all twin gestations. Dizygotic twins always are diamniotic, dichorionic. The rate of dizygotic twinning varies between populations secondary to differing incidences of double ovulation among different population groups. Elevated gonadotropin levels result in increased rates of double ovulation. Gonadotropin levels are high in Western Nigerian women, who consequently have very high dizygotic twinning rates (49 per 1000 births). In contrast, Japanese women, with low gonadotropin levels, have a dizygotic twinning rate of 1.3 per 1000 births.

There is also a genetic basis to dizygotic twinning, the incidence reported as 1 in 58 in families with a history of dizygotic twins on the maternal side. The frequency of dizygotic twinning is related to age, increasing up to age 37 and then decreasing. Women with higher parity have higher rates of twinning, as do tall women. Black women have a higher dizygotic twinning rate than white women. Increased rates of twinning have also been reported to occur with conceptions in the first 3 months of marriage (thought to be a consequence of elevated gonadotropin levels associated with frequent sexual relations). Malnutrition can decrease dizygotic twinning rates.

Superfecundation

Fertilization of 2 ova can occur either at the same coitus or at separate episodes within a short time. Fertilization of 2 ova at different times is known as superfecundation. (Cases of women with multiple sexual partners giving birth to twins of different racial composition have occurred as a result of this phenomenon.)

PLACENTA

Dichorionic placentas account for 80% of all placentas in twinning, and monochorionic placentas account for the other 20% (Figure 38–2). Dichorionic placentas arise either from dizygotic or monozygotic twinning, whereas monochorionic placentas always result from monozygotic twinning. Placentas from monozygotic twins may be single, fused double, or 2 separate placentas. There are often vascular anastomoses between monochorionic placentas. The placentas of dizygotic twins may be separate or fused, but vascular communication between the placentas occurs only in extremely rare cases.

The increased competition for space in the uterus leads to an increased incidence of marginal and velamentous cord insertion in twins. The umbilical cords of monoamniotic-monochorionic twins can arise widely separated or near each other; rarely, the cord arises from a single origin then branches to the twin pairs. There is an increased incidence of single umbilical artery in twin gestations.

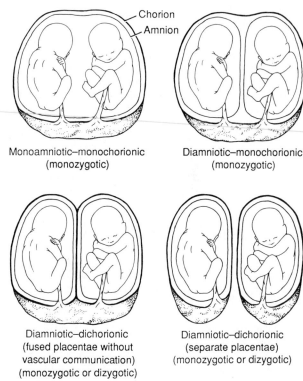

Monoamniotic–monochorionic
(monozygotic)

Diamniotic–monochorionic
(monozygotic)

Diamniotic–dichorionic
(fused placentae without
vascular communication)
(monozygotic or dizygotic)

Diamniotic–dichorionic
(separate placentae)
(monozygotic or dizygotic)

Figure 38-2. Possible configurations of the chorion and amnion during a twin gestation.

DIAGNOSIS

Until recently, one-half of twin gestations were not detected until the time of birth. Now, with ultrasonography available, the vast majority of twin gestations are identified early, enabling patients to receive the close surveillance necessary during their pregnancy.

Other factors that suggest the possibility of twin gestation are as follows: a family history of twins; a pregnancy achieved through ovulation induction; fundal height measurements larger than expected for gestational age; the auscultation of 2 fetal heart beats; or an elevated serum alpha-fetoprotein level, which may be secondary to a twin pregnancy.

Chorionicity can often be diagnosed using ultrasonography in the following ways. First, the membranes are counted. If 3 or 4 membranes are seen on the ultrasonogram, the twins are diamniotic-dichorionic; if 2 membranes are seen, the twins are diamniotic-monochorionic; and if membranes are not visible on repeated ultrasonograms, the twins are probably monoamniotic-monochorionic. Second, if the sex of each twin is different, the twins are diamniotic-dichorionic. Third, if separate placentas are seen, the twins are diamniotic-dichorionic.

MORBIDITY & MORTALITY

Twin gestations are high-risk pregnancies with elevated maternal and perinatal morbidity and mortality. The perinatal mortality rate of twin gestations is 10–15%, about 5 times the rate of singleton gestations. The risk is greatest for the second twin of the pair.

The type of twin is a major determinant of fetal risk. The perinatal mortality rate is 2–3 times higher in monochorionic twins than in dichorionic twins. The mortality rate is highest for monoamniotic-monochorionic twins. These twins account for only 1–2% of monozygotic twins but carry a mortality rate of 50–60%. The high death rate arises from encircling of cords and knotting. In addition, many monoamniotic-monochorionic twins have interfetal placental anastomoses, which can result in twin-twin transfusion syndrome and increased mortality.

The mortality rate for diamniotic-monochorionic twins ranges from 25–50%, secondary to the high frequency of twin-twin transfusion syndrome. The placentas are fused, and usually there are interfetal blood vessel communications. The majority are arterial-arterial or venous-venous anastomoses, which usually do not cause problems, whereas arterio-venous anastomoses can lead to twin-twin transfusion syndrome. A simple method for identifying the type of vascular communication after delivery is to inject milk into an umbilical artery and follow its course across the placenta.

Diamniotic-dichorionic twins have a 9% mortality rate.

COMPLICATIONS

Prematurity

Prematurity is responsible for the majority of fetal and neonatal morbidity and mortality in twin gestations. Approximately 10% of all preterm deliveries are secondary to twin gestation, and these account for 25% of all deaths due to prematurity. Approximately 50% of twins deliver before 37 weeks of gestation.

The risk of maternal pulmonary edema associated with treatment in premature labor with beta mimetics for tocolysis and steroids for promotion of fetal lung maturation is increased in twin gestations.

Twin-Twin Transfusion Syndrome

Twin-twin transfusion is a serious complication seen in monochorionicity. It is caused by arterio-venous shunting and occurs when a placental cotyledon is fed by the artery of one twin and drained by the vein of the other. If this transfer is not accompanied by arterio-arterio or venous-venous anastomoses, then one twin constantly donates blood to the other. The recipient becomes plethoric, hypervolemic, and hypertensive. The donor becomes anemic and hypotensive. Cardiac compensation (hypertrophy) occurs in the recipient. Large differences in size between the fetuses may occur. Polyhydramnios occurs in the recipient as a result of increased volume of fetal urine output secondary to the hypervolemia. The donor often develops oligohydramnios. The syndrome usually begins in the second trimester.

Approximately 5–15% of monochorionic twins have twin-twin transfusion syndrome. Suspicion is increased if ultrasonography shows a single placenta and single chorion, a disparity in fetal size, and polyhydramnios in the larger twin, with or without oligohydramnios in the smaller twin. If oligohydramnios develops in the smaller twin, it is crowded against the uterine wall by the larger twin and its movement greatly decreases ("stuck twin"). Hydrops secondary to congestive heart failure is a terminal sign of twin-twin transfusion syndrome.

Acute polyhydramnios in twin-twin transfusion syndrome is usually first seen at 21–28 weeks of gestation. Conservative treatment of acute polyhydramnios consists of bedrest. However, this therapy is ineffective, with fetal mortality approaching 100%, usually because of prematurity. More aggressive treatment options consist of serial amniocenteses and indomethacin therapy. Unfortunately, serial amniocenteses are often followed by rapid reaccumulation of amniotic fluid. The risk of infection, preterm labor, and abruption increases with serial amniocenteses. Another option is indomethacin therapy, either alone or in combination with serial amniocenteses. Indomethacin, a prostaglandin synthetase inhibitor, decreases fetal renal perfusion, thereby decreasing urine output. The fetal ductus arteriosus must be carefully monitored because of the risk of in-utero closure of the ductus with indomethacin therapy.

Because of the high mortality rate in both twins in twin-twin transfusion syndrome, some authorities advocate selective termination of the donor twin in order to salvage one viable fetus. Alternatively, in-utero obliteration of the anastomotic site through the use of Nd:YAG-laser cauterization has been reported to interrupt and reverse the process of twin-twin transfusion, allowing the survival of both twins.

Acardiac twin, an extremely rare complication of monochorionicity, occurs in 1 of every 48,000 pregnancies. In this condition one twin does not develop a heart, and the normal twin perfuses the acardiac twin through 2 vascular anastomoses, one being arterio-arterio and the other being venous-venous.

Growth Discordancy

Approximately 25% of twin gestations are complicated by intrauterine growth retardation, which can occur in one or both of the twins.

Growth discordancy, most commonly defined as an intertwin difference of >20% in ultrasonographically calculated weights, may be caused by intrauterine growth retardation, twin-twin transfusion syndrome, or genetically determined constitutional differences in the twin pair. (Some clinicians have used a difference of greater than 6 mm in biparietal diameters as a sign of growth discordancy; however, because of the decreased accuracy of biparietal diameter measurements in twins, this difference does not correlate well with growth discordancy. Differences of greater than 20 mm in abdominal circumference appear to correlate much better with growth discordancy.) In general, growth-discordant twins have increased morbidity and mortality, although if both fetuses, even though discordant, are appropriate size for gestational age, their risks are similar to those for concordant twins. The outcome of growth-discordant twins depends on the degree of discordancy, the time of diagnosis and initiation of close antepartum surveillance, and the birth order of the twins. Outcomes are worse if the second twin is smaller. The incidence of congenital anomalies in the smaller twin is elevated.

Possible causes of growth discordancy include site of placental implantation, the anatomic relationship of the uterus and the growing gestation, unequal crowding of the twins, fetomaternal transfusion, single umbilical artery, and abnormal cord insertion.

Determining whether growth discordancy is secondary to intrauterine growth retardation or twin-twin transfusion may be difficult. Seeing 2 placentas or 2 chorions during an ultrasonographic examination excludes the diagnosis of twin-twin transfusion, except in extremely rare cases. Both Doppler studies and cordocentesis have been used with mixed success in attempts to differentiate these 2 disorders.

Death of One Twin

The risk of intrauterine fetal demise in twins is 0.5–6.8%. The prognosis depends on the cause of death of the dead twin, the degree of shared fetal circulation, the gestational age, and the time between the death of the first twin and delivery of the second. A single fetal death is usually well tolerated if it occurs by the early second trimester. The risks to the remaining fetus become much higher if death of one twin occurs later in pregnancy, when as many as 46% of surviving fetuses have been reported to suffer major morbidity or death. A recent report showed an incidence of major morbidity or mortality of 17% in surviving monochorionic twins, whereas no major morbidity or mortality was seen in surviving dichorionic twins.

Early death and absorption of one twin is common; less than 50% of twins diagnosed by ultrasonography in the first trimester will go on to deliver as twins. The **vanishing twin phenomenon,** in which twins are seen on first-trimester ultrasonograms but only a singleton is seen later, carries a good prognosis for the surviving twin.

Fetus papyraceous is usually caused by a single fetal death in the second trimester and generally has a good prognosis. This condition occurs when one twin dies, its tissue fluid is absorbed, and its amniotic fluid disappears. The fetus then becomes compressed and incorporated into the membranes. This condition can occur in both monozygotic and dizygotic twins.

Death of one twin in the third trimester carries the worst prognosis.

Disseminated intravascular coagulation (DIC) in the surviving twin or mother is rare but possible. DIC may occur in up to 25%

of intrauterine fetal demises retained longer than 4 weeks. Tissue thromboplastin from the dead twin invades the circulation of the other twin, activating the extrinsic clotting pathway in the live twin or the mother. DIC must be treated immediately. Maternal DIC with the death of a single fetus is one of the only instances in which treatment of DIC with heparin may be considered.

An increase in structural abnormalities in the surviving monochorionic twin has been reported. This type of abnormality results from embolization of thromboplastic material from the dead twin and can lead to abnormalities in the central nervous system, gastrointestinal tract, and renal system, as well as terminal limb defects, aplasia cutis congenita, and hemifacial microsomia.

Another complication related to shared circulation in twins after one twin dies is relaxation of the vascular bed of the dead fetus. This condition results in the transfusion of blood from the living fetus into the dead fetus with subsequent anemia of the living fetus.

The condition of the surviving twin must be assessed with frequent nonstress tests or biophysical profiles (twice weekly). In addition, serial ultrasonography should be performed every 2–3 weeks, and maternal coagulation studies should be performed weekly. Delivery of the surviving twin should be solely for obstetric indications.

Other Complications

Polyhydramnios occurs in 12% of twin gestations. It is often transient, with onset in the second trimester with subsequent spontaneous resolution. This transient polyhydramnios is usually associated with normal fetuses, whereas nonresolving polyhydramnios is associated with abnormal fetuses.

Most reports show an increased incidence of preterm labor secondary to polyhydramnios, although this has been disputed. Acute polyhydramnios occurs in approximately 2% of twin gestations, usually in monochorionic twins.

The stillbirth rate in twins is 2–3 times that of singletons, and spontaneous abortion is twice as common in twin pregnancies.

Twinning is associated with an increased incidence of fetal malformation, disruption, and deformity, reflected by a rate of congenital anomalies in twins that is twice that of singletons. Monozygotic twins have twice the rate of anomalies as dizygotic twins. The incidence of chromosomal abnormalities is no higher in twins than in singletons.

If one abnormal fetus is identified on genetic amniocentesis, selective termination of this fetus is possible, and, if the abnormal fetus is terminated in the first or early second trimester, the probability that the remaining genetically normal twin will survive is excellent.

Other complications seen with increased frequency in multiple gestation are hyperemesis, anemia, abruption, and placenta previa. The risk of velamentous insertion of the cord and vasa previa is 6–9 times higher in twin pregnancies. Preeclampsia is 3–5 times more common in multiple than in single pregnancies. There is also an increase in malpresentation, cord prolapse, cord entanglement, dysfunctional labor, fetal distress, and surgical intervention. The incidence of uterine atony and postpartum hemorrhage increases with twin gestations as does the incidence of cerebral palsy.

ANTENATAL MANAGEMENT

Once multiple gestation is diagnosed, patients should be counseled regarding their increased risks and the need for frequent surveillance during the pregnancy. The increased nutritional needs of these patients must be addressed early, and it is essential to stress the importance of an adequate social support system for the parents.

Prevention of prematurity and decreasing the associated morbidity and mortality are the most important factors in the management of twin gestations. The critical period for preterm birth prevention is between 26–32 weeks. Various modalities to prevent preterm labor in twins have been advocated. Among them are prophylactic cerclage; prophylactic tocolysis; home uterine monitoring; decreased physical activity; and bedrest, either at home or with hospitalization.

There is no evidence that prophylactic cerclage or prophylactic beta agonists improve outcome in twin pregnancies.

Some studies have shown home uterine monitoring to be of value in preventing preterm labor, although there is disagreement on this issue.

Bedrest appears to be valuable in preventing preterm labor and increasing fetal weights, though this has also been debated. A study in the third trimester comparing hospitalized patients at bedrest to nonhospitalized patients not at bedrest showed the average gestational age at delivery in the hospitalized patients was 37.4 weeks with an average weight at birth of 2581 g. In the nonhospitalized patients, the average gestational age at delivery was 35 weeks, and the average birth weight was 1972 g. The perinatal mortality in the hospitalized group was 54:1000 compared to 217:1000 in the nonhospitalized group.

Bedrest is thought to improve placental blood flow and take pressure off the cervix. If bedrest is to improve outcome it must be initiated at 25–26 weeks of gestation, before the critical period for preterm labor. Bedrest at home, or simply decreasing physical activity significantly by 25–26 weeks, may be just as effective as hospitalization in decreasing preterm labor incidence without the additional cost and inconvenience of hospitalization. In the USA, patients with uncomplicated twin gestations are rarely hospitalized solely for bedrest.

Concordant twins are evaluated for growth with ultrasonography every 3–4 weeks beginning at 26 weeks of gestation and with twice weekly nonstress tests (often accompanied by biophysical profiles) beginning about 34 weeks.

Discordant twins are followed with frequent antenatal testing. Nonstress tests (often accompanied by) biophysical profiles are initiated at the time of diagnosis and repeated twice weekly; serial ultrasonograms are performed every 2–3 weeks. The twins are delivered when fetal lung maturity is documented or sooner, in cases of severe discordancy or fetal distress. (An attempt should be made to perform an amniocentesis on both sacs to determine pulmonary maturity in growth discordant twins. If this is not possible, the sac of the larger twin should be tapped because the smaller twin is more likely to be mature when discordancy is due to intrauterine growth retardation. This relationship may not exist if the difference in size is due solely to constitutional factors.)

Antepartum management of monoamniotic twins consists of intensive monitoring because of the heightened risk of perinatal mortality in these pregnancies. Hospitalization with bedrest with daily nonstress tests or biophysical profiles may be initiated as early as 25–26 weeks of gestation in an effort to detect early evidence of cord accidents in these pregnancies. Serial ultrasonograms are performed every 2–3 weeks. Delivery is usually by cesarean section at the time of pulmonary maturity or evidence of fetal distress.

MANAGEMENT OF LABOR & DELIVERY

The intrapartum period is a time of heightened risk for twin gestations and must be carefully managed. The latent phase of labor in twin gestations tends to be shorter than in single pregnancies, whereas the active phase and second stage of labor are lengthened. Dysfunctional labor patterns are seen with increased frequency in twins.

Both twins must be monitored closely during labor. Initially, separate external fetal heart monitors for each twin are used. When possible, the membranes of the presenting twin are artificially ruptured to allow internal monitoring of this twin. Twin pregnancy is not a contraindication to labor induction. Before the introduction of continuous electronic fetal monitoring, an interval of more than 15 minutes between the delivery of the 2 twins was associated with increased risk of poor outcome. However, with continuous monitoring, there is no absolute limit on the interval between delivery as long as the second twin can be adequately monitored, is tolerating labor, and labor is progressing. (There have been cases in which one twin has been born prematurely and the delivery of the second twin was delayed for weeks with a good outcome.)

All twins should be delivered in secondary or tertiary care hospitals. It is essential that 2 obstetricians, 2 pediatricians, sufficient nursing personnel, and an anesthesiologist are immediately available during labor and are in attendance at the delivery. If vaginal delivery is anticipated, the delivery should take place in a delivery room equipped for immediate cesarean section should complications arise.

PRESENTATION & ROUTE OF DELIVERY

The presentation and weights of the twins are major factors in determining the route of delivery. Previous low transverse cesarean section is not an absolute contraindication to vaginal delivery in twins. The rates of occurrence of the various types of twin presentations are summarized in Table 38–1.

Vertex-Vertex Presentations

Vertex-vertex twins should always be delivered vaginally regardless of weight, except for obstetrical indications. After delivery of the presenting twin, the cord is clamped and the position of the second fetus is determined. It is important to keep the cord of the first twin clamped until after the second twin has been delivered because the second twin can exsanguinate through the unclamped

Table 38-1. Rate of occurrence of various types of twin presentation.

Twin A	Twin B	Rate of Occurrence (%)
Vertex	Vertex	40
Vertex	Breech	26
Breech	Vertex	10
Breech	Breech	10
Vertex	Transverse	8
Other	Other	6

cord of the first if placental anastomoses exist. (The two cords are differentiated for postpartum studies by clamping one cord with a straight clamp and the other with a curved clamp.)

The second twin is closely monitored after delivery of the first, and as soon as possible, amniotomy is performed and a scalp electrode is emplaced. If labor is inadequate, oxytocin augmentation is started. If fetal distress or change in presentation of the second twin is encountered, cesarean section may be performed, or the infant may be delivered with forceps, vacuum, internal podalic version (turning the fetus to breech presentation by intrauterine manipulation and delivering by breech extraction) by an obstetrician experienced in these procedures.

Vertex-Breech Presentations

The route of delivery of vertex-breech twins depends on their estimated weights. If the estimated weight of the breech twin is less than 1500 g, most authors advocate cesarean delivery because of the increased morbidity in a breech fetus weighing less than 1500 g when delivered vaginally. If the estimated weight of the breech twin is greater than 1500 g, vaginal delivery can be attempted as long as there are no other contraindications to vaginal breech delivery. After the first twin is delivered, the second twin can either be delivered breech, or an external version can be attempted; if successful, the second twin can be delivered vertex.

Nonvertex Presenting Twin

Because of the increased risks associated with vaginal delivery of twins when the presenting twin is not vertex, most authors recommend cesarean section.

GESTATIONS OF THREE OR MORE FETUSES

Gestations with 3 or more fetuses are uncommon, although their incidence is increasing in proportion to the increased number of pregnancies achieved through ovulation induction, in vitro fertilization, and embryo transfer. The incidence of spontaneous triplets is 1 in 8100, whereas that of guadruplets 1 in 700,000. The mean gestational age at delivery of triplets is 33–34 weeks and that of guadruplets is 29–30 weeks.

These pregnancies can also be monozygotic, multizygotic, or any combination of these and this is reflected in the placentation.

The complications associated with twin gestation also apply to these multiple gestations and occur with much greater frequency. As with twins, the major complication is prematurity and the incidence of this increases with increasing fetal number.

These pregnancies are managed with frequent antenatal testing and bedrest is usually instituted at 25–26 weeks gestation. With close surveillance the outcome of triplet gestations can approach that of twins.

Most authorities recommend delivery by cesarean section for gestations of three or more fetuses.

Because of the poor prognosis associated with multifetal gestations of four or more, early selective reduction has been employed. With this procedure, fetal number is decreased, usually to two, in an effort to lower the probability of very premature delivery which is common in these pregnancies. Ethical controversies obviously exist over this issue.

SUGGESTED READINGS

Cunningham FG, MacDonald PC, Gant NF: Multifetal pregnancy. Chapter 34 in: *Williams Obstetrics,* 18th ed. Appleton & Lange, 1989.
Porreco RP (guest editor): Twin gestation. *Clin Obstet Gynecol* 1990;**33**:1.

39 | Third-Trimester Bleeding

C. Andrew Combs, MD, PhD

Vaginal bleeding at any time during pregnancy demands prompt and thorough investigation. At prenatal visits, in childbirth preparation classes, and in educational literature, patients are repeatedly warned to report bleeding of any amount or duration. Bleeding before 20 weeks of gestation is usually called **threatened abortion.** Bleeding after 20 weeks is generally called **third-trimester bleeding** even though the third trimester technically begins at 26 weeks of gestation. Third-trimester bleeding complicates about 5–10% of pregnancies.

Several distinct entities can cause third-trimester bleeding, and the significance of bleeding to the mother and the fetus depends on the precise cause. **Placental abruption** (complete or partial separation of the placenta before delivery of the fetus) accounts for about half of the cases, has significant potential for serious maternal complications, and is associated with perinatal mortality rates of 20–50%. **Placenta previa** (implantation of the placenta over the cervical os) is found in one-fourth to one-third of cases of third-trimester bleeding, carries a high risk of maternal hemorrhage, and is associated with perinatal mortality rates of 5–25%. **Vasa previa** (rupture of a fetal vessel that courses over the cervical os) is responsible for only about 1% of cases but often leads to rapid fetal exsanguination, with fetal or neonatal death in about 80% of cases. The remainder of cases are due to extrauterine lesions (cervix, vagina, vulva) and are not generally associated with substantially increased risk of maternal or perinatal death.

Optimal management of third-trimester bleeding involves an orderly sequence of steps to stabilize the mother, to arrive efficiently at an etiologic diagnosis, and to construct a subsequent management plan appropriate for both maternal and fetal wellbeing. As in many emergencies, however, the clinician does not follow the usual sequence of history taking, then physical examination, then laboratory testing. In particular, the clinician should *not* perform a pelvic examination before an ultrasound evaluation to exclude placenta previa because inserting a finger into a placenta previa can precipitate life-threatening hemorrhage.

INITIAL MANAGEMENT & DIAGNOSIS

A patient who reports vaginal bleeding in late pregnancy must be evaluated immediately in the hospital labor and delivery unit.

Assessment of Severity

When the patient arrives, maternal vital signs should be taken immediately, and the perineum and clothing should be quickly inspected to assess the severity of bleeding. Care should be taken to keep the mother in the lateral decubitus position to avoid the **supine hypotension syndrome** that can result from compression of the vena cava by the gravid uterus.

If there is brisk, ongoing bleeding or if there are signs of maternal hypovolemia (pallor, cold-clammy skin, diaphoresis, confusion, tachycardia, hypotension), a large-bore intravenous line should be started without delay and initial volume resuscitation begun with crystalloid solution. Oxygen should be given. At the same time, blood specimens can be sent to the blood bank for type and crossmatch and to the laboratory for determination of hematocrit and for other tests outlined below. Urine output should be monitored hourly, preferably with an indwelling catheter.

Allied personnel should be notified as soon as possible about the condition of the patient. The anesthesiologist and the labor-room nursing staff can be helpful in evaluating and stabilizing the mother. The neonatal staff should be alerted to the possibility of delivery of a compromised infant.

Fortunately, in most cases, the mother does not present with rapid hemorrhage or shock.

As soon as the mother is stable, the fetal heart rate should be recorded, and continuous electronic fetal monitoring can be started. If there are signs of fetal distress, the mother should be repositioned, the vital signs rechecked, and oxygen given. Fetal distress unresponsive to these interventions is frequently an indication for immediate delivery.

Review of Prenatal Record

Gestational age should be determined based on a review of menstrual dating, early examinations, and early sonograms. Any pregnancy complications or medical complications should be noted.

History

The events surrounding the bleeding episode can provide important clues to the cause. Although frequently imprecise, the patient can often give an order-of-magnitude estimate of the volume of bleeding (1 tsp = 5 mL, 1 tbs = 15 mL, 1 cup = 250 mL). Particular attention should be given to the activities immediately preceding the bleeding, especially the presence of pain or uterine contractions. A clear watery discharge may suggest ruptured membranes. The clinician should inquire about the occurrence of any recent trauma (motor vehicle accidents, blows to the abdomen, or falls). Other questions that should be asked specifically include the following: time of most recent coitus, recent drug or tobacco use, and the recent general health of the patient.

Physical Examination

The fundal height should be measured; a significant size-for-date discrepancy may indicate that the uterus is distended by concealed blood. It is important to note the presence of uterine contractions or tenderness. The perineum should be carefully inspected to determine whether there is any vulvar lesion that could explain the bleeding. The presence of hemorrhoids should also be noted, because these may occasionally be the source of bleeding. Of course, a brief but thorough physical examination should be performed to determine the presence of any other complicating condition.

Ultrasound Examination

Of particular importance is the relation of the placenta to the cervical os. If during the ultrasound scan the placenta can be seen to impinge on the os, the diagnosis is placenta previa, and pelvic examination should not be performed. It is important to remember that a fundal location of the placenta does not necessarily exclude the possibility of previa, because the placenta can occasionally have a distant, extra lobe (succenturiate placenta). In placental abruption, experienced sonographers can often demonstrate the presence of concealed blood within the uterus. Any other abnormalities of the placenta should be noted, the fetal position and age should be determined, and a survey of the fetus for anomalies should be performed.

Pelvic Examination

Speculum examination is essential *if there is no evidence of placenta previa* on the sonogram. A sterilized speculum should be gently inserted, and the cervix and vaginal walls should be inspected for any source of bleeding. It is important to note whether any blood within the vaginal vault is fresh, red blood or old, brown blood. Any cervical dilation should be noted. If there is a pool of blood, it can be aspirated into a syringe for later testing to determine whether it is of fetal or maternal origin. If there is a pool of clear fluid or dilute blood, rupture of membranes should be suspected. Cervical cultures should be obtained because cervicitis can result in a friable cervix that bleeds easily. *Trichomonas* and *Chlamydia* are common organisms in this setting. Cervical neoplasia may also produce a friable cervix, and a cytologic smear should also be obtained if there is not an excessive amount of blood. Digital examination of the cervix, to determine dilation, effacement, and station should be performed last.

Laboratory Tests

For third-trimester bleeding, laboratory tests should include, at a minimum, a determination of the hematocrit or hemoglobin. A tube of clotted blood should be sent to the blood bank for type-and-crossmatch or at least type-and-blood-group screening if there is any suspicion that the mother will need a transfusion, if there is a placenta previa, or if it seems likely that she will be delivered in the immediate future.

A coagulation profile may be considered, depending on the diagnosis. As discussed later, severe placental abruption will occasionally be followed by disseminated intravascular coagulation. Coagulopathy is rarely a cause of third-trimester bleeding.

Origin of Blood

Blood from the vaginal vault can be tested to determine whether it is of fetal or maternal origin. The popular Apt test involves mixing the supernatant of lysed, centrifuged blood with 0.25 N NaOH. A yellow-brown color results from the conversion of maternal blood to alkaline globin-hematin; fetal blood remains pink because it is resistant to alkali. In practice, however, this test is often subjective and difficult to interpret. Probably a better method is to simply prepare a standard Wright-stained smear and to examine for the presence of nucleated red cells. These constitute the majority of fetal cells but are rare in the maternal circulation.

However, in practice, the issue of fetal-versus-maternal bleeding relates only to the diagnosis of vasa previa. If there is significant fetal bleeding, there will almost always be accompanying evidence of fetal distress.

Fetomaternal Bleeding

The passage of fetal erythrocytes into the maternal circulation is fairly common with placental abruption and probably also with placenta previa. If fetomaternal bleeding is massive, there will be evidence of fetal distress on the heart rate monitor. The occurrence of fetomaternal bleeding is especially important in the *Rh-negative mother* because the passage of Rh-positive cells can result in isoimmunization, possibly complicating the current pregnancy but especially subsequent pregnancies. In Rh-negative women with third-trimester bleeding, a dose of Rh-immune globulin should be given in an amount adequate for the amount of fetal cells that have passed. The *Kleihauer-Betke acid elution test* can be used to detect and quantify fetal cells in the maternal circulation. One 300-μg ampule of Rh-immune globulin is sufficient coverage for up to 15 mL of fetal cells. For larger volumes of fetomaternal bleeding, the appropriate dose must be calculated.

Provisional Diagnosis

At this point, it is often possible to determine whether the bleeding is due to placenta previa, placental abruption, extrauterine bleeding, or vasa previa. Subsequent management will depend on the precise diagnosis, the gestational age, and the stability of the mother and fetus.

In many cases (up to 50% in some series), no definite cause for bleeding can be identified. Sometimes these cases are called **marginal sinus ruptures** because of a presumption that they represent bleeding from a venous sinus coursing around the margin of the placenta. However, such a sinus can rarely, if ever, be demonstrated on direct examination of the placenta, and the term is probably best abandoned. Most of these cases are probably due to mild degrees of placental abruption and should be managed accordingly, as discussed below.

PLACENTAL ABRUPTION

Other terms for placental abruption are **abruptio placentae** and **accidental hemorrhage.** In the United Kingdom, abruption is called "premature separation of the normally implanted placenta" to emphasize the distinction from placenta previa.

Definition & Spectrum

Abruption is defined as the complete or partial separation of the placenta from its uterine implantation site before the delivery of the fetus. Although abruption is probably always accompanied by some degree of uterine bleeding, in as many as half the cases the blood is retained within the uterus and there is no external bleeding (Figure 39-1). Abruption can range from a mild, self-limited event discovered incidentally when the placenta is examined after a normal delivery to a catastrophic complete separation with immediate fetal death and fatal maternal hemorrhage.

Incidence

Depending on the diagnostic criteria, abruption occurs in 0.5-4% of pregnancies. As mentioned previously, many cases of vaginal bleeding of undetermined cause probably represent mild degrees of placental abruption.

Risk Factors

Several clinical risk factors for abruption have been identified. Abdominal trauma, ranging from a high-speed motor-vehicle accident to a seemingly minor fall, is associated with a high incidence of abruption, but accounts for only a minority of cases. Women with preeclampsia, chronic hypertension, and other vascular disorders have an increased incidence of abruption. Sudden decompression of the uterus from preterm premature rupture of the membranes or from therapeutic amniocentesis for hydramnios is followed by a 2- to 3-fold increased incidence of abruption. Other known or suspected risk factors include poor weight gain, cigarette smoking, cocaine use, diabetes, amnionitis, fetal anomalies, male fetus, and high parity. Women with a history of abruption in a previous pregnancy have a 10-20% risk of abruption in the subsequent pregnancy.

Pathophysiology

It must be remembered that separation of the placenta from the uterus is a normal process that usually occurs after delivery of the fetus. The precise mechanisms involved in this separation, either normally or in abruption, are incompletely understood. Uterine contractions are probably important. Classic severe

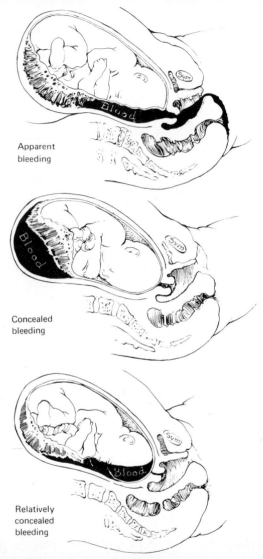

Apparent
bleeding

Concealed
bleeding

Relatively
concealed
bleeding

Figure 39–1. Spectrum of placental abruption. Sym, symphysis.
(Redrawn and reproduced with permission from Beck and Ro-
senthal: Obstetrical Practice, *7th ed. Williams & Wilkins, 1957.)*

abruption is associated with painful, hypertonic contractions, although it is not always clear whether these contractions are the cause of the abruption or a response to it. Uterine contractions may explain abruptions that occur after preterm premature rupture of membranes or sudden decompression with therapeutic amniocentesis.

There is a natural **zone of separation** or **basal plate** in the decidual lining of the endometrium. Poor nutrition or oxygenation may lead to necrosis of the decidua and predispose patients to early placental separation. This mechanism may explain the association of abruption with maternal vascular disease, diabetes, smoking, cocaine use, and poor weight gain.

Whatever the mechanism, when all or part of the maternal surface of the placenta frees itself from the endometrium, the underlying spiral arteries are free to pump maternal blood into the space so created. These vessels will continue to bleed until either contraction of the myometrium occludes them or until intrauterine pressure exceeds spiral arterial pressure. Platelet plugging and blood coagulation are relatively unimportant in stopping the bleeding from the large spiral arteries.

The course of the abruption depends on the location and amount of the initial separation. When the separation is at the placental margin, the episode is typically self-limited. Maternal blood from the spiral arteries dissects along the "path of least resistance" between the fetal membranes and the endometrium and may or may not escape through the cervix.

When the separation is near the center of the placenta, maternal blood must either remain trapped or must dissect more of the placenta away from the uterus. Such abruptions are typically severe and rapidly progress to complete separation of the placenta with resultant fetal death.

The placenta contains a high concentration of thromboplastic substances. Disruption of the normal placental attachments can result in release of these substances into the maternal circulation, resulting in disseminated intravascular coagulation.

Symptoms & Signs

The presentation of placental abruption is extremely variable and depends on the location and the extent of placental separation. In about one-fourth of cases, the diagnosis is not suspected antenatally, but is made as an incidental finding after an otherwise normal delivery.

Vaginal bleeding is the most common symptom and is reported in 50–80% of cases. The bleeding can range in amount from scant spotting to frank hemorrhage.

Uterine contractions are commonly reported. Classically, these are remarkably painful and tumultuous. However, contractions may be mild, rare, or absent. The uterus may be tender to palpation, especially over the region of the placenta. Unremitting low-back pain is occasionally the only presenting symptom, especially with concealed hemorrhage from a posterior placenta.

Maternal hypotension or shock occurs rarely and is usually preceded by significant, obvious blood loss. Anemia is a late finding. Disseminated intravascular coagulation occurs in about one-third of abruptions that are severe enough to kill the fetus and is vanishingly rare in mild abruptions.

Evidence of fetal distress may be found on external monitoring. Signs include baseline tachycardia, prolonged bradycardia, loss of baseline variability, repetitive late decelerations, or severe variable decelerations.

Diagnosis

The diagnosis of abruption can be based on clinical findings, ultrasonographic findings, or pathologic findings.

Clinically, the diagnosis is based on some combination of significant vaginal bleeding without evidence of placenta previa, hypertonic painful uterine contractions, tenderness to uterine palpation, and evidence of fetal distress. There are no universally accepted absolute diagnostic criteria, and the diagnosis depends on the vigilance of the examiner.

Ultrasonic examination may clarify the diagnosis in one-fourth to one-half of the cases. Skilled sonographers can demonstrate a separation of the placental margin or the presence of retained blood within the uterus. There is a spectrum of sonographic findings, just as there is a spectrum of clinical findings. Blood can be trapped between the fetal membranes and uterus (**subchorionic bleeding**), between the placenta and uterus (**retroplacental bleeding**), or, rarely, within the substance of the placenta. Of course, in many cases, the blood may completely escape through the cervix and thus not be demonstrable by sonography at all.

There may be an evolution of sonographic findings over days to weeks. Initially, retained blood appears hyperechoic. As the blood clot organizes, there is a period when it has the same echogenicity as the placenta, and it is thus difficult or impossible to detect. At this stage, the placenta may appear thickened and heterogeneous or may appear normal. Later, the organized clot appears hypoechoic. Over the next several weeks, the clot may be resorbed, leaving only large maternal venous lakes. Ultimately, the sonographic abnormalities disappear altogether. On the other hand, there may be further placental separation over time, with the appearance of fresh blood clots within the uterus.

Pathologic diagnosis is based on gross and microscopic examination of the placenta after delivery. The findings depend on the time elapsed between abruption and delivery of the placenta. If delivery is accomplished within a few minutes of the abruption, the placenta may appear completely normal. If sufficient time has elapsed (minutes to hours), clotted blood may adhere to the maternal surface of the placenta. After several days, the clot begins to organize and then resorb. Findings include pale areas of fibrin deposition and infarction. Even with skilled placental examination, the pathologic diagnosis does not agree with the clinical diagnosis in more than half the cases.

Management

The first goal of management is to prevent shock, organ failure, and death of the mother. Considerations of fetal well-being are secondary if the mother is acutely ill. However, maintenance of adequate maternal blood volume and oxygenation is clearly beneficial to both mother and fetus. Once the mother is stable, attention can be turned toward optimizing the fetal condition. The second goal of management is to prevent perinatal asphyxia and, ultimately, to deliver an infant with the best probability of intact survival.

It is generally agreed that immediate delivery is indicated if any of the following conditions are present: term pregnancy, ongoing brisk bleeding, maternal disseminated intravascular coagulation, or persistent evidence of fetal distress.

It is controversial whether vaginal delivery should be considered or whether all mothers with placental abruption should be delivered by cesarean. Clearly, if there is brisk bleeding or evidence of fetal distress, cesarean section is indicated. However, in most cases, the mother is not in shock, and the fetal heart rate pattern appears normal. In these cases, induction of labor is reasonable if the labor unit is equipped to provide continuous fetal monitoring and immediate cesarean section. It must be remembered that the abruption may extend unexpectedly, with rapid deterioration of the maternal and fetal condition.

In preterm gestations, the decision to deliver the fetus or to attempt to gain more time in utero involves weighing the risks of premature delivery versus the risk that the abruption itself may compromise the fetus. A growing body of evidence shows that the majority of perinatal deaths after placental abruption are due to complications of premature delivery and not to direct complications of the abruption, such as hypoxia or hypovolemia. Thus, in the absence of maternal compromise or fetal distress, it is most reasonable to attempt to delay delivery until fetal maturity is attained.

Amniocentesis should be performed to test for fetal lung maturity. If the fetus is immature, betamethasone or dexamethasone (12 mg intramuscularly in 2 doses 12 hours apart) can reduce the risk of infant respiratory distress syndrome. If the fetus is mature, delivery is indicated.

Tocolysis can be considered if there are persistent uterine contractions. Magnesium sulfate is generally preferred over beta-sympathomimetics (ritodrine, terbutaline) because the latter cause maternal tachycardia and may mask this important sign of unsuspected concealed hemorrhage. The risk that tocolysis will overly relax the uterus and promote further hemorrhage is small compared with the risk that contractions will result in preterm delivery. Further, contractions are an added stress to a fetus already potentially compromised by the abruption itself.

Once the initial episode has abated, the mother should be observed at hospital bedrest until she has been stable for at least a week. Transport to a tertiary center should be considered once the mother is stable.

Fetal surveillance (nonstress test or biophysical profile) should be performed to assess the possibility of fetal hypoxia. Contraction stress testing is contraindicated; uterine contractions can provoke an extension of the abruption. Serial ultrasonograms (every 3–4 weeks) should be performed to evaluate the possibility of intrauterine growth retardation resulting from an inadequately functioning placental surface area.

In the majority of abruptions managed expectantly, delivery occurs within 2 weeks despite the use of tocolysis and hospital bedrest. Most of these early deliveries are due to repeated episodes of bleeding and contractions. Some are due to spontaneous rupture of membranes, and most of the remainder are the result of evidence of fetal distress.

Management of Disseminated Intravascular Coagulation (DIC)

Release of placental thromboplastin into the maternal circulation can initiate DIC, defined as the activation of the clotting cascade within the maternal vasculature. The resulting consumption of platelets and fibrinogen causes a state of impaired coagulation. DIC occurs in about 3% of severe abruptions, but is rare in milder episodes.

Diagnosis is based on laboratory tests of coagulation. The most useful tests are platelet count (less than $100,000/\mu L$), fibrinogen (less than 200 mg/dL), and fibrin degradation products (high-range elevation). These abnormalities will peak about 12 hours after the onset of the abruption and typically resolve spontaneously after delivery.

Patients with abnormal coagulation tests should be observed closely for bleeding from the site of the intravenous line, and gastrointestinal mucosa. Intra-abdominal and intracerebral hemorrhage are possible, but rare.

Therapy depends on the magnitude of the abnormality and the occurrence of bleeding complications.

Treatment of thrombocytopenia is indicated in the following situations: if the platelet count falls below $50,000/\mu L$; if there are bleeding complications; or if surgery is contemplated. Transfusion of a 6-unit pack of random-donor platelets should raise the platelet count by about $30,000/\mu L$. However, continued DIC can consume the transfused platelets, so counts should be checked 1 hour and 6 hours after transfusion.

Treatment of hypofibrinogenemia is indicated only if there are bleeding complications. Either cryoprecipitate (rich in fibrinogen and factor VIII; 1–2 units/10 kg of body weight) or fresh-frozen plasma (10–20 mL/kg of body weight) may be given.

Uteroplacental Apoplexy (Couvelaire Uterus)

Extravasation of blood into the myometrium results in a mottled, ecchymotic appearance of the uterine surface. This complication is found occasionally at cesarean section after severe abruptions. After delivery of the placenta, the uterus may be flaccid and dysfunctional, resulting in postpartum hemorrhage. In most cases, the hemorrhage will respond to oxytocic stimulation and surgical hemostasis; hysterectomy is rarely required.

PLACENTA PREVIA

Placenta previa is defined as implantation of the placenta over the internal cervical os. Three types are recognized, depending on the amount of overlap of the placenta and the os (Figure 39–2). **Complete previa (central previa** or **total previa,** 25% of cases) occurs when the os is completely covered by placenta; **partial previa** (25% of cases), when the os is partially covered by placenta; and **marginal previa** (50% of cases), when the edge of the placenta just touches the internal os. **Low-lying placenta** (Figure 39–3) is diagnosed when the placenta does not touch the internal os, but the examiner can palpate the placental margin with a finger inserted

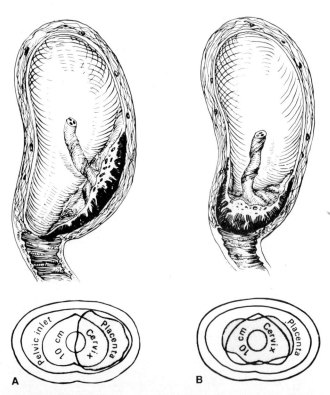

Figure 39–2. Placenta previa. **A:** partial. **B:** complete. *(Reproduced, with permission, from Benson RC: Handbook of Obstetrics & Gynecology, 8th ed. Lange, 1983.)*

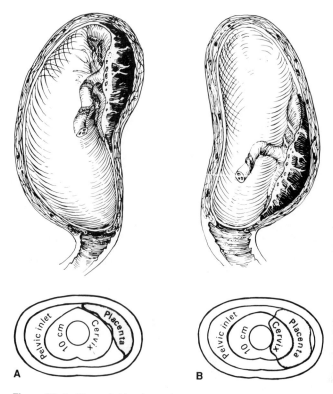

Figure 39-3. Placental implantation. **A:** normal placenta. **B:** low implantation. *(Reproduced, with permission, from Benson RC: Handbook of Obstetrics & Gynecology, 8th ed. Lange, 1983.)*

through the cervix. This condition is probably unimportant as a cause of either bleeding or preterm delivery.

Incidence

Ultrasonography at about 16 weeks of gestation will show placenta previa in up to 15% of pregnancies. Most of these are marginal previas and will resolve spontaneously into low-lying placentas as the uterus enlarges. The incidence of placenta previa in the third trimester is about 0.5–1%.

Etiology

It is not known precisely what mechanisms determine the placental implantation site of the developing embryo; thus, it is not known why the placenta occasionally implants at or near the os. Clinical associations with placenta previa include increasing parity, advanced maternal age, previous abortions, previous cesarean sections, fetal anomalies, male fetus, and uterine leiomyomata distorting the endometrial cavity. The recurrence risk is about 5–10%.

Symptoms & Signs

In the overwhelming majority of cases, the presenting symptom is painless vaginal bleeding. The bleeding may vary in amount from scant spotting to copious hemorrhage. In most cases, no precipitating event can be identified. Often, bleeding will be precipitated by uterine contractions. Occasionally, bleeding will follow coitus.

The timing of the first bleeding episode is variable. The first episode typically occurs at 28–32 weeks but can occur as early as the middle of the second trimester. Occasionally, no bleeding will occur until the patient presents in labor at term.

The usual course is for a bleeding episode to be followed by a few days or weeks of quiescence. Each successive episode typically involves greater volumes of blood loss, although the course can be unpredictable.

Diagnosis

Ultrasonography is the mainstay of diagnosis. As mentioned previously, the important finding is the relation of the placenta to the internal cervical os. If the placenta is implanted over the cervical os, the diagnosis is made. Ultrasonography will successfully establish the diagnosis in more than 95% of cases.

In the rare case in which ultrasonography cannot clearly define the placental margins, magnetic resonance imaging can be performed.

Diagnosis by pelvic examination can precipitate brisk bleeding and must be avoided.

Management

As with abruption, the first goal of management is to stabilize the mother and prevent hypovolemic shock, organ failure, and death. With appropriate management, these complications are rare. The second goal is to deliver a fetus with an optimal chance of intact survival. The high perinatal mortality rate associated with placenta previa (5–25%) is almost entirely attributable to preterm delivery.

Because most previas begin bleeding long before term, the usual approach is expectant management with hospital bedrest, volume resuscitation, and blood transfusion as needed. If bleeding episodes are associated with uterine contractions, tocolytic agents are often useful. Once the mother is stable, transport to a tertiary center should be considered because preterm delivery can be anticipated. Betamethasone or dexamethasone can be given to accelerate fetal lung maturity.

Because previas can lead to sudden and copious bleeding, at least 2 units of blood for transfusion should be immediately available to all women hospitalized for placenta previa. Packed red cells are a more efficient use of scarce blood bank resources than whole blood. Hematocrit should be measured weekly, and transfusion given for values less than 30%. On average, over the course of several weeks, women with complete previa may require as many as 5 units of blood; with partial previa, 4 units; and with marginal previa, 2–3 units.

Serial ultrasonograms (every 3–4 weeks) should be performed to reevaluate placental location and to assess fetal growth. As the uterus enlarges with advancing gestation, marginal previas are often "pulled up" away from the internal os, becoming low-lying placentas.

Weekly fetal surveillance (nonstress test, biophysical profile) should be performed. The contraction stress test is contraindicated because it may precipitate further bleeding.

Home bedrest, with strict instructions to avoid sexual activity, may be considered if a patient meets all of the following criteria: (1) no previous heavy bleeding requiring blood transfusion; (2) round-the-clock caretaker available to handle emergencies; (3) patient and caretaker are judged to be reliable and compliant; (4) telephone in home; (5) home is less than 5 minutes from the hospital; and (6) transportation to the hospital is always available. Few patients will meet all of these criteria.

Beginning at about 36 weeks, amniocentesis for fetal lung maturity should be performed. If mature, the fetus should be delivered.

Route of Delivery

With complete previa and most partial previas, cesarean delivery is the only acceptable route. Attempts at vaginal delivery can result in placental laceration and abruption with resultant fetal and maternal death.

Blood loss during cesarean delivery for previa is often greater than normal. Hemostasis after delivery of the placenta is often difficult because the lower uterine segment contracts poorly. It is frequently necessary to place hemostatic sutures in the bleeding implantation site. Placenta accreta (growth of the placenta into the myometrium) is common. The incidence approaches 25% when previa occurs with a history of previous cesarean section. The patient should be counseled preoperatively about the possible need for hysterectomy. Because of the potential for extreme blood loss, most anesthesiologists prefer general anesthesia rather than regional anesthesia for cesareans with placenta previa.

With marginal previa, vaginal delivery is sometimes possible. As the cervix dilates, the fetal head may tamponade the placental margin and prevent excessive bleeding. To assess whether vaginal delivery is feasible in a patient who is not bleeding and shows no signs of fetal distress, a *double set-up examination* can be performed to determine the precise placental location. The patient is taken to the operating room, placed in low lithotomy position, and prepared and draped for cesarean section. The anesthesiologist is in attendance, and the neonatologist is alerted. The scrub nurse and surgeons are scrubbed, gowned, and gloved. A skilled examiner then performs a gentle digital examination. If the placenta does not completely cover the internal cervical os and the examination does not cause bleeding, induction of labor should follow. Otherwise, a cesarean section should be performed.

VASA PREVIA

Bleeding from the fetal umbilical artery or vein can result in rapid fetal exsanguination, fetal distress, and death. This rare circumstance occurs when there is a *velamentous insertion of the cord.* In this unusual condition, the umbilical cord is attached to the fetal membranes rather than to the fetal surface of the placenta. The umbilical vessels must therefore course through the membranes for a distance before they reach the placenta. If this course takes them in front of the fetal presenting part, near the cervical os, they are at risk for rupture and bleeding or compression by the presenting part.

The most common scenario is bleeding after spontaneous or

artificial rupture of the membranes. Signs of fetal distress rapidly ensue (fetal tachycardia with persistent severe variable decelerations or late decelerations). Fetal survival depends on rapid recognition and prompt cesarean section. The pediatrician should be informed of the diagnosis and should be prepared for the need for fluid resuscitation and transfusion of the newborn. Unfortunately, even the fastest of operations may not save the fetus. The perinatal mortality rate is about 50–80%. Fortunately, vasa previa is rare, occurring in only 0.03–0.05% of deliveries.

BLEEDING FROM EXTRAUTERINE SOURCES

In 10–20% of cases, third-trimester bleeding is caused by a lesion in the lower genital tract (Table 39–1). Careful examination usually leads to the correct diagnosis. With the exception of the carcinomas, these lesions do not generally pose a grave risk to the mother or fetus.

Table 39–1. Extrauterine causes of third-trimester bleeding.

Cervical lesions
  Cervicitis (especially *Trichomonas, Chlamydia*)
  Endocervical polyps
  Erosions
  Lacerations
  Cervical intraepithelial neoplasia
  Carcinoma
Vaginal lesions
  Varicosities
  Traumatic lacerations
  Foreign bodies
  Adenosis or carcinoma
Vulvar lesions
  Varicosities
  Ulcerative lesions (especially herpes simplex)
  Traumatic lacerations
  Carcinoma
Rectal lesions
  Hemorrhoids
  Fissures
  Traumatic lacerations
  Carcinoma

BLEEDING OF UNKNOWN CAUSE

In as many as 30–50% of cases, no definite cause of third-trimester bleeding can be determined. Most of these are probably mild placental abruptions and should be managed accordingly with bedrest and observation. In up to half of these cases, bleeding will recur and may lead to early delivery.

Bloody show is the term used to describe the passage of a plug of cervical mucous. The mucous is typically streaked with minute amounts of blood, far less than 1 mL, probably representing bleeding from small cervical vessels as the cervix begins to dilate and efface. Labor usually ensues within 48 hours. Patients at term who report bloody show do not necessarily need immediate evaluation if the history is typical and there is no further bleeding. Before term, there is obviously a risk of preterm labor, and immediate evaluation is indicated.

SUGGESTED READINGS

Knab DR: Abruptio placentae. An assessment of the time and method of delivery. Obstet Gynecol 1978;**52:**625.

Sholl JS: Abruptio placentae: Clinical management in nonacute cases. *Am J Obstet Gynecol* 1987;**156:**40.

Silver R et al: Placenta previa: Aggressive expectant management. *Am J Obstet Gynecol* 1984;**150:**15.

Section VII:
Fetal Assessment

Antepartum Fetal Assessment | 40

Anne C. Regenstein, MD

The new technologies of ultrasonography and electronic fetal heart rate monitoring have fostered the development of antepartum fetal assessment. The goal of antepartum fetal assessment is to identify fetuses at risk, screen them with an appropriate test, and intervene when fetal health appears to be in jeopardy.

Situations in which the fetus is at risk include maternal medical illnesses, such as hypertension, diabetes, and sickle cell anemia, and complications of pregnancy, such as postterm pregnancy, premature rupture of the membranes, and preeclampsia. In these and other situations, the health of the fetus and the uteroplacental unit is suspect. Antepartum testing is used to detect the compromised fetus before a permanent insult has occurred.

The type of test and frequency of testing are based on the nature and severity of the condition. Protocols vary from institution to institution with respect to when to begin testing, frequency of testing and which single test or combination of tests are to be used for a given complication.

When antepartum test results are abnormal, more information may be obtained from other antenatal tests. Management is tailored to the individual patient based on multiple clinical factors.

FETAL HEART RATE MONITORING

The mainstay of antepartum fetal assessment is electronic fetal heart rate (FHR) monitoring. The aim of electronic FHR monitoring is to assess the physiologic state of the fetus and the uteroplacental unit. For antenatal assessment an external FHR monitor is used. Most electronic external FHR monitors use Doppler ultrasonography to assess the FHR. For information regarding internal FHR monitors, please refer to Chapter 41, Fetal Assessment During Labor.

A monitor placed on the abdomen measures the FHR, which is recorded as beats/min on a continuously moving strip of paper. The features assessed are the baseline FHR and the variability of the FHR as well as the nonperiodic and periodic changes.

Basal Fetal Heart Rate

The normal FHR is between 110 and 160 beats/min. The baseline FHR is best ascertained between contractions during a 10- to 20-min observation period. The most common cause of fetal tachycardia (> 160 beats/min) is maternal fever; other causes include betamimetic drugs, fetal hypoxia, and maternal thyrotoxicosis. Fetal bradycardia (< 110 beats/min) may be due to acute hypoxia, congenital heart block, or local anesthesia.

Fetal Heart Rate Variability

Beat-to-beat variability is the difference between successive R-R intervals. When normal beat-to-beat variability is present, the tracing of the FHR appears as a jiggly line, whereas when beat-to-beat variability is absent, the tracing of the FHR appears as a straight line.

Variations in FHR are controlled by the autonomic nervous system and related cardiac innervation. The presence of beat-to-beat variability reflects an intact pathway from the cerebral cortex, through the midbrain, and the vagus nerve, to the conducting system of the heart.

Beat-to-beat variability can be classified as **short-term variability,** the difference between adjacent beats or several beats, and **long-term variability,** irregular and crude waves occurring 3–6 times/min. The FHR tracing shown in Figure 40–1 demonstrates both types of variability. Assessment of variability is based primarily on long-term variability.

The presence of beat-to-beat variability is a reassuring sign because it indicates an adequately oxygenated fetus. However, an important caveat is that beat-to-beat variability detected with an external FHR monitor may be artifactual.

Normal beat-to-beat variability is defined as an amplitude of at least 6 beats/min. Less than 6 beats/min is called **diminished**

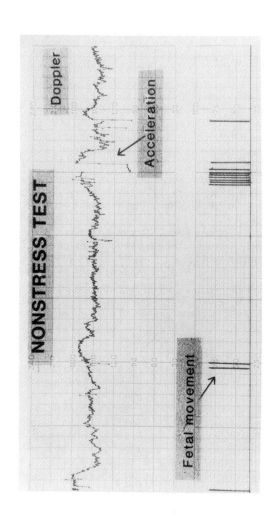

Figure 40-1. Reactive nonstress test. Notice increase of fetal heart rate to more than 15 beats/min for longer than 15 seconds following fetal movements, indicated by the vertical marks on the lower part of the recording. *(Photo courtesy of Dr. K. Leveno.)*

483

beat-to-beat variability, and less than 2 beats/min is called **absent** beat-to-beat variability. Absent or diminished FHR variability, irrespective of the type of monitoring, may be an ominous sign. However, it is also associated with fetal sleep and drug effects. **Saltatory** beat-to-beat variability is defined as amplitudes greater than 25 beats/min and may be an early sign of fetal hypoxia.

A. FHR Acceleration: An acceleration is defined as an elevation in the FHR of 15 beats/min above the baseline FHR for 15 seconds (Figure 40–1). Accelerations in the FHR are often associated with fetal movement. Accelerations are reassuring signs because they require the integration of peripheral neuronal receptors and an intact myocardium.

B. FHR Decelerations: Three types of FHR decelerations described as early, variable, and late are helpful in assessing fetal well being (Figure 40–2). An **early deceleration** is a gradual deceleration that mirrors the timing and the recorded shape of a contraction. When the contraction is complete, the FHR has returned to baseline FHR. With its curved shape, it somewhat resembles a U. This pattern is frequently seen late in labor and is associated with compression of the fetal head. There is no correlation between early decelerations and adverse fetal outcome.

In contrast, a **variable deceleration** is variable in timing, and it may or may not be associated with a contraction. These deceleration patterns are V- or W-shaped with a sharp slope downward and upward. Variable decelerations can occur as a result of compression of the umbilical cord.

Variable decelerations are further divided by their nadir and length into mild, moderate, and severe. **Mild variable decelerations** are less than 30 seconds in duration or less than 30 beats/min below the baseline FHR, whereas **moderate variable decelerations** are 30–60 seconds in duration and less than 60 beats/min below the baseline FHR. Mild and moderate variable decelerations do not indicate fetal compromise. However, **severe variable decelerations** represent insufficiency of umbilical blood flow. Severe variable decelerations are longer than 60 seconds or are more than 60 beats/min below the baseline FHR or at a rate of 60 beats/min. Persistence of this pattern is cause for concern and is associated with fetal acidosis.

Late decelerations are similar in configuration to early decelerations. However, the decrease in the FHR occurs after the contraction begins, and the FHR does not return to baseline FHR for 10–30 seconds after the contraction ends. Persistent late decelerations are of great concern because they imply uteroplacental insufficiency.

During a contraction, myometrial pressure exceeds collapsing pressure for the vessels coursing through the myometrium. Therefore, the contraction is a time of impaired oxygen exchange. If uteroplacental insufficiency is present, contractions will lead to a transient decrease in oxygen tension. The low oxygen tension is sensed by the fetal chemoreceptors, leading to vagal discharge and a decrease in the FHR. Late decelerations may also arise from myocardial hypoxia, as is seen with prolonged fetal hypoxia.

In summary, the following steps should be followed to assess a FHR recording, whether antepartum or intrapartum:

(1) Obtain a recording of at least 20 minutes duration that has good tracings of both the FHR and the uterine activity. The placement of the monitors may need to be adjusted if there are gaps in the tracing.
(2) Ascertain what the baseline FHR is by looking at the periods between contractions. A normal FHR ranges between 110 and 160 beats/min.
(3) Ascertain how frequently the contractions occur either by counting the number of contractions within a given time period or by measuring the elapsed time between the peaks of contractions. Usually the graph paper is set to move at a rate of 3 cm/min, so that the thick vertical lines divide 1-min intervals and the lighter, thinner, vertical lines divide 10-second intervals.
(4) Assess the presence or absence of beat-to-beat variability.
(5) Note any periodic changes (early and late decelerations).
(6) Note any nonperiodic changes (variable decelerations).

NONSTRESS TEST

The nonstress test (NST) is the first-line test used in most institutions to assess fetal well being. A reactive NST in which FHR accelerations are noted is a reassuring test. Criteria vary as to what constitutes a reactive tracing. The most common criterion is that 2–3 accelerations must occur within 10–20 minutes. Most clinicians define an acceleration as 15 beats/min above the baseline FHR for more than 15 seconds. However, some clinicians require the whole acceleration to be 15 beats/min above baseline FHR, whereas others require only the apex to reach this point. The NST has good specificity; in other words, the false-negative rate is low. Except

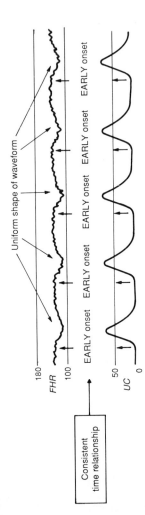

A. Early deceleration (head compression): uniform shape – early timing

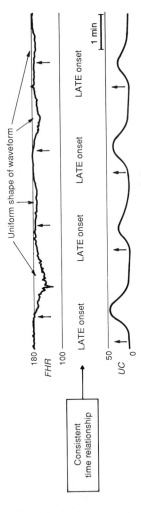

B. Late deceleration (uteroplacental insufficiency): uniform shape – late timing

486

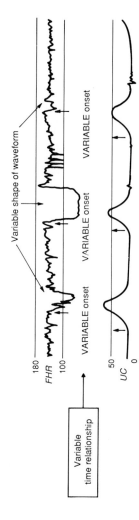

C. Variable deceleration (cord compression): variable shape – variable timing

Figure 40-2. Fetal heart rate (FHR) decelerations in relation to the time of onset of uterine contraction (UC). (*From Hon:* An Atlas of Fetal Heart Rate Patterns. *New Haven, CT, 1968.*)

487

for the fetus of a woman with diabetes mellitus, the postterm fetus, or a fetus suffering from intrauterine growth retardation, a reactive NST assures fetal well being for 1 week.

When a NST is nonreactive, the test period may be extended to see if the fetus becomes reactive. After 80 minutes of observation, it is highly unlikely that a fetus that has had a nonreactive NST will demonstrate a reactive NST. There is no evidence that maternal ingestion of food or manipulation of her abdomen increases reactivity. The vibroacoustic stimulus, or artificial larynx, can be used to stimulate the fetus. A 3-second stimulus is applied with the apparatus positioned over the fetal head. Although the overall incidence of nonreactive tests remains unchanged, the time to reactivity decreases, thereby decreasing overall test time.

Less than 5% of NSTs are nonreactive. Unfortunately, the sensitivity of the NST is poor. Only about 40% of patients with a nonreactive NST demonstrate fetal distress during labor. Depending on the clinical situation, either the test should be repeated the following day, or more information should be obtained using other methods of fetal assessment. Decelerations of the FHR during an NST may signify an abnormality of the umbilical cord and therefore may also require further evaluation.

CONTRACTION STRESS TEST

During the contraction stress test (CST), uteroplacental function is evaluated by assessing the fetal response to the stress of contractions. If satisfactory contractions are not occurring spontaneously, contractions can be stimulated using exogenous oxytocin or nipple stimulation. Three contractions within 10 minutes are required for a CST to be considered adequate. Results are defined as follows:

(1) **Positive:** repeated, uniformly late decelerations. Some clinicians define a positive test as late decelerations associated with more than half of the uterine contractions. A CST may be considered positive with fewer than 3 contractions in 10 minutes if there are repetitive late decelerations with uterine activity.

(2) **Negative:** stable FHR with no late decelerations.

(3) **Equivocal:** late decelerations that do not persist throughout the recording.

(4) **Hyperstimulation:** excessive uterine activity leading to fetal bradycardia.

(5) **Unsatisfactory:** FHR not monitored adequately or inability to stimulate uterine activity.

A negative CST is an indicator of adequate uteroplacental function. The number of false negatives is very low. A positive CST is associated with an increased rate of fetal distress during labor and cesarean section. However, the false-positive rate for the CST is high. For the most part, when a mature fetus demonstrates a positive CST, it should be delivered by induction or cesarean section, depending on the clinical situation. The immature fetus with a positive CST may pose a dilemma. Other information, such as a detailed sonogram, the presence of reassuring FHR patterns, a biophysical profile, or in some cases, cordocentesis, may help in the management of these patients.

Indications for CST include postterm pregnancies, hypertension, and intrauterine growth retardation; a CST is also used as a diagnostic test after a nonreactive NST is obtained. Contraindications for a CST are preterm labor, a risk of preterm labor (eg, as indicated by multiple gestation or incompetent cervix), previous vertical uterine scar, other previous uterine surgery that would preclude labor, and placenta previa. The main drawbacks of this test are that it has a high false-positive rate and it is time consuming to perform.

BIOPHYSICAL PROFILE

This antepartum test is commonly referred to as an intrauterine Apgar score. An NST and an ultrasound assessment of the fetus constitute this test. In some institutions, the biophysical profile is the primary test, whereas in other institutions, it is used as a backup test when more information is desired. Five variables are assessed and a score of 0 or 2 is given for each. Thus, 10 is most commonly the highest possible score and 0 the lowest. The fetus is observed ultrasonographically for a maximum of 30 minutes (Table 40–1).

A score of 10 or 8 is considered normal. A score of 6 is considered equivocal, and a management plan is based on the clinical situation. A score of 4 suggests fetal asphyxia, and unless a repeat test shows improvement, delivery should probably be undertaken. A score of 0 or 2 indicates almost certain fetal asphyxia, and the fetus should be delivered.

As with the previous tests, the biophysical profile (BPP) has

Table 40-1. Intrauterine Apgar score.

Variable	Score 2	Score 0
Nonstress test	Reactive	Nonreactive
Fetal breathing movements	30 s of sustained fetal breathing movements	< 30 s of fetal breathing movements
Fetal tone	One motion of a limb from a position of flexion to extension and a rapid return to flexion	Fetus in a position of partial or full limb extension with no return to flexion
Fetal movement	3 or more gross body movements	2 or less gross body movements
Amniotic fluid	A pocket of amniotic fluid that measures at least 2 × 2 cm in 2 perpendicular planes	Largest amniotic fluid pocket measures less than 2 × 2 cm

good specificity. The specificity is more than 80% for neonatal morbidity, and more than 90% for neonatal mortality. However, its sensitivity is approximately 50% for neonatal morbidity.

AMNIOTIC FLUID INDEX

Decreased amniotic fluid volume is associated with growth-retarded infants and has been shown to be predictive of poor outcome in postterm pregnancies. The amniotic fluid index is a measurement used to quantify the adequacy of amniotic fluid volume.

An amniotic fluid index is obtained by ultrasonographically measuring the vertical "depth" of the largest pocket of amniotic fluid in four quadrants of the maternal uterus and then adding the 4 measurements together. The dividing lines of the quadrants are a transverse line through the umbilicus and the linea nigra. The ultrasound transducer is held longitudinally and perpendicular to the maternal abdomen. A vertical measurement of the largest pocket is taken. Fetal parts or cord that occupy the space are not considered part of the pocket.

A score of 5 cm or less represents diminished amniotic fluid and may be an indication for delivery. Serial measurements of the amniotic fluid index may be used to ascertain whether there is a trend toward diminishing fluid.

DOPPLER ULTRASONOGRAPHY

Doppler ultrasonography is another diagnostic tool for assessing the fetal-placental unit. However, its clinical usefulness in obstetrics remains to be determined. In general applications of Doppler ultrasonography, the movement of red blood cells in a vessel is detected. The Doppler effect is used to calculate the velocity of blood flow and to estimate the volume of flow. However, in obstetrics, the diameters of the maternal uterine arteries, the fetal cerebral arteries, and the fetal umbilical arteries are small so that the flow and velocity measurements cannot be accurately determined. Therefore, the Doppler waveforms are described by the relationship between systolic velocity and diastolic velocity. This relationship is a reflection of the impedence of blood flow within the placenta because an increase in impedence results in a decrease in diastolic flow relative to systolic flow.

Some of the more common formulas used to describe the Doppler ultrasound measurements are as follows: systolic/diastolic ratio; the Pourcelet index, calculated as $(S - D)/S$; or the pulsatility index, calculated as $S - D/mean$.

As normal pregnancy advances, uterine blood flow and diastolic velocity increase. Therefore, the above indices decrease as the pregnancy matures. When an elevation in the ratio of the systolic velocity to diastolic velocity of the umbilical artery for a given gestational age is noted, intrauterine growth retardation is suspected.

Clearcut abnormalities in Doppler measurements are absent or reversed diastolic flow. Preliminary studies have shown that abnormal Doppler measurements are associated with intrauterine growth retardation, but that biometric ultrasound measurements are more sensitive and selective for this diagnosis. Preeclampsia and postterm pregnancy not complicated with intrauterine growth retardation may not be associated with abnormal Doppler measurements.

FETAL MOVEMENT MONITORING

Maternal recognition of fetal movement is first noted between 16 and 20 weeks of gestation (often referred to as "quickening").

A normal fetus has sleep-wake cycles with periods of activity and rest. Each fetus has its own rhythm and rate of movement, and each woman varies in her ability to perceive movement. A decrease in fetal movement sometimes heralds fetal death. Therefore, it is useful to record fetal activity.

The pregnant woman should be instructed to count fetal movements at least once a day. She should note at least 4 movements in 1 hour.

SUGGESTED READINGS

Gabbe SG: Antepartum fetal evaluation. In: *Obstetrics: Normal and Problem Pregnancies,* 2nd ed. Gabbe SG, Niebyl JR, Simpson JL (editors). Churchill Livingstone, 1991.

Leveno KJ, Cunningham FG: Forecasting fetal health. In: *Williams Obstetrics,* Supplement No. 19 (Aug/Sept). Appleton & Lange, 1988.

Rutherford SE et al: The four quadrant assessment of amniotic fluid volume. *Obstet Gynecol* 1987;**70:**353.

Thacker SB, Berkelman RL: Assessing the diagnostic accuracy and efficacy of selected antepartum fetal surveillance techniques. *Obstet Gynecol Surv* 1986;**41:**121.

Fetal Assessment During Labor | 41

Patricia A. Robertson, MD

Because the stress of labor can affect fetal well being, the assessment of the fetus is critical in the intrapartum period. This chapter discusses different approaches to intrapartum fetal assessment and the benefits and risks of each method. The benefits include the diagnosis of a sudden intrapartum asphyxial event or the occurrence of persistent fetal distress. The risks include the risk of infection to the mother or fetus if internal monitoring is used, and the possible misinterpretation of the fetal heart rate monitor strip which might lead to an unnecessary Cesarean section.

FETAL HEART RATE MONITORING

Techniques

The most traditional method of intrapartum fetal assessment is evaluation of the fetal heart rate. Intermittent auscultation by fetoscope or Doppler ultrasound on a regular basis is the minimum amount of fetal heart monitoring recommended for low-risk pregnancies. Pregnancies in the high risk-category (eg, maternal diabetes or hypertension, postterm gestation, breech presentation) are frequently monitored continuously throughout active labor. Because of the serious problem of litigation in the field of obstetrics, some hospitals and health practitioners monitor all labors with continuous fetal heart rate monitoring. It must be emphasized that it is important to have an appropriately trained health care provider available to interpret monitor strips if continuous monitoring is used.

The fetal heart rate can be continuously monitored by either an external, noninvasive Doppler technique (Figure 41–1) or by an internal electrode (Figure 41–2). The external Doppler technique can measure fetal heart rate and periodic changes in the pattern of the fetal heart rate (accelerations and decelerations). Because this technique depends on the reflected ultrasound signal, if the fetus

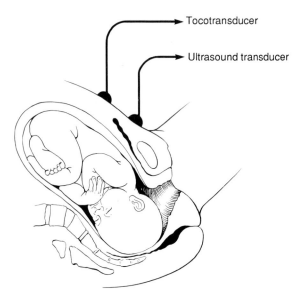

Tocotransducer

Ultrasound transducer

Figure 41-1. External fetal heart rate monitoring. *(Redrawn, with permission, from Hon EHG:* Hosp Pract *[Sept] 1970;5:1.)*

changes position, the signal can be lost at different intervals until the monitor is readjusted. The internal electrode requires ruptured membranes and cervical dilation of at least 1–2 cm. The internal fetal electrode is applied to either the scalp, if the fetus is in a vertex presentation or to the buttock if the fetus is in a breech presentation. The internal electrode records not only the fetal heart rate and periodic changes but also short-term and long-term variability, which is important information in fetal assessment.

In general, unless there is a specific indication, the noninvasive external Doppler monitor, rather than the internal electrode, is used if continuous monitoring of the fetus during labor is elected. Indications for placement of the internal electrode include an external monitor tracing that suggests fetal distress or inability to monitor the fetus adequately by external Doppler monitor. Contraindications to the placement of an internal fetal electrode include active maternal genital herpes, maternal HIV infection or a fetal condition that involves a fetal coagulopathy (eg, hemophilia).

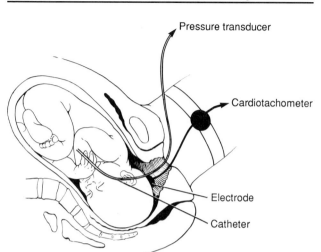

Figure 41–2. Internal fetal heart monitoring. *(Redrawn, with permission, from Hon EHG:* Hosp Pract *[Sept] 1970;5:91.)*

To interpret the fetal heart rate monitor strip, it is necessary to document the timing of uterine contractions. Uterine contractions can be palpated or recorded by external tocotransducer or internal transducer. An external pressure transducer can record the frequency and the duration of uterine contractions. An internal transducer requires ruptured membranes and cervical dilation of at least 1–2 cm. The internal transducer is either a standard water column intrauterine pressure catheter or a solid transducer catheter. The catheter is placed transvaginally and threaded through the cervix into the uterus. Risks of the internal transducer include increasing the risk of chorioamnionitis due to the presence of the catheter in the uterus. Uterine perforation has rarely been reported as a risk. The advantage of the internal transducer is an accurate measurement of the strength of the uterine contractions, which is critical when considering a diagnosis of cephalopelvic disproportion. An additional advantage to the internal catheter is the ability to infuse a saline solution for the treatment of fetal distress (amnio-infusion).

Interpretation

Fetal distress can be diagnosed intrapartum by an abnormal fetal heart rate or the presence of periodic changes in the fetal heart rate pattern. Normal fetal heart rate during labor is 110–160 beats/ min. Tachycardia of the fetal heart greater than 160 beats/min can indicate chorioamnionitis, maternal dehydration, fetal distress, or fetal supraventricular tachyarrhythmia. Bradycardia of the fetus can indicate fetal distress or congenital heart block of the fetus.

Periodic changes in the fetal heart rate include accelerations and variable and late decelerations. Accelerations of the fetal heart rate with fetal movement or uterine contractions are associated with fetal well being. Variable decelerations can be mild, moderate, or severe, depending on the depth and length of deceleration, and have a "block-like" configuration (Figure 41–3). Variable decelerations may or may not be associated with uterine contractions; that is, they are variable in their occurrence. Tolerance of the fetus to

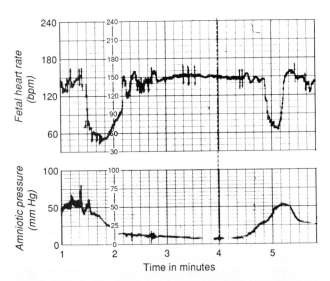

Figure 41–3. Fetal heart rate tracings: variable decelerations. *(Reproduced, with permission, from Babson SG et al:* Management of High-Risk Pregnancy and Intensive Care of the Neonate, *3rd ed. Mosby, 1975.)*

variable decelerations differs according to the amount of fetal reserve. For instance, a full-term, well-oxygenated fetus often tolerates mild to moderate decelerations well during the second stage of labor, whereas a preterm, growth-restricted fetus might not tolerate the same decelerations. Late decelerations are decelerations that are mirror images of contractions, often delayed in relation to the contraction, in contrast to the block-like variable decelerations. Persistent late decelerations are frequently associated with significant fetal distress (Figure 41–4).

Good long-term and short-term variability reflects fetal well being. The external monitor technique for determining fetal heart rate variability is not always reliable. Thus, if the results obtained with an external monitor are of concern, an internal electrode is usually recommended. Decreased variability can be associated with fetal distress or medications (eg, narcotics or magnesium sulfate). The most ominous sign for significant fetal asphyxia is the combination of persistent late decelerations and lack of variability in the fetal heart rate tracing.

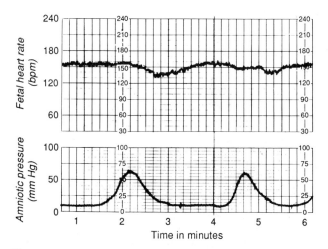

Figure 41–4. Fetal heart rate tracings: late decelerations. *(Reproduced, with permission, from Babson SG et al:* Management of High-Risk Pregnancy and Intensive Care of the Neonate, *3rd ed. Mosby, 1975.)*

FETAL STIMULATION

Two methods have recently been used to assess fetal well being by stimulating the fetus. The first method is acoustic stimulation of the fetus. A horn, or artificial larynx stimulus, is applied directly to the maternal abdomen. A resultant increase in fetal heart rate secondary to the stimulus is interpreted as indicating fetal well being. The second method is fetal scalp stimulation by pelvic examination during labor. An increase in the fetal heart rate with direct massage of the fetal scalp or buttock usually reflects a nonacidotic fetus.

FETAL SCALP BLOOD SAMPLING

Acidosis in the fetus can be directly measured during labor with the technique of fetal scalp or buttock sampling. This sampling method is often used to provide additional information when a suspicious fetal monitor tracing has been obtained. The technique of fetal sampling requires ruptured membranes and a cervical dilation of at least 3 cm. A plastic cone is placed in the vagina to directly see the presenting part. A small incision is made with a scalpel, and blood is collected in a heparinized glass tube. If the pH is less than 7.20, fetal distress is confirmed. If the pH is 7.20–7.24, possible fetal distress is present, and the fetal scalp sampling should be repeated every 20–30 minutes if the monitor tracing continues to suggest fetal distress. A pH of more than 7.24 is a reassurance of fetal well being. However, if further periodic changes occur, further fetal samplings may need to be performed because the result of the fetal scalp sample is but a reflection of an instant in time.

TREATMENT OF FETAL DISTRESS

Once fetal distress is diagnosed, specific measures are taken to alleviate the distress. If oxytocin is being administered, it is stopped. Additional measures include the following: (1) placing the mother on her left or right side to increase uterine blood flow, (2) adjusting the bed to a Trendelenberg position to alleviate pressure on a possible prolapsed umbilical cord, (3) administering oxygen by mask, and (4) administering fluids intravenously. Amnio-infusion can be administered through an intrauterine catheter if needed. If fetal distress continues, terbutaline (a tocolytic) can be administered intravenously or subcutaneously to slow or stop the contractions that may be causing the fetal distress. If severe fetal distress continues despite these measures, a cesarean section should be considered unless a spontaneous or operative vaginal delivery is possible.

UMBILICAL CORD GAS SAMPLING AT THE TIME OF BIRTH

Umbilical cord gas sampling at the time of birth provides an objective means to assess the neonatal condition and to retrospectively assess the intrapartum monitor strip. At the time of birth, a segment of umbilical cord is doubly clamped and cut. Two blood samples are drawn up in heparinized syringes from the cord: a sample from the umbilical artery and a sample from the umbilical vein. These samples are then analyzed for pH, HCO_3, Po_2, Pco_2, and base deficit. Different types of acidemia can be defined with this information (eg, respiratory, metabolic, or mixed). In general, fetal distress is confirmed if the umbilical venous sample pH is less than 7.20 and if the umbilical arterial sample pH is less than 7.10.

SUGGESTED READINGS

Parer JT: *Handbook of Fetal Heart Rate Monitoring.* Saunders, 1983.
Cunningham FG, MacDonald PC, Gant NF: *Williams Obstetrics.* 18th ed. Appleton & Lange, 1989.

Section VIII:
Labor, Delivery, & Postpartum Care

The Course & Conduct of Normal Labor & Delivery | 42

Patricia L. Collins, MD, PhD

PHYSIOLOGY OF INITIATION OF PARTURITION

Human parturition, or the birth process, is not thoroughly understood. There are several theories in the literature, 2 of which are the progesterone withdrawal theory and the fetal-maternal communication system theory. Animal models are available to study the initiation of labor, but they do not completely explain initiation of parturition in humans.

Progesterone Withdrawal Theory

In some species (eg, the rat or rabbit), progesterone is maintained at elevated pregnancy levels by the corpus luteum. Labor can be induced at any time during gestation by withdrawing the progesterone, that is, by removing the corpus luteum. In these species, labor begins when there is a physiologic withdrawal of progesterone and a concomitant increase in estrogen. However, in humans, there is no demonstrable decrease of progesterone nor is there an increase in estrogen at the time of the initiation of labor.

In the sheep, initiation of parturition comes about after maturation of the fetal hypothalamic-pituitary-adrenal axis. The fetal adrenal then produces more cortisol, which causes the placenta to synthesize a 17α-hydroxylase enzyme. With synthesis of this enzyme, the placenta alters the pathway of steroid biosynthesis such that less progesterone (progesterone withdrawal) but more estrogen is produced. However, in humans, the 17α-hydroxylase enzyme is not expressed in the placenta, and an increase in fetal cortisol does not have the same role as in the sheep model.

Fetal-Maternal Communication System Theory

This theory says that human parturition is triggered by a maturational event in the fetus, producing a molecular signal(s) that is then transmitted through the amniotic fluid to the fetal membranes. This results in increased prostaglandin production by the fetal membranes and the maternal decidua, which, in turn, causes increased myometrial activity. The human fetal maturational event is unknown. Because of clinical evidence that abnormalities of the pituitary-adrenal axis, such as anencephaly or fetal adrenal hypoplasia, can prolong gestation, there is speculation that these fetal endocrine organs may be involved. The intermediate signal from the fetus to cause increased fetal membrane prostaglandin production is not completely understood.

It is known that prostaglandins, particularly PGE_2 and $PGF_{2\alpha}$, can cause uterine contractions at any time during human gestation. However, other substances, such as leukotrienes, endothelin, and oxytocin, also cause uterine contractions. Whether these compounds are involved in the initiation of human parturition is not known.

STAGES OF NORMAL LABOR

Labor is divided into 3 stages, as described by Friedman in 1978 (Figure 42-1):

First stage-This stage is defined as from the onset of labor until the complete dilation of the cervix. The first stage begins with the onset of regular uterine contractions that are of sufficient frequency and strength to cause effacement (shortening) and dilation (opening) of the cervix and descent of the fetus. The first stage ends when the cervix is completely effaced (100%) and completely dilated (10 cm).

The first stage is divided into the latent phase and the active phase. The latent phase begins with the onset of labor and is the period when the cervix softens, slowly effaces and dilates, usually to about 4-5 cm. The active phase is the period beginning at about 4-5 cm of dilation when the cervix begins to change more rapidly and the fetus is descending in the pelvis. The active phase ends when the cervix is completely dilated.

Second stage-This stage extends from complete effacement and dilation of the cervix to the complete birth of the fetus.

Third stage-The third stage of labor is the period from delivery of the fetus to delivery of the placenta and fetal membranes.

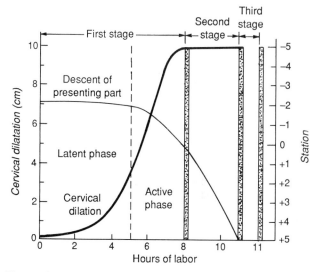

Figure 42-1. Freidman curve, showing a typical time course for 3 stages of normal labor.

MECHANISM OF NORMAL LABOR

Lie, Presentation, & Position of the Fetus

The **fetal lie** refers to the relationship of the long axis of the fetus to the long axis of the mother and can be **longitudinal, transverse,** or **oblique.** The majority of fetuses at term gestation are in a longitudinal lie (Figures 42–2 through 42–4).

The **presentation** refers to that part of the fetus that enters the pelvis first. Most fetuses (96%) at term gestation are in a vertex or occiput (head first) presentation (Figures 42–2 and 42–3). The next most common presentation is breech (3.5%) (Figure 42–4). Rare presentations are face, brow, or shoulder.

Position refers to the relationship of a reference point of the presenting part of the fetus to the maternal pelvis. For vertex presentations, the reference point is the occiput. For breech presentations, the reference point is the sacrum; for the face, the chin (mentum); and for the shoulder, the acromion. Thus, the reference point for any presentation may be either to the right (R) or left (L)

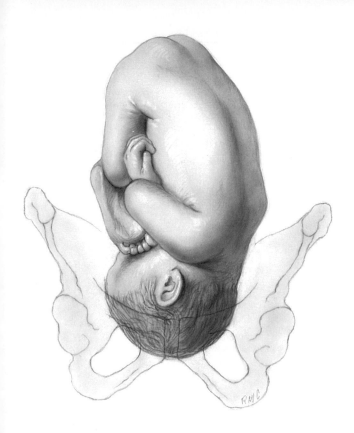

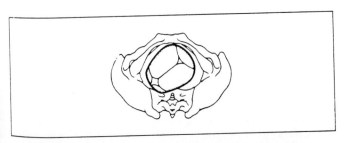

Figure 42–2. Longitudinal lie and vertex presentation: left occiput anterior (LOA) position. *(Reproduced, with permission, from Cunningham FG, MacDonald PC, Gant NF: Williams Obstetrics, 18th ed. Appleton & Lange, 1989.)*

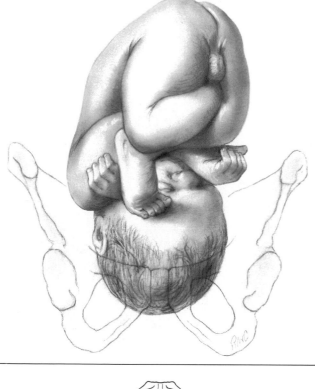

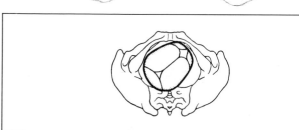

Figure 42–3. Longitudinal lie and vertex presentation: right occiput posterior (ROP) position. *(Reproduced, with permission, from Cunningham FG, MacDonald PC, Gant NF: Williams Obstetrics, 18th ed. Appleton & Lange, 1989.)*

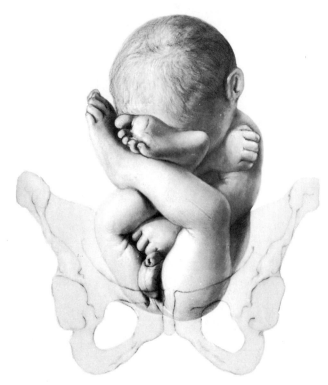

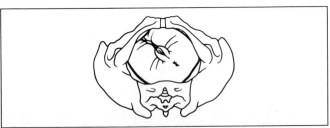

Figure 42-4. Longitudinal lie and breech presentation: left sacrum posterior (LSP) position. *(Reproduced, with permission, from Cunningham FG, MacDonald PC, Gant NF:* Williams Obstetrics, *18th ed. Appleton & Lange, 1989.)*

side in the maternal pelvis as well as anterior (A), posterior (P), or transverse (T) in the maternal pelvis. Examples of positions are LOA for left occiput anterior (Figure 42–2), ROP for right occiput posterior (Figure 42–3) and LSP for left sacrum posterior (Figure 42–4).

Cardinal Movements of Labor: Vertex Presentation

The process by which the fetus adapts and moves through the bony pelvis are described by the cardinal movements of labor: **engagement, descent, flexion, internal rotation, extension, external rotation** and **expulsion** (Figure 42–5). These are arbitrary divisions, because the movements of the fetus through the pelvis are continuous and often simultaneous processes.

Engagement is defined as the passage of the largest part of the fetal head, the biparietal diameter, through the pelvic inlet. This criterion is usually met when the bony part of the fetal vertex is at the level of the ischial spines. The fetal vertex usually enters the pelvis in the occiput transverse position.

With adequate uterine contractions and the ability of the fetal head to change its shape (**molding**) to adapt to the bony pelvic contours and axes, there is descent of the fetal vertex. As the vertex descends and meets resistance, there is flexion of the fetal head.

The fetus next undergoes internal rotation such that the vertex is in the occiput anterior position. This is accompanied by further descent until the vertex reaches the perineum. Extension of the head brings the vertex under the symphysis until the head is born.

External rotation then occurs and brings the vertex back to the position it was in at the time of internal rotation. This rotation is also called restitution. The fetal body also rotates such that the fetal shoulders are now in the anterior-posterior diameter of the pelvis. Expulsion occurs as the anterior and posterior shoulders and body of the fetus are born.

MANAGEMENT OF EARLY LABOR

Admission for Labor

The following recommendations for admission history and physical examination are meant as guidelines only, since they should be tailored to the individual patient. They are also streamlined for patients who have had prenatal care and who are otherwise healthy with normal pregnancies.

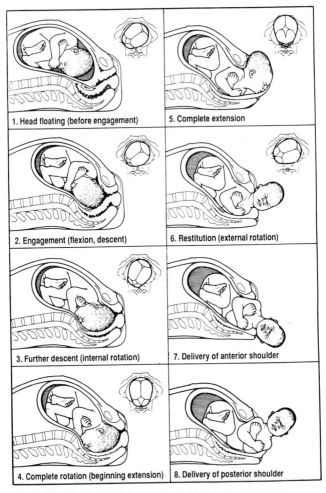

1. Head floating (before engagement)

2. Engagement (flexion, descent)

3. Further descent (internal rotation)

4. Complete rotation (beginning extension)

5. Complete extension

6. Restitution (external rotation)

7. Delivery of anterior shoulder

8. Delivery of posterior shoulder

Figure 42–5. Cardinal movements of labor in the left occiput anterior position. *(Reproduced, with permission, from Cunningham FG, MacDonald PC, Gant NF:* Williams Obstetrics, *18th ed. Appleton & Lange, 1989.)*

The decision of when to admit a laboring patient to the hospital is individual to both the patient and physician. For example, a primiparous patient in very early labor with intact membranes can often labor at home until her contractions become more regular and intense. At times it is difficult to differentiate between **false labor** and **true labor.** The contractions of true labor are usually more regular, become more frequent and intense over time, and persist through bed rest, hydration, and sedation.

A. History: On admission, a history should be obtained of the onset, frequency, duration, and amount of discomfort of uterine contractions. Inquiry should be made as to whether there is vaginal bleeding or discharge consistent with loss of a mucous plug or consistent with rupture of the fetal membranes and when this occurred. It is also important to ask if the fetus is moving normally. If the patient has any medical problems, inquiry should be made as to any changes in the medical condition since the last clinic visit.

B. Physical Examination: The physical examination should begin with vital signs and general appearance. A brief, general physical examination is performed. The obstetrical part of the physical examination includes abdominal and pelvic examinations.

1. Abdominal examination–An abdominal examination is performed to estimate the size of the fetus and to assess the lie, presentation, position, and degree of engagement of the fetus by Leopold's maneuvers (Figure 42–6). These maneuvers are described below. The first 3 maneuvers are done facing the patient.

The **first maneuver** consists of palpating the top of the uterus to assess whether the breech (round, softer, nodular) or vertex (round, hard, freely movable) is in the uterine fundus.

The **second maneuver** is performed by putting one hand on either side of the maternal abdomen to assess which side of the uterus contains the fetal back (firm, curved) or small parts (small, nodular, often movements).

The **third maneuver** consists of grasping the presenting part with one hand to again assess the presentation (breech or vertex) and also to assess the degree of descent into the pelvis. A fetus with a presenting part that is freely movable is not engaged.

The **fourth maneuver** is performed facing away from the patient. The examiner places both hands on the lower abdomen with the tips of the fingers pointing toward the symphysis to assess position and descent by palpating the cephalic prominence.

2. Pelvic examination–*Caution:* Do not conduct a pelvic examination if there is excessive vaginal bleeding or if there is a

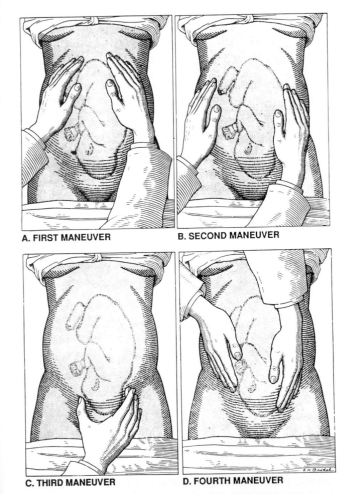

A. FIRST MANEUVER

B. SECOND MANEUVER

C. THIRD MANEUVER

D. FOURTH MANEUVER

Figure 42–6. Leopold's maneuvers for determining fetal presentation (**A,B**), position (**C**), and engagement (**D**). *(Reproduced, with permission, from Cunningham FG, MacDonald PC, Gant NF: Williams Obstetrics, 18th ed. Appleton & Lange, 1989.)*

known history of placenta previa or vasa previa. If the patient has a history consistent with rupture of the fetal membranes, a sterile speculum examination should be performed first. When membranes have ruptured, there is a pool of amniotic fluid in the posterior vaginal fornix, which, when dried on a microscope slide and examined under the microscope, shows a typical ferning pattern. Amniotic fluid turns nitrazine pH indicator paper from yellow (more acidic due to vaginal secretions) to blue (more basic due to amniotic fluid). If a patient is in early labor with ruptured membranes, a digital cervical examination should be deferred because, the more often vaginal examinations are performed with ruptured membranes, the greater the likelihood of infection.

In a patient with intact membranes or one who is in active labor, an initial cervical examination should be performed to assess the position (posterior, mid, anterior), consistency (firm, moderate, soft), effacement (shortening, 0–100%), and the dilation (0–10 cm) of the cervix. Also, the station of the presenting part should be assessed. When the presenting part is at the level of the ischial spines, the station is zero. The pelvis is then divided into centimeters above (−1 to −5) and below (+1 to +5) the level of the ischial spines. Another method is to divide the true pelvis into thirds above (−1 to −3) and below (+1 to +3) the level of the ischial spines.

The bony pelvis should also be reexamined to assess the pelvic type (clinical pelvimetry).

C. Laboratory Assessment: A clean-catch urine specimen, complete blood count, and a blood bank tube for type and screen should be obtained.

D. Monitoring: An initial external fetal heart rate monitoring strip of at least 20 minutes should be obtained (see Chapter 41).

A tocodynamometer is an external monitor to assess the frequency and duration of uterine contractions. An external monitor does not give any information about the strength of uterine contractions. If accurate assessment of uterine tone or strength of contractions is necessary, an internal intrauterine pressure catheter (IUPC) can be placed.

MANAGEMENT OF THE FIRST STAGE OF LABOR

The following areas need to be addressed during the first stage of labor:

Intravenous access–The need for intravenous access during a normal labor is individual to the patient, physician, or hospital.

Diet–The patient can be given clear liquids while in active labor.

Activity–Patients need not be at bedrest during a normal labor, particularly if the fetus has descended well into the pelvis, thus decreasing the chance of umbilical cord prolapse.

Monitoring–The need for external or internal electronic fetal heart rate monitoring should be individually assessed. All viable fetuses should be monitored in some way during labor.

Assessment of labor progress–The patient should be examined as frequently as necessary to assure adequate progression of labor. Such examinations are usually performed every 3–4 hours during the latent phase if the membranes are intact and about every 1–2 hours during the active phase.

Pain management–Narcotics can be given either subcutaneously, intramuscularly, or intravenously. An appropriate antiemetic is usually given with the narcotic. Epidural anesthesia, a regional anesthesia, is a widely used method of pain control. Ideally, epidural anesthetics are placed at the beginning of the active phase of labor. Nitrous oxide is an inhaled anesthetic that can be used for pain relief during labor. Many couples prefer "natural childbirth" methods of pain control, which involve breathing and psychological techniques (eg, the Lamaze method).

MANAGEMENT OF THE SECOND STAGE OF LABOR

Normal Spontaneous Vertex Delivery

After the cervix is completely dilated (10 cm), with each contraction, the patient is instructed to bear down as though she were straining at stool. This "pushing" aids in the descent of the fetal vertex. Eventually, the perineum and vulva will bulge as they are distended by the fetal head. The patient should be encouraged to seek a comfortable position in order to push effectively. Most patients are in dorsal lithotomy position, but lateral Sims', semi-Fowler's, or squatting positions are also acceptable. If the patient is on her back, the uterus should be displaced to the left or right to aid in blood return from the lower extremities and to improve placental blood flow.

As the delivery becomes eminent, the perineum should be cleansed with a surgical soap. The person assisting the birth should wear a water-resistant gown and should have eye protection as part of universal blood and body fluid precautions.

A. Episiotomy: As the vulva and perineum are distended further by the fetal head, a decision is made as to whether an episiotomy is necessary. An episiotomy is a surgical incision of the perineum that begins midline and extends directly posteriorly (median or midline episiotomy) or extends laterally to the right or left (mediolateral episiotomy). The incision also extends into the vaginal mucosa. The purpose of an episiotomy is to increase the diameter of the perineum to prevent ragged tears of the vagina and perineum, to ensure sufficient room for an operative vaginal delivery (forceps or vacuum extractor), or to shorten the second stage of labor. Adequate anesthesia should be administered before attempting episiotomy.

B. Delivery of the Fetal Head: When the biparietal diameter of the fetus distends the perineum and vulva (**crowning**), the birth of the head is eminent. The person assisting the birth should control the extension of the head slowly into the palm of one hand and give support to the posterior perineum with the other hand. As the head is extending in a controlled manner, to further decrease the chance of perineal lacerations, the operator can maneuver the perineum around the fetal chin, a movement called the modified Ritgen maneuver.

Once the head is born, the fetal nose and mouth should be cleared with a bulb aspirator. Next, palpate around the neck of the infant to assess whether there is a nuchal cord (umbilical cord around the fetal neck). If a nuchal cord is present, reduce it by gently maneuvering the cord over the head. If the nuchal cord is too tight to reduce, doubly clamp the umbilical cord, cut the cord between the clamps and unwrap the cord from around the infant's neck.

C. Delivery of the Shoulders: The infant will externally rotate, bringing the shoulders into the anteroposterior diameter of the pelvis. To assist the delivery of the shoulders, grasp the fetal head between the palms of your hands and apply gentle, steady downward traction until the anterior shoulder clears the symphysis. Then apply gentle, steady traction directly upward until the posterior shoulder has cleared the posterior perineum.

D. Delivery of the Body: The infant's body usually follows spontaneously but can be assisted by maternal expulsive effort or by gentle traction. *Note:* do not hook your fingers into the axilla because you can damage nerves and do not grasp and tract on the fetal abdomen because you can damage internal organs.

After delivery of the infant, the cord is doubly clamped and cut between the clamps. Another section of cord can be doubly clamped and cut if cord blood gases are indicated. Cord blood specimens can also be collected at this time.

Operative Vaginal Delivery

Operative vaginal delivery refers to the use of forceps or vacuum extractor to deliver the fetus.

There are many different types of forceps, but all of them have the following features (Figure 42–7):

(1) A **blade** that fits around the fetal head.
(2) A **shank** that connects the blade to the handle.
(3) A **handle** that is used for traction.

A vacuum extraction device is either a small metal or Silastic cup that fits on the fetal head and is held in place by a vacuum. The operator applies traction to the fetal head by a string or chain attached to the cup.

A. Indications: Operative vaginal delivery can be used for the following indications:

(1) An operative vaginal delivery is undertaken to shorten the second stage of labor, for example, because of a prolonged second stage of labor or because of maternal exhaustion.
(2) A second stage of labor is contraindicated. An example of this would be any medical condition in which continued valsalva maneuver would be harmful to the mother, such as a berry aneurysm.
(3) Fetal distress is present, such as a prolonged, unresolving fetal bradycardia.

B. Classification: Operative vaginal deliveries are categorized by the level and position of the fetal vertex at the time the instrument is applied. These deliveries are classified as outlet, low, or mid forceps or outlet, low, or mid vacuum extraction. Both high forceps and high vacuum extraction deliveries are contraindicated in modern obstetrical practice.

1. Prerequisites–Before forceps or the vacuum extractor is used, the cervix must be completely dilated, the maternal bladder must be empty, the fetal head must be engaged in the pelvis, and the position of the vertex must be precisely known. For both procedures, there should be adequate anesthesia.

2. Anesthesia–The choice of anesthesia for an operative deliv-

RIGHT

LEFT

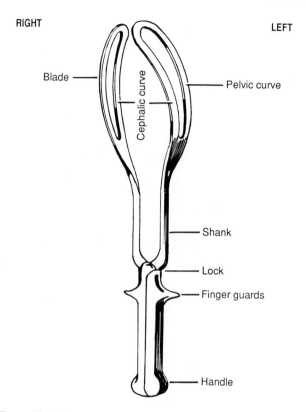

Blade

Cephalic curve

Pelvic curve

Shank

Lock

Finger guards

Handle

Figure 42-7. Forceps used for operative vaginal delivery. *(Reproduced, with permission, from Benson RC:* Handbook of Obstetrics & Gynecology, *8th ed. Lange, 1983.)*

ery depends somewhat on the type of instrument used and how high in the pelvis the fetal vertex is at the time the instrument is applied. The most common choices are regional anesthesia: pudendal nerve block, spinal block, or epidural analgesia.

Abdominal Operative Delivery

A cesarean section is delivery of a fetus after incision through the abdominal wall and uterus (hysterotomy). The type of cesarean section refers to the incision on the uterus not the incision on the skin. The most common and most desirable type is the low segment transverse incision, which refers to a hysterotomy made in the lower uterine segment. A classical incision refers to a vertical incision on the uterus that extends into the active segment (fundal portion).

The type of anesthesia used for a cesarean delivery depends on the preferences and condition of the patient, the indication for cesarean section, the anesthesiologist, and the hospital. Options include general anesthesia with endotracheal intubation or regional anesthesia such as epidural or spinal anesthesia.

MANAGEMENT OF THE THIRD STAGE OF LABOR

The third stage of labor begins immediately after the delivery of the fetus and ends with the delivery of the placenta and fetal membranes. Usually the placenta separates within several minutes after delivery of the infant but can take as long as 30 minutes.

Delivery of the Placenta

It is important to wait for signs of placental separation before gently pulling on the umbilical cord. Excessive traction before placental separation can cause evulsion of the cord and may cause bleeding or uterine inversion. Clinical signs of placental separation include an apparent lengthening of the umbilical cord as the placenta descends, a gush of blood, and a rounding upward of the uterine fundus as the placenta is extruded into the lower uterine segment and vagina.

The placenta is delivered by *gently* pulling on the umbilical cord with one hand while the other hand is above the symphysis. Delivery of the placenta can be aided by having the patient bear down. As the placenta is being extruded, lift it upward to clear the vagina. If the membranes have not completely delivered, grasp

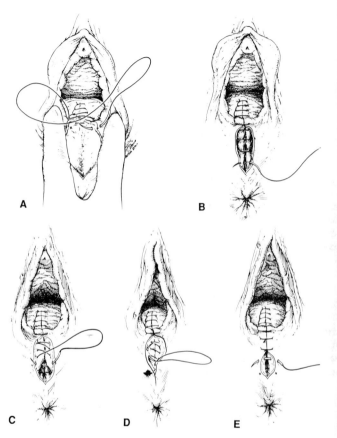

Figure 42–8. Repair of a miline episiotomy. *(Reproduced, with permission, from Cunningham FG, MacDonald PC, Gant NF:* Williams Obstetrics, *18th ed. Appleton & Lange, 1989.)*

them with a clamp and gently apply traction. Immediately after the delivery of the placenta, massage the uterine fundus until it is firm and bleeding is minimal. At this point, oxytocin can be given intravenously or intramuscularly to help maintain the uterus in a contracted state and thus minimize bleeding. If oxytocin is not effective in controlling uterine atony, methylergonovine maleate (Methergine) or 15-methyl prostaglandin $F_{2\alpha}$ may be used in appropriate patients.

The cervix and vagina should be inspected for lacerations. Lacerations are described as first, second, third, or fourth degree. A **first-degree laceration** involves the skin or vaginal mucosa but does not include the underlying muscle or fascia. A **second-degree laceration** also includes the fascia and muscles of the perineal body. A **third-degree laceration** involves the capsule and muscles of the anal sphincter. A **fourth-degree laceration** extends through the rectal mucosa.

Episiotomy Repair

Adequate anesthesia should be administered before attempting episiotomy or laceration repair. The choices of anesthesia include injection of a local anesthetic, such as lidocaine, a perineal dose of local anesthetic administered through the epidural catheter, a pudendal nerve block, or a saddle block.

Repair of a midline episiotomy is illustrated in Figure 42–8. The vaginal wall is first reapproximated to the level of the hymeneal ring (Figure 42–8A). The underlying deep fascia and submucosal layers of the perineum are repaired (Figures 42–8B and -8C). The skin is closed with a subcuticular stitch (Figure 42–8D). Rarely, the remainder of the incision may also be closed with interrupted sutures through the skin and subcutaneous fascia (Figure 42–8E).

SUGGESTED READING

Cunningham FG, MacDonald PC, Gant NF: *Williams Obstetrics,* 18th ed. Appleton & Lange, 1989.

Complications of Labor & Delivery | 43

Carol A. Major, MD

Abnormal labor is defined as any variation in the normal pattern of cervical dilatation or descent of the presenting fetal part. An abnormality in labor may be caused by the following: (1) dysfunctional uterine contractions, (2) fetal malpresentation or excessive size, or (3) abnormalities in the structure of the birth canal. Abnormalities of the first stage of labor complicate approximately 8–11% of all cephalic deliveries. Second-stage abnormalities are almost as common.

PATHOGENESIS

The identification of an abnormal labor requires an assessment of the **powers** (uterine function and expulsive efforts), the **passenger** (the fetus), and the **passage** (the pelvis).

Abnormalities of the Powers

An assessment of the power of the first stage of labor involves an evaluation of the force of the uterine contractions. The pressures generated with uterine contractions can be quantified with the introduction of an intrauterine pressure catheter. Uterine force may be measured by measuring the absolute amplitude of each contraction or by using Montevideo units (MVUs). Montevideo units are calculated by subtracing the baseline uterine pressure (8–12 mm Hg) from the peak contraction pressure for each contraction in a 10-minute period. The pressures generated for each uterine contraction are added and for a normal labor should be greater than 200.

Hypertonic uterine dysfunction is characterized by pain that is out of proportion to the intensity of the uterine contractions. The uterine contractions are uncoordinated and lack the fundal dominance that is a feature of normal contractions. They are ineffective in effacing or dilating the cervix. The management of this problem can involve the use of low-dose oxytocin or sedation.

Hypotonic uterine dysfunction occurs when the uterine contractions are less than 25 mm Hg in amplitude above baseline or if the MVUs are less than 200. If this is the case, oxytocin augmentation is indicated. The fetus should be continuously monitored during such augmentation.

Abnormalities of the Passenger

Assessment of the passenger consists of an evaluation of the fetus's presentation, position, and estimated fetal weight. Abnormal presentations account for a significant proportion of labor abnormalities.

A. Persistent Occiput Posterior: This is the most common cause for delay in the second stage of labor. Spontaneous rotation of the occiput to the anterior position occurs in approximately 95% of labors. Persistent occiput posterior usually occurs in a patient with transverse narrowing of the midplane of the pelvis, as in the anthropoid pelvis. It is also more common with conduction anesthesia. Management includes awaiting spontaneous delivery; manual rotation; forceps rotation (Scanzoni maneuver); and lower midpelvic delivery by forceps, vacuum extraction or cesarean section.

B. Transverse Arrests: This disorder occurs when the fetal head descends to the midpelvis with the widest diameter of the fetal head in the transverse position. It occurs more often in a platypelloid or android pelvis. Kielland's or Barton forceps may be used for traction to the vertex in the transverse diameter until the pelvic floor is reached. At this point, anterior rotation can be accomplished. Another option is cesarean section, when indicated.

C. Brow Presentation: This complication is rare. It is caused by inadequate flexion of the head. The usual course of labor with a brow presentation is conversion to an occiput or a face presentation (67%). If spontaneous conversion does not occur, then delivery by cesarean section may be indicated.

D. Face Presentation: Face presentations occur in approximately 1 in 500 deliveries. The cause for face presentation is essentially the same as for a brow presentation. A mentum posterior position in most cases can not be delivered vaginally. However, in many cases, a mentum posterior will spontaneously rotate to a mentum anterior and can be delivered vaginally.

E. Compound Presentation: Compound presentations occur when an extremity prolapses alongside the presenting part and both enter the pelvis simultaneously. The cause is unknown, although it is more common with premature infants. Cord prolapses occur in approximately 10% of these cases. The prolapsed extremity usually moves out of the way spontaneously. Extremity elevation may be done under double set up conditions.

F. Fetal Macrosomia: Macrosomia is defined as a fetal weight of greater than 4000 g. The major complication associated with macrosomia is arrested labor secondary to cephalopelvic disproportion. Arrested labors associated with this condition lead to an increased incidence of shoulder dystocia, operative vaginal deliveries and post partum complications.

G. Shoulder Dystocia: This complication occurs in 1.5 of every 1000 deliveries. When fetuses weigh more than 4000 g, the incidence increases to 17 in 1000 deliveries. The diagnosis is made when the anterior shoulder is wedged behind and obstructed by the pubic bone. The head is applied tightly to the perineum as if it were being pulled back by the shoulders. The management consists of proceeding immediately to delivery. All initial attempts to suction the infant's mouth and nose before delivery of its shoulders should be bypassed in an effort to prevent the baby from restituting and permitting the anterior shoulder to be wedged behind the pubic bone. Suprapubic pressure should be applied to dislodge the shoulder from behind the pubic bone, and the patient's hips should be flexed in an exaggerated fashion bringing the knees towards the chest (McRobert's maneuver) in an attempt to further open the pelvic outlet. A corkscrew maneuver (Wood's maneuver) may be attempted by applying pressure to the infant's back, and finally, the posterior arm may be delivered or deliberate clavicular fracture attempted. A last-effort maneuver is the Zavenelli maneuver, which involves replacement of the vertex back up through the vagina into the uterus and then subsequent delivery by cesarean section.

Abnormal development of the fetus may also contribute to abnormal labor patterns. Fetal tumors (eg, sacrococcygeal teratomas and fetal abdominal tumors) and fetal malformations (eg, hydrocephalus and cystic hygromas) may all lead to significant dystocia requiring cesarean section.

Abnormalities of the Passage

Pelvic abnormalities may be secondary to an actual narrowing in the dimensions of the pelvis or due to external compression of the passage way.

An **inlet contraction** should be suspected in cases of malpresentation and failure of the presenting part to engage. The antero-posterior diameter of the pelvis in such cases is usually less than 10 cm, and the transverse diameter is less than 12 cm.

A **midpelvic contraction** is characterized by converging side-walls and prominent spines. There is also a narrow sacrosciatic notch. The anteroposterior diameter is usually less than 11.5 cm and the transverse diameter is less than 9.5 cm.

An **outlet contraction** is almost always associated with a mid-pelvic contraction. This exists when the intertuberous diameter is less than 8 cm.

ABNORMALITIES OF THE FIRST STAGE OF LABOR

Each phase of labor can be complicated by faster than normal progress (**precipitous disorder**), slower than normal progress (**pro-traction disorder**), or complete cessation of progress (**arrest disor-der**). The diagnostic criteria and the management of various abnor-malities of the first stage of labor are described in detail below.

Precipitous Labor

Precipitous labor is defined as the completion of both the first and second stages of labor in 3 hours or less. The maximum slope of dilatation and descent in this labor abnormality is defined as being 5 cm/hour or more. There is no known cause of precipitous labor; however, it is known that its incidence increases with subse-quent pregnancies. The management of this labor abnormality in-cludes treatment with tocolytic agents, such as $MgSO_4$ or terbuta-line, to decrease the frequency and intensity of the uterine contractions. The hyperactive uterine contractions associated with precipitous labor may predispose patients to uterine rupture. Also the rapid passage of the fetus down the birth canal may lead to an increased incidence of intracranial bleeding in the fetus, postpar-tum hemorrhage, and shoulder dystocia.

Prolonged Latent Phase

Prolonged latent phase is defined as a latent phase that lasts longer than 20 hours in a primiparous patient and longer than 14 hours in a multiparous patient. Causes of this labor abnormality include the following: (1) an unfavorable cervix at the onset of labor, (2) ineffective contractions, (3) excessive sedation, (4) receiv-ing conduction anesthesia too early, and (5) being in false labor.

The management of a prolonged latent phase of labor may consist of artificial rupture of membranes (amniotomy); however, the beneficial effect of amniotomy is unproven and may predispose patients to amnionitis. Oxytocin, as well as prostaglandin E$_2$ gel, may also be beneficial in ripening the cervix and stimulating regular uterine contractions. Sedation with morphine or secobarbital for persistent ineffective contractions is sometimes helpful with this type of prodromal labor activity in that it provides a rest period and allows for relaxation for a few hours. The pediatricians should be notified at the time of delivery if these agents have been used.

Complications of labor associated with prolonged latent phase include amnionitis, postpartum hemorrhage, and water intoxication. The incidence of amnionitis is increased with increased duration of rupture of membranes and an increased number of cervical examinations. Both postpartum hemorrhage and water intoxication (due to the antidiuretic hormone effect of oxytocin) are usually secondary to prolonged oxytocin use. Contraindications to oxytocin use include fetal distress, placenta previa, placenta abruptio, and previous uterine surgery, which may predispose a patient to uterine rupture (eg, classical cesarean section or extensive myomectomy).

Protraction Disorders

A protracted active phase of dilatation is described when dilatation of the cervix occurs at a rate of less than 1.2 cm/hour in the primiparous patient and at a rate of less than 1.5 cm/hour in the multiparous patient. A **protracted descent** is defined when the descent of the presenting part occurs at rates of less than 1 cm/hour and 2 cm/hour in the primiparous and multiparous patients, respectively. Some of the most common causes of these protraction disorders are listed below:

(1) Fetopelvic disproportion (occurs in approximately one-third of patients).
(2) Malpresentation (eg, occiput posterior).
(3) Excessive sedation.
(4) Early rupture of membranes.
(5) Tumor (fetal or maternal) blocking the birth canal.
(6) Over distension of the uterus, secondary to multiple gestation or hydramnios.

The management of these disorders includes a systematic evaluation of the uterine forces, the fetal presentation, and the pelvic adequacy. The uterine forces are assessed in terms of the frequency, the intensity, and the duration of the uterine contractions. If the patient is in active labor and the presenting part is engaged, an amniotomy may sometimes improve the quality of the uterine contractions. An intrauterine pressure catheter is used to measure the forces of the uterine contractions. If these forces are found to be inadequate, the use of oxytocin is recommended. A careful pelvic examination is useful in determining the fetal position, presentation, and lie as well as in assessing the various pelvic dimensions that may be responsible for the labor abnormality. The complications of the protraction disorders are similar to those of a prolonged latent phase.

Arrest Disorders

An **arrest of dilatation** and **arrest of descent** in the patient are defined as the cessation of cervical dilatation for 2 hours or more in the active phase and the cessation of progressive descent for 1 hour or more after the beginning of the descent process of labor. Fetopelvic disproportion accounts for 50% of arrested labors. Malpresentations of the fetus, such as persistent occiput posterior, brow, and face presentations, may also be responsible for arrests during labor. The use of regional anesthesia and excessive sedation, which sometimes lead to ineffective pushing efforts, have also been shown to be responsible for a small percentage of arrests during labor.

The management of this labor abnormality again includes an evaluation of the powers, the passenger, and the passage. An amniotomy, as well as the use of oxytocin, may improve the quality of the uterine contractions and thus may be an appropriate treatment for this labor abnormality. An assisted operative vaginal delivery with vacuum extraction or forceps may be attempted for arrests of descent if all of the criteria for a safe operative vaginal delivery are met (see below).

ABNORMALITIES OF THE SECOND STAGE OF LABOR

Full dilatation signifies the second stage of labor. Abnormalities of this stage are often the result of abnormalities of descent of the presenting part. During the second stage, normal descent occurs at a rate of greater than 1 cm/hour in primiparous patients. The mean duration of the second stage in a primiparous patient is

50 minutes. Normal descent during the second stage of labor in a multiparous patient is greater than 2 cm/hour with the mean being 20 minutes. An epidural anesthetic may appreciably reduce maternal expulsive efforts and forces and, as a result, lead to a delay in the descent of the presenting part and spontaneous rotation. As a consequence, epidural anesthesia may lead to an overall increase in the length of the second stage of labor. Occasionally, in cases such as these, the pain relief effects of the epidural are allowed to diminish before the patient is allowed to push. Also, in certain cases, the patient is allowed an extended time to complete the second stage of labor as long as the fetus continues to make some progress in descent. Because of the increase in extended second stages of labor, there is an increased incidence of deliveries by forceps, vacuum and cesarean sections.

Forceps & Vacuum Extraction

Forceps and the vacuum extractor are designed to facilitate delivery. Indications for an operative vaginal delivery include the presence of inadequate expulsive forces secondary to maternal exhaustion or the use of regional anesthesia. Abnormal presentations of the fetus can also result in the need for forceps or a vacuum extractor. In many cases, the second stage of labor needs to be shortened because of maternal medical problems, such as heart disease or vascular diseases or because of fetal problems, such as fetal distress.

The following criteria must be met before forceps or vacuum extraction is used:

(1) The fetal weight and the pelvic size must be adequately estimated.
(2) The fetal head must be engaged.
(3) The cervix must be completely dilated.
(4) The position and station of the fetus must be correctly identified.
(5) The bladder must be emptied.
(6) The patient must have adequate anesthesia.
(7) An appropriate indication for an operative vaginal delivery must exist.
(8) The operator must be experienced with and knowledgeable of the procedure.

Several complications are associated with the use of forceps and vacuum extraction. However, as long as the above conditions are met and the operator is skilled in the use of the instruments, these complications are rare. The maternal complications include lacerations of the vagina, vulva, and cervix as well as injury to the bladder or rectum. Rupture of the uterus has also been reported. The fetal complications associated with operative vaginal deliveries include cephalohematomas, skull fractures, and intracranial injuries. Soft tissue lacerations and peripheral nerve injuries are also potential complications.

Breech Presentation

Breech presentation occurs in approximately 25% of deliveries that take place at 28 weeks of gestation, whereas at term, the incidence of breech presentation is 3–4%. It is the most common abnormal presentation. Predisposing fetal factors that may lead to a breech presentation include hydrocephaly, anencephaly, prematurity, polyhydramnios, multiple gestation, and congenital anomalies. In fact, congenital anomalies are associated with approximately 6% of all breech presentations. The maternal factors associated with a breech presentation include placenta previa, uterine anomalies, and pelvic anomalies. The overall perinatal mortality rate is 3 times higher with a breech presentation compared with a vertex presentation.

The 3 different types of breech presentations are described below:

(1) **Frank breech** (70% of all breech presentations): They are characterized by flexion at the hips and extension at the knees with the lower extremities adjacent to the abdomen and thorax.
(2) **Complete breech** (5% of all breech presentations): They are characterized by flexion at the hips and flexion at the knees.
(3) **Footling breech** (25% of all breech presentations): They are characterized by flexion at the hips with extension at one or both of the knees. In these cases, the presenting part is either one or both of the feet.

The management of a breech presentation may include performing an external version, awaiting for spontaneous conversion to a vertex presentation, performing cesarean section, or attempting a vaginal breech delivery. The risks of a vaginal breech delivery include cord accidents, head entrapment, birth injury, and birth asphyxia. Cord prolapse occurs 20 times more often in footling breech presentations than in vertex presentations. Frank breech and vertex presentations have a comparable rate of cord prolapse. The criteria for performing a vaginal breech delivery are as follows:

(1) The pelvic adequacy must be determined by either a clinical evaluation or preferably by computed tomographic (CT) pelvimetry. Adequate CT pelvimetry measurements include an anteroposterior (inlet) diameter of 11–12 cm, a transverse (inlet) diameter of 11–12 cm, and an interspinous (midpelvis) diameter of 10 cm.

(2) The estimated fetal weight must be between 2500 and 3500 g.

(3) The fetal head must not be hyperextended.

(4) There must be normal progress in labor.

(5) The fetal heart rate tracing must be reactive without any signs of fetal distress.

(6) Adequate anesthesia (preferably a regional anesthetic) must be available.

(7) An experienced obstetrician should be present.

(8) Oxytocin augmentation is not contraindicated.

External version is a maneuver for converting breech or any other abnormal presentation to cephalic presentation. It is performed before the onset of labor, usually between 36 and 38 weeks of gestation. Ultrasonography is necessary to determine the fetal position, the absence of congenital anomalies, the amount of amniotic fluid, and the location of the placenta. The procedure is usually performed under intermittent ultrasonographic assessment.

Before the procedure begins, a tocolytic agent is given to relax the uterus. Thereafter, gentle abdominal pressure is used to elevate the breech and deflect the head towards the pelvis. The fetal cardiac motion and rate are evaluated intermittently during the procedure with the use of ultrasound. External version must be performed in a location where a rapid operative delivery can be performed if necessary.

The presence of a multiple gestation, a placenta previa, an anomalous fetus, a uterine anomaly, a previous classical cesarean section, a macrosomic fetus, or a fetus with intrauterine growth retardation is a contraindication to external version. Previous uterine surgery (eg, simple myomectomies and low transverse cesarean sections), oligohydramnios, and active labor are relative contraindications to external version. The complications associated with external versions include placental abruption, premature rupture of the membranes, cord accidents, fetal injuries, and fetal distress.

ABNORMALITIES OF THE THIRD STAGE OF LABOR

Postpartum hemorrhage occurs in approximately 5-8% of all term deliveries. The most common causes are listed below:

(1) Uterine atony, which may be secondary to prolonged labor, uterine distention, or excessive anesthesia. Atony accounts for more than 90% of the cases of postpartum hemorrhage.
(2) Laceration of the birth canal.
(3) Complications with separation of the placenta (accreta).
(4) Retained fragments of placenta.
(5) Placenta previa.
(6) Inversion or rupture of the uterus.
(7) Tumors of the uterus or cervix.
(8) Hematologic disorder.

Postpartum hemorrhage is usually diagnosed when the amount of blood lost is equivalent to 1% or more of the body weight. Generally accepted standards for blood loss include 500 mL for a vaginal delivery and 1000 mL for a cesarean section. Management includes identification and repair of any visible lacerations; manual removal of the placenta, if indicated; bimanual uterine massage; the use of oxytocin, methylergonovine maleate, or prostaglandin, and curettage of the uterus if necessary.

The cause of a retained placenta is usually unknown. Separation of the placenta, or the third stage of labor, normally occurs within 30 minutes after delivery, secondary to forceful uterine contractions. The management of a retained placenta consists of gentle cord traction with suprapubic pressure or manual removal. If either of these techniques fails, the placenta may be removed with curettage. Rarely, placenta accreta occurs, a condition in which the villi are attached directly to the myometrium, thus preventing separation. This condition may require a hysterectomy to control the bleeding.

Uterine inversion may occur secondary to excessive traction on the umbilical cord when the placenta is implanted in the fundus. The incidence increases when marked uterine relaxation occurs as a result of administration of tocolytics or anesthetic agents. It occurs in approximately 1 in 15,000 deliveries. The diagnosis can be established by recognition of the following events:

(1) Protrusion of the inverted uterus out of the vagina with the placenta still attached.
(2) Profuse vaginal bleeding.

(3) Profound maternal shock secondary to vagal stimulation.

(4) Severe abdominal pain.

The management of a uterine inversion involves the removal of the placenta and the repositioning of the uterus. The uterus is usually replaced by using the fist or the fingers to replace the uterus. Adequate anesthesia is recommended. An inhalation anesthetic, such as halothane, will also relax the uterus. Infusion of intravenous fluids should be at maximum. Atropine can be beneficial in relieving the shock. After the uterus has been replaced, the patient is given either oxytocin or methylergonovine maleate. An abdominal approach may be necessary in replacing the uterus.

SUGGESTED READINGS

American College of Obstetricians and Gynecologists. Dystocia. *ACOG Technical Bulletin* No. 137, 1989.

Bottoms SF, Hirsch VJ, Sokol RJ: Medical management of arrest disorders of labor: A current overview. *Am J Obstet Gynecol* 1987;**156**:935.

Friedman EA: *Labor: Clinical Evaluation and Management,* 2nd ed. Appleton-Century-Crofts, 1978.

Sokol RJ et al: Normal and abnormal progress: I. A quantitative assessment and survey of the literature. *J Reprod Med* 1977;**18**:47.

44 | Postpartum Care

Thomas J. Musci, MD

The **puerperium** is defined as the period of time immediately after childbirth through the sixth week postpartum. This period is marked by dramatic changes in the anatomy and physiology of the postpartum patient. Providing optimal care for the obstetric patient during the puerperium depends on a thorough understanding of these changes. In addition to the anatomic restructuring of various organ systems, the postpartum period presents new demands on maternal physiology in order, for example, to accommodate lactation, restore maternal iron stores, and reestablish the pituitary-ovarian axis. Along with special attention to physiologic changes, the obstetrician must also be aware of the social and psychological adaptations required of the patient and her family during the postpartum period.

INVOLUTION

Involution is the process of regressive change in the anatomy of the female genital organs and other systems from the maximally altered term pregnant state to a condition that resembles a nearly prepregnant state.

Uterine Changes
A. Placental Site: Rapid decrease in volume of the uterine cavity after delivery causes shearing off of the placenta. The placental attachment site in the decidual bed shrinks to approximately one-half its original diameter. Contraction of arterial smooth muscle and uterine smooth muscle causes compression of the vessels supplying the placental bed, thereby achieving mechanical hemostasis. Vessels become thrombosed and a classic inflammatory response occurs in the arteries and veins. Obliterated veins are sloughed with the remainder of the necrotic decidua.
B. Endometrium: Between 7 and 10 days after delivery,

several characteristic events take place that lead to the regeneration of the endometrium:

(1) Inflammatory (normally not infectious) infiltration (polymorphonuclear leukocytes, lymphocytes) of the placental site, endometrium, and superficial myometrium.
(2) Decidual necrosis (superficial layer).
(3) Proliferation of endometrial gland remnants from basal decidua.

C. Corpus: A 10-fold reduction in the mass of the uterus takes place in approximately 6 weeks as the uterus decreases from the pregnant weight of 1000 g to the normal nonpregnant weight of 100 g. Although the total number of muscle cells does not diminish, other aspects of this process of cytoplasmic reduction are poorly understood. The uterine fundus is still palpable abdominally 2 weeks after delivery. Following this time, it recedes into the true pelvis and is palpable only on bimanual examination. By 6 weeks, the uterus should be about prepregnant size.

D. Cervix: After vaginal delivery, the cervix is thin, and floppy, and the os remains open. Restoration of a cervical isthmus, and internal os and thickening of the cervix require approximately 1–2 weeks. The hyperplasia and hypertrophy of the glands of the cervical epithelium regress within 6 weeks. The bruising and lacerations seen in the immediate postpartum examination result in a permanent change in the appearance of the parous cervix. It is characterized by a somewhat thicker outer surface and lateral depressions on visual examination.

Vagina

The vaginal epithelium seen in the pregnant vagina is smooth and has diminished ruggae compared with the epithelium in the nonpregnant state. After vaginal delivery the vaginal vault itself is enlarged and probably does not revert to its prepregnant dimensions. However, the vaginal epithelium does resume its ruggated appearance by approximately 2–3 weeks.

Urinary System

A. Urinary Tract: The anatomic changes of the urinary tract that accompany pregnancy are predominantly marked by the dilatation of the ureters and renal pelves, thought to occur as a consequence of compression of the ureters by adjacent vessels and not by the enlarging uterus. Progesterone, which becomes markedly elevated above nonpregnant levels, may contribute to this to a small degree because of its effects on decreasing smooth muscle tone. On the basis of ultrasound studies of postpartum patients performed 6 weeks after delivery, the pregnancy-related dilatation of the collecting system returns to the prepregnant state by the sixth week in most patients. The specific details of this change over time are unknown. It is also generally accepted that the immediate postpartum bladder is in a relative state of hypotonia. Whether this condition is due solely to trauma and resulting edema from labor and delivery or to additional factors is not known. It is thought that the inhibitory effects of conduction anesthesia may leave the postpartum patient at higher risk for urinary retention and urinary tract infection. The use of epidural anesthesia and prolonged labor have been found to transiently diminish bladder function.

B. Renal Function: The characteristic changes seen in renal function during pregnancy are as follows: a 50% increase in glomerular filtration and in creatinine clearance and a biphasic change in renal plasma flow (25% increase in early pregnancy diminishing toward term and dropping below normal for up to several months). Glomerular filtration rate and creatinine clearance return to normal by the eighth week.

Ovarian Function

Elevated serum prolactin levels in postpartum patients who are lactating delay the resumption of ovulation. In nonlactating patients, elevated postpartum prolactin levels fall into the normal range by about 3 weeks postpartum, and ovulation has been shown to occur as early as 27 days postpartum (mean time to ovulation = 70 days). Estrogen levels drop significantly immediately after delivery and, in those patients who are lactating, remain suppressed throughout the period of nursing. Although follicle-stimulating hormone (FSH) levels are identical in both lactating and nonlactating patients, it is thought that the ovary is unresponsive to FSH in the presence of high prolactin levels. It has long been recognized that lactation, in terms of its suppression of ovulation, can work as a ''natural contraceptive'' for postpartum patients. However, pregnancy can occur while lactating in as many as 25% of patients within 12 months of delivery and can occur without a preceding menstrual period.

Hematologic & Cardiovascular Changes

The puerperal period is associated with an increased risk of thromboembolism, especially in patients having undergone cesarean section. The pregnancy-associated changes in the coagulation system (the so-called hypercoagulable state) combined with factors such as vessel wall injury and venous stasis contribute to this increased risk. Increased levels of fibrinogen and of factors VII through X, gradually return to normal levels by approximately 2 weeks postpartum.

During pregnancy the average increase in maternal blood volume above nonpregnant levels is about 45–50%. This increase results from an increase in both plasma and erythrocyte volume. In spite of this augmentation in erythrocyte production, the mean concentration of hemoglobin and the hematocrit decrease slightly during normal pregnancy (average hemoglobin concentration is 12.1 g/dL). This decrease has been referred to as the physiologic anemia of pregnancy. Unless the patient has had an unusually large amount of blood loss associated with delivery, postpartum hemoglobin and hematocrit values in a patient who has taken iron supplements during pregnancy should follow a predictable course. Immediately after delivery, total blood volume decreases, resulting in an overall blood loss with a subsequent mild hemodilution caused by mobilization of extravascular fluid. Hematocrit and hemoglobin values significantly lower than labor admission values probably indicate a considerable intrapartum blood loss. Within one week of delivery, plasma volume decreases to levels approximating nonpregnant values. At this point hemoglobin values should accurately reflect the maternal state. Any excess circulating hemoglobin above nonpregnant levels are used for iron stores. Conversely, low levels indicate the net result of pregnancy, and specific therapy may need to be instituted (see below).

CLINICAL MANAGEMENT

Immediate Postpartum Care

The period of observation immediately after delivery is directed at assuring a stable maternal physiologic state. First and foremost is the assessment of consciousness, airway and respiration, blood pressure, and amount of vaginal bleeding. To a certain degree, this level of monitoring in the postpartum recovery period will depend on whether the delivery was achieved operatively with the use of anesthesia or whether complications occurred during delivery. After delivery of the placenta, the uterus must remain firm, and its fundus should be palpable approximately at the level of the umbilicus. A firm (compressed) uterus will ensure a minimal amount of continued uterine blood loss, and if compression is not maintained spontaneously, it should be achieved by manual massage through the abdomen or by intravenous or intramuscular administration of oxytocin. Excess bleeding resulting from atony of the uterus will require additional measures, such as the administration of uterotonic agents (eg, methylergonovine maleate or prostaglandins) and in some cases surgical intervention.

In-Hospital Care

Most patients spend the immediate postpartum period in the hospital. The period of rest and observation in the hospital after an uncomplicated vaginal delivery has been reduced in recent years to about 24–48 hours. In cases of cesarean section, an uncomplicated postoperative course usually necessitates at least a 3-day stay. Shortening of the postpartum hospital stay has mostly been inspired by economic factors; however, in the majority of cases a prolonged hospital stay is not warranted.

In recent years, an important part of in-hospital postpartum care has focused on facilitating parent-infant bonding and establishing rudimentary breast feeding and infant care skills in the primipara. Consequently, many postpartum units now provide infant rooming-in with the parent unless either patient requires special care or observation.

A. Perineal Care: Because many patients either have episiotomy or vulvar or perineal lacerations at delivery, special attention to the care of the perineum is necessary. The major yet simple goal of puerperal perineal care is cleanliness and maintenance of intact sutures at repair sites. The perineum should be inspected periodically throughout the stay for wound breakdown or early infection. Patients should be instructed on methods of frequent cleaning, and in the immediate period after delivery, application of ice packs can help minimize swelling and discomfort. In the USA most episiotomies performed are the midline variety, and provided there is no hematoma or extensive bruising, complete healing should require about 3 weeks. Analgesics, such as acetaminophen with codeine, are usually all that is required in the first few days for pain control. In patients that have third- or fourth-degree extension of midline episiotomies or mediolateral episiotomies, more potent analgesics may be needed in the immediate postpartum period. In addition, the use of stool softeners helps diminish pain on defecation and may minimize anal mucosal trauma in cases of fourth-degree lacerations. Excess perineal pain that is unresponsive to previously instituted measures of cold sitz baths and analgesics may signal a hemorrhagic or infectious complication and necessitates a careful examination of the vagina, perineum, and rectum.

B. Vaginal Bleeding or Lochia: The continued sloughing of decidual tissue from the uterine cavity is evident as vaginal bleeding and is known as lochia. Immediately postpartum vaginal flow may be moderate, mimicking the flow of a menstrual period, and it is bloody **(lochia rubra).** The amount of lochia should be carefully followed during the first day postpartum, and excess flow should alert the clinician to the possibility of unnoticed vaginal or cervical lacerations. Three to 5 days postpartum the lochia becomes less frankly bloody and is called **lochia serosa.** Malodorous or purulent vaginal discharge is a hallmark of postpartum genital tract infection and may precede any other objective findings. Several days after delivery the lochia usually becomes pale and is referred to as **lochia alba.** Patients should be told that lochia may persist for up to 5 weeks in total. A short episode of increased bleeding at about 2 weeks may merely indicate a sloughing of material from the old placental site and is generally not indicative of any problem.

C. Uterine Cramping: Within the first 3 days after delivery, increased uterine tonicity may be appreciated as pain, especially in the multiparous patient. The uterus often contracts vigorously at intervals, and even if these contractions are not associated with retained products of conception or infection, analgesia may be required. If the patient is breast feeding, she may perceive increased uterine cramping at the time of suckling. This cramping is common and is probably caused by the release of oxytocin with the milk letdown reflex.

D. Early Ambulation: Unless there is a concomitant medical condition that contraindicates ambulation, patients should be strongly encouraged to walk soon after delivery. Early ambulation postpartum is important because it has been shown to decrease the incidence of thrombosis and pulmonary embolism during the puerperium, which is the period of highest risk associated with pregnancy.

Postpartum Follow-Up

The postpartum visit is usually scheduled 4–6 weeks after delivery, unless there has been an antenatal or postpartum complication. In certain instances, home visits by visiting nurses may be required for monitoring and assistance with procedures such as wound care, blood pressure checks, or insulin management, but these are special circumstances. More important, patients should be educated to report problems by telephone and should not be given the sense that they have no medical recourse for 4–6 weeks. Problems such as delayed postpartum bleeding, late puerperal infection, and severe depression will be evident long before the first postpartum visit.

A. Physical Activity: Provided that delivery has been uncomplicated, there is no reason to medically limit physical activity or exercise at discharge. Fatigue is a common experience when caring for a newborn infant, and patients will certainly self-limit activity within their own capacity. However, prolonged lethargy and fatigue may be associated with depression or thyroid dysfunction and should not necessarily be dismissed as normal.

B. Sexual Activity: Little scientific evidence is available to help with recommendations for resumption of intercourse postpartum. In general, most practitioners recommend that reestablishment of sexual relations should be guided by the extent of vaginal and perineal trauma at delivery and by the duration of postpartum vaginal bleeding. It is unlikely that there is increased risk associated with intercourse within a few weeks of delivery, although in practice only a small percentage of patients resume intercourse within 6 weeks of delivery. The length of time until normal libido returns varies considerably. In addition, women who choose to breast feed may experience vaginal atrophy (associated with decreased estrogen levels), leading to vaginal dryness and discomfort during intercourse. If this is the only reason for decreased interest, vaginal lubricating modalities can be safely used. For some patients a convenient and effective method of contraception will alleviate some of the hesitancy to resume normal sexual activity.

C. Weight Loss and Dietary Considerations: On average the immediate postpartum period is associated with a 5.2-kg (12-lb) weight loss, accounted for by infant, uterine contents, and fluid loss. There is a gradual loss of body fluid over the next several weeks. In general, a normal diet is recommended with the added nutritional considerations specific to breast feeding. In practice, most patients are continued on iron and vitamin supplementation for at least a month postpartum, longer if breast feeding. Excess weight gained during pregnancy in the form of fat requires special dietary attention and can be addressed even while breast feeding.

LACTATION

Over the last 20 years the attitudes toward breast feeding in Western countries has dramatically shifted from one of little interest and even negativism to one of enthusiasm and encouragement of its practice. Now there is little doubt about the overwhelming advantages of breast feeding, not only for the health of the infant and enhancement of maternal-infant interaction but also for its practical attributes, such as decreased expense and increased convenience over formula feedings. The increased popularity of breast feeding is greatest among upper income and highly educated groups. It has now become the responsibility of the entire health care team to educate and encourage new mothers in the practice.

Milk Production

Nursing can begin as soon after delivery as practicality permits. Early suckling is beneficial in achieving successful breast feeding and maternal-infant bonding and provides the newborn with the immunological benefits of colostrum. Successful breast feeding does not necessarily come naturally to infant or mother, so attention to proper techniques and scheduled suckling within the first few days is important. One such schedule would be as follows: 5 minutes per breast per feeding on day 1, 10 minutes on day 2, and 15 minutes or more thereafter. **Colostrum** secretion generally lasts for the first 2–5 days postpartum. In addition to antibodies, colostrum contains complement, macrophages, lymphocytes, lactoferrin, lactoperoxidase, and lysozyme, all of which are beneficial for host resistance. Production of colostrum or milk may appear to be minimal or insufficient early on. Patients should be encouraged to persist with breast feeding because continued suckling increases production. They should be reassured that lack of colostrum or milk production within the first few days is not a problem for the newborn.

Gradually there is a conversion to mature milk production. Human milk has a high content of lactose and contains unique proteins, amino acids (essential and nonessential), fatty acids, vitamins, and minerals. All vitamins except vitamin K are present in human milk. Vitamin K administration to the newborn shortly after delivery is therefore beneficial. While human milk has a relatively low concentration of iron, it seems to be more readily absorbed than does cow milk. The regulation of iron content in milk takes place in the mammary glands and is not reflective of maternal stores. Table 44–1 compares the level of nutrients in human colostrum, in human milk, and in cow milk.

The initial breast engorgement seen in early postpartum patients is due to vascular and lymphatic congestion and increased tension in the milk ducts. This normal physiologic state of lacta-

Table 44-1. Approximate concentrations (per mL) of components of human colostrum, human mature milk, and cow milk.[1]

	Human Colostrum	Human Mature Milk	Cow Milk
Water (g)	—	88	88
Lactose (g)	5.3	6.8	5.0
Protein (g)	2.7	1.2	3.3
Casein:lactalbumin ratio	—	1:2	3:1
Fat (g)	2.9	3.8	3.7
Linoleic acid	—	8.3% of fat	1.6% of fat
Potassium (mg)	55	55	58
Sodium (mg)	92	15	138
Chloride (mg)	117	43	103
Calcium (mg)	31	33	125
Magnesium (mg)	4	4	12
Phosphorus (mg)	14	15	100
Iron (mg)	0.09[2]	0.15[2]	0.10[2]
Vitamin A (μg)	89	53	34
Vitamin D (μg)	—	0.03[2]	0.06[2]
Thiamine (μg)	15	16	42
Riboflavin (μg)	30	43	157
Nicotinic acid (μg)	75	172	85
Ascorbic acid (μg)	4.4[3]	4.3[3]	1.6[3]

[1] Reproduced, with permission, from Edwards (editor): Res Reprod, vol 6, 1974.
[2] Poor source.
[3] Just adequate. *From Edwards (ed): Res Reprod, vol 6, 1974.*

tion is often associated with pain. In most cases, this engorgement occurs within 2–4 days postpartum and, in the common situation in which hospital discharge is early, occurs at home. Patients can be advised to practice round-the-clock demand feedings and to apply hot compresses before nursing to help alleviate discomfort.

Milk production in a normal healthy mother engaged in breast feeding a healthy infant ranges from 600 to 900 mL per day. This level of production requires about 600 kcal per day from maternal stores or diet. It is for this reason that normal women who have been well nourished store about 5 kg of excess fat during pregnancy. A well-balanced diet should, with the exception of calcium and iron, provide all the recommended nutrients for a mother during lactation. The composition of breast milk is minimally influenced by maternal diet, except for fat content. A diet rich in animal fat will be reflected in breast milk with a high content of saturated fats. The converse is also true with a diet that contains predominantly polyunsaturated fats. The levels of specific vitamins can be affected in cases of severe maternal vitamin deficiencies. However, in the case of a well-balanced diet, breast milk vitamin content is not influenced by maternal ingestion, and the need for vitamin supplementation is not well established.

Contraindications

Contraindications to breast feeding are few. The high chance of transmitting infectious viral agents through breast milk make certain disease or carrier states contraindications to breast feeding, for example, human immunodeficiency virus positivity, active hepatitis B infection (eg, e antigenemia) and acute hepatitis. In addition, the maternal use of certain medications, their transfer into breast milk, and potential effects on the newborn contraindicate breast feeding. Examples of such drugs are cyclophosphamide, radiopharmaceuticals, tetracycline, chloramphenicol, warfarin, and lithium. This list is not exhaustive, and each case needs to be evaluated using a current reference on the effects of specific drugs on nursing infants. In general, the concentration of a drug in breast milk, while influenced by many factors, is usually less than or equal to that in the maternal plasma. Thus, the amount ingested by the infant through the breast milk is small in most cases.

Of the few complications of breast feeding, **peurperal mastitis** is the most common. Among all pregnancies, its incidence is low, although accurate data are not available. Mastitis occurs in two forms: epidemic, which occurs in hospitalized women during a nursery staphylococcal outbreak, and the more common form, endemic, which occurs sporadically in nonhospitalized nursing mothers. The disease is characterized by a lobular cellulitis of the periglandular tissue with or without irritation or fissures of the nipple. The common constellation of signs and symptoms include fever, myalgias, area of pain and redness in a V-shape on the breast, and cracking of the nipple. The most common pathogens are *Staphylococcus aureus,* and group A and group B streptococci. Recent data indicate that early treatment with antibiotics helps resolve mastitis within 24–48 hours with a low incidence of abscess formation. In untreated patients breast abcess develops often. In early mastitis, oral antibiotic therapy should be initiated with a penicillinase-resistant penicillin. Additional measures should include analgesics, ice packs, and breast support. Mastitis is not a contraindication to continued breast feeding, and patients often need to be reassured that the newborn will not develop a systemic infection. The continued expression of milk may even help resolve the infection more promptly. Because the nipple and breast on the affected side may be tender, attention to adequate analgesia is important.

Inhibition & Suppression of Lactation

A consideration of lactation suppression is necessary for those patients who cannot or will not breast feed. For whatever reason, when a patient is not going to breast feed, specific measures are used to eliminate the possibility of painful engorgement of the breasts. The simplest initial method is to avoid suckling or expression of milk, thereby allowing the natural inhibition of prolactin secretion to cause breast gland involution. In about half of patients, this method is effective, and painful engorgement is not encountered. For those that develop symptoms, breast binding, ice packs, and analgesics are required. The key is not to stimulate the breasts to produce more milk. Alternative pharmacologic methods can be used to suppress lactation. The currently preferred drug is bromocriptine. Bromocriptine, a peptide ergot alkaloid, is a dopamine receptor agonist that inhibits the release of prolactin. The usual regimen is 2.5 mg twice a day for 2 weeks and is effective in eliminating painful breast engorgement. Less than 10% of patients experience a rebound lactation when the drug is discontinued. However, this rebound reaction is more frequent when the duration of therapy is shorter than 14 days. Mild side effects seen in less than 5% of patients include nausea, headache, and nasal congestion. **Orthostatic hypotension,** a more serious effect, is rare but has been seen with the use of higher doses. Bromocriptine is effective in suppressing lactation once lactation has been initiated and remains the drug of choice for women who must discontinue nursing for any reason.

POSTPARTUM COMPLICATIONS

Although the immediate postpartum period is usually uneventful, with normal physiologic and anatomic changes proceeding smoothly, this period can be marked by serious medical complications. The more common complications are discussed below.

Postpartum Hemorrhage

Postpartum hemorrhage is defined as a total blood loss of more than 500 mL at delivery or within the first 24 hours postpartum. Given that the placental bed receives about 600 mL/min of blood flow, acute and excess blood loss can occur rapidly with any significant delay of uterine contraction following placental separation. Uterine atony, or failure of the uterus to contract effectively after delivery, is the most common cause of postpartum hemorrhage. In addition, incomplete or partial separation of the placenta, with portions retained within the uterus, also contribute to this life-threatening complication. Other causes of postpartum hemorrhage include soft tissue lacerations (cervical, vaginal, or perineal), uterine rupture, and uterine inversion.

Initial medical management should include a rapid infusion of intravenous fluid with 20–40 units of oxytocin per liter of isotonic saline solution. The second drug of choice is an intramuscular injection of ergonovine, an ergot alkaloid and potent myometrial constrictor, unless the patient is hypertensive, which is a contraindication to using this drug. If further medical management is required, 15-methyl prostaglandin $F_{2\alpha}$ intramuscularly or intramyometrially, can be used in patients with no history of bronchospasm. Uterine atony and persistent bleeding refractory to medical management often require surgical intervention, which usually involves ligation of the uterine or hypogastric arteries.

Puerperal Infections

Classically, postpartum febrile morbidity is defined as an oral temperature of 38 °C or greater on any 2 of the first 10 days after delivery, exclusive of the first 24 hours. While the most common cause of febrile morbidity in the postpartum period is infection of the genital tract, most commonly endometritis, other causes include infection of the urinary tract or episiotomy site, mastitis, or complications of anesthesia. Currently, the overall incidence of endomyometritis approaches 2% after vaginal deliveries and approximately 30% after cesarean sections, with the severity of infection highest after abdominal delivery.

Predisposing factors that increase the chance of puerperal infection have been studied and reported extensively. These factors include length of labor and duration of rupture of membranes, retained products of conception, vaginal colonization with group A or group B streptococci, abdominal delivery, and socioeconomic status. Other factors that may be important include number of vaginal examinations during labor, intrauterine manipulation of fetus or placenta, anemia, and lower genital tract lacerations.

The principle clinical features of endomyometritis are fever, malaise, abdominal pain, uterine tenderness, and purulent or foul-smelling lochia. Not all patients will have the complete clinical picture. Additional laboratory work should include white blood cell count, blood cultures, and, if possible, a uterine culture obtained through a catheter designed to eliminate vaginal or cervical contamination. With appropriate antibiotic therapy, the majority of patients with endomyometritis after vaginal delivery will improve within a few days, and overall response rate to initial drug therapy should be at least 95%. Although many drug regimens are available, those that address the polymicrobial nature of the disease, including anaerobic organisms, should be used. A second- or third-generation cephalosporin alone is usually effective, with a minority of patients requiring a multiple antibiotic regimen.

In patients with uterine infection after cesarean section, there may be a larger contribution from anaerobic organisms that underscores the need for an antibiotic regimen that treats both aerobic and anaerobic bacteria. In practice, this means treatment with drugs such as clindamycin with gentamicin or a later-generation cephalosporin or a penicillin derivative that has extended anaerobic coverage; the response rates of these drugs is about 90%. If therapy with drugs from these categories are not successful, the clinician must then search for known causes of failure such as pelvic abscess, pelvic hematoma, or septic pelvic thrombophlebitis.

In addition to the uterus, the abdominal incision is another common site of infection. Low-grade fever and local skin erythema around the wound should alert the clinician to the possibility of early wound abscess with or without cellulitis. Should infection be identified, the incision should be reopened widely, debrided, and treated with local cleaning measures. Intravenous antibiotics are usually not needed in these circumstances unless advanced cellulitis or necrotizing fasciitis has developed. In this latter rare occurrence, extensive surgical debridement is required.

Thromboembolic Disease

The incidence of venous thromboembolism is more than 5 times greater during pregnancy than in the nonpregnant state. It is the leading nonobstetrical cause of postpartum death but is a disease in which early detection and treatment can greatly improve outcome. The incidence in the postpartum period is about 3 times greater than in the antepartum period. It is thus important to know the signs and symptoms of deep vein thrombosis so that early diagnosis can be achieved.

In the puerperium the appearance of deep venous thrombosis is most often seen within 3 days postpartum but may occur as late as one month after delivery. The progression to pulmonary embolism, an event associated with a 15% mortality rate, occurs in about 24% of patients that are not treated. In patients that have recognized deep vein thrombosis and receive anticoagulant therapy, pulmonary embolism occurs in only 4–5%, with a less than 1% mortality rate. The need for early detection and treatment cannot be overstated.

The most accurate and precise test for deep vein thrombosis is the venogram. Venography can detect at least 95% of venous thromboses and provides information about exact location and size. Initial management steps include elevation of the extremity to improve venous flow and to alleviate discomfort. Most important, however, is the institution of continuous intravenous heparin anticoagulation therapy. Heparin has the advantage of allowing rapid adjustments in dose to achieve therapeutic levels and its structure prevents it from entering the breast milk, which is an advantage for patients wishing to continue breast feeding. Continuous intravenous heparin therapy is continued for 7–10 days or until symptoms have abated and there is no evidence of recurrence. Thereafter, long-term anticoagulation is continued generally for about 4 weeks with either subcutaneous heparin or oral sodium warfarin therapy.

Pulmonary embolism is heralded by the onset of dyspnea and tachypnea. In many patients pleuritic chest pain, cough, tachycardia, and apprehension may also be evident. Additionally, about one-third of patients experience hemoptysis or fever. In the patient already being treated for deep vein thrombosis, the onset of these signs signal embolization, usually of small clots to the lung periphery. In the patient without symptoms of deep venous clot, the above clinical picture will require a workup to find a thrombus or perfusion defects in the lung. Diagnosis of pulmonary embolism requires full anticoagulation in a manner outlined above for deep vein thrombosis.

CESAREAN SECTION

The postpartum care of the patient after cesarean section requires not only attention to normal puerperal changes but also special attention to general issues of care after any major abdominal procedure. The most commonly performed cesarean section uses a low transverse abdominal incision (Pfannenstiel) and a transverse lower uterine segment incision.

Patients require careful observation in the immediate post-operative period. Vital signs, urine output, and amount of vaginal bleeding is assessed every 15 minutes. Special attention should be payed to the degree of uterine tone and the presence of heavy vaginal blood loss. Deep breathing and cough is encouraged especially if a general anesthetic was used.

Most patients are kept from taking anything by mouth for at least the first 24 hours. Intravenous administration of fluids is therefore continued until adequate oral fluids are taken. Because many patients will mobilize large quantities of extracellular fluid within the first 24–48 hours after delivery, careful monitoring of urine output is important.

Encouragement to take deep breaths is part of the postoperative regimen to minimize the risk of atelectasis and postoperative pneumonia. Incentive spirometry can be effective during this period. Early mobilization of patients after surgery can significantly reduce the risk of developing thrombosis or embolism. Ambulation should begin the day of surgery.

It is important to remember that abdominal incisions are painful. Adequate pain medication will help the patient deal with early ambulation, deep breathing, and early maternal-infant bonding. Morphine sulfate, for example, is an effective narcotic. When taking fluids by mouth, medications such as acetaminophen with codeine are often effective.

As occurs with many abdominal procedures, ileus is not uncommon after cesarean section. Normal peristalsis generally returns within a few days, at which time a normal diet is resumed.

The abdominal incision should be inspected and the dressing changed on the first postoperative day. Many surgical incisions are currently closed with skin staples, and these can be safely removed and surgical tape applied on the third postoperative day.

PSYCHOLOGICAL ADAPTATION

Depression is the most common psychiatric disorder observed during or after pregnancy and may afflict as many as 10% of patients. The primary cause of postpartum depression tends to be lack of emotional support from the biologic father or partner. In addition, severe complications of pregnancy requiring prolonged bedrest or hospitalization or concurrent underlying chronic or acute illness may precipitate a depressed state. The presence of the following 5 features in a patient should suggest the possibility of clinical depression: (1) sleep disturbance, (2) altered eating habits, (3) loss of interest in usual activities, (4) prolonged fatigue, and (5) depressed mood or mood swings. It is also important to remember that some of the above symptoms may be seen in thyroid disorders, which need to be ruled out as well.

The most common form of postpartum depression is a mild form termed the "blues." It most often occurs within the first 1–2 weeks after delivery and tends to be self-limited within a 6-week period. The specific emotions experienced include the following: loneliness, anger at the newborn or oneself, fear, or a sense of defeat. In addition, complaints such as headache, confusion, sleeplessness, or apathy may surface. If this state interferes with the patient's ability to care for the newborn, psychiatric consultation is required.

True postpartum depression is a much more severe condition relative to the "blues" and may be associated with a patient's desire to do harm to the newborn or a severe inability to bond with the child. Psychiatric consultation and in some cases antidepressant medication are needed.

Symptoms of postpartum psychosis include those seen in depression but tend to be more severe and long lasting and have associated psychotic behavior. Often hospitalization in addition to mandatory psychotherapeutic measures is needed.

BIRTH CONTROL

The immediate postpartum period is an excellent time to continue discussion of contraceptive choices with the patient. The obstetrician has a responsibility to inform the patient about her options and, most important, to ascertain whether her knowledge of pregnancy prevention is sufficient to ensure adequate family planning choices. Contraceptive methods are discussed at length in Chapter 6; however, some specific methods warrant attention in the postpartum period.

If adequate prenatal counseling has occurred, the immediate postpartum period is an appropriate time to accomplish permanent sterilization. Tubal ligation can be performed at the time of cesarean section or within the first 2 days after vaginal delivery. A small periumbilical incision is used in most cases to access the uterine tubes for ligation and cutting. This procedure rarely prolongs the patient's hospital stay. The failure rate of postpartum sterilization is approximately 0.5%.

Many patients who have used oral contraceptives before pregnancy and have found it a convenient method will desire to resume taking them postpartum. Two issues related to the resumption of oral contraceptives are important. First, since the risk of thromboembolic disease is increased in the postpartum period, waiting at least 2 weeks after delivery to prescribe a low-dose oral contraceptive (35 μg or less of ethinyl estradiol) is generally recommended. Second, in mothers who wish to breast feed, there has long been concern over the amount of hormone present in the breast milk and what its effect may be on the infant. Currently, there is no known harmful effect of the small amount of hormone on the growth and development of infants. Contraceptive agents with high amounts of estrogen are thought to suppress lactation. Even the use of oral contraceptives with lower doses of estrogen during lactation has been associated with a small reduction in milk production. If oral contraceptives are chosen by the breast-feeding mother, it is best to wait until lactation and feeding patterns are thoroughly established before oral contraceptives are initiated.

SUGGESTED READINGS

Andolsek KM: *Obstetric Care: Standards of Prenatal, Intrapartum, and Postpartum Management.* Lea & Febiger, 1990.

Briggs GG, Freeman RK, Yaffe SJ: *Drugs in Pregnancy and Lactation: A Reference Guide to Fetal and Neonatal Risk,* 2nd ed. Williams & Wilkins, 1986.

Bullough VL, Bullough B: *Contraception: A Guide to Birth Control Methods.* Prometheus Books, 1990.

California Department of Health Services, Maternal and Child Health Branch, WIC Supplemental Food Branch: *Nutrition During Pregnancy and the Postpartum Period: A Manual for Health Care Professionals.* 1989.

Cunningham FG, MacDonald PC, Gant NF: *Williams Obstetrics,* 18th ed. Appleton & Lange, 1989.

Zuspan FP, Quilligan EJ: *Douglas-Stromme's Operative Obstetrics,* 5th ed. Appleton & Lange, 1988.

Index

Page numbers followed by n, t, and f indicate footnotes, tables, and figures, respectively. Page numbers in **boldface** type indicate major discussions.